Foundations for
Health Promotion

For Elsevier

Content Strategist: *Alison Taylor*
Content Development Specialist: *Veronika Watkins*
Project Manager: *Umarani Natarajan*
Designer: *Christian Bilbow*
Illustration Buyer: *Amy Naylor*

Foundations for
Health Promotion

FOURTH EDITION

Jennie Naidoo

Principal Lecturer, Health Promotion and Public Health,
University of the West of England, Bristol, UK

Jane Wills

Professor of Health Promotion, London South Bank
University, London, UK

ELSEVIER

ELSEVIER

First edition 1994
Second edition 2000
Third edition 2009

ISBN 978-0-7020-5442-6

British Library Cataloguing in Publication Data
A catalogue record for this book is available from the British Library

Library of Congress Cataloging in Publication Data
A catalog record for this book is available from the Library of Congress

Contents

Preface

Health promotion is a core aspect of the work of a wide range of healthcare workers and those engaged in education and social welfare. It is an emerging area of practice and study, still defining its boundaries and building its own theoretical base and principles. This book aims to provide a theoretical framework for health promotion, as this is vital to clarify practitioners' intentions and desired outcomes. It offers a foundation for practice which encourages practitioners to see the potential for health promotion in their work, to be aware of the implications of choosing from a range of strategies and to be able to evaluate their health promotion interventions in an appropriate and useful manner.

This fourth edition of *Health Promotion: Foundations for Practice* has been comprehensively updated and expanded to reflect recent research findings and major organizational and policy changes over the last decade. Our companion volume, *Public Health and Health Promotion: Developing Practice* (Naidoo and Wills, 2010), discusses in more detail some of the challenges and dilemmas raised in this book, e.g. partnership working, tackling inequalities and engaging the public.

The book is divided into four main parts. The first part provides a theoretical background, exploring the concepts of health, health education and health promotion. Part One concludes that health promotion is working towards positive health and well-being of individuals, groups and communities. Health promotion includes health education but also acknowledges the social, economic and environmental factors which determine health status. Ethical and political values inform practice, and it is important for practitioners to reflect upon these values and their implications. Part One embraces the shift towards well-being rather than a narrow interpretation of health, and the move away from a simple focus on lifestyle changes as the goal of health promotion. Its aim is to enable readers to understand and reflect upon these theoretical drivers of health promotion practice within the context of their own work.

Part Two explores strategies to promote health, and some of the dilemmas they pose. Using the Ottawa Charter (World Health Organization, 1986) framework to identify the range of strategies, the potential, benefits and challenges of adopting each strategy are discussed. Examples of interventions using the different strategies are presented. What is reflected here is how health services have not moved towards prioritizing prevention, although there is much greater acceptance and support for empowerment approaches in work with individuals and communities. While policies that impact on health still get developed in isolation from each other, there is a recognition of the need for health in all policies, and for deliberative democracy and working methods that engage with communities as the ways forward.

Part Three focuses on the provision of supportive environments for health, identified as a key strategy in the Ottawa Charter. Part Three explores how a range of different settings in which health promotion interventions take place can be oriented towards positive health and well-being. The settings discussed in this part – schools, workplaces, neighbourhoods, health services and prisons – have all been targeted by national and international policies as key for health promotion. Reaching specific target groups, such as young people, adults or older people, within these settings is also covered in Part Three. There is much debate about the need for systems thinking and seeing such settings more broadly as environments where physical, social and economic drivers come together, and not just as places in which to carry out health education and lifestyle behaviour interventions.

Part Four focuses on the implementation of health promotion interventions. Each chapter in this part discusses a different stage in the implementation process, from needs assessment through planning to the final stage of evaluation. This part is designed to help practitioners to reflect on their practice through examining what drives their choice of practical implementation strategies. A range of real-life examples helps to illustrate the options available and the criteria that inform the practitioner's choice of approach.

This book is suitable for a wide range of professional groups, and this is reflected in the choice of examples and illustrative case studies, which have been completely updated for this edition. In response to reader feedback about the ways to engage with a textbook, we have changed the format for this edition. Each chapter has between 6 and 15 learning activities which encourage readers to engage with the text and extend their learning. Indicative feedback about the points that a reader or student might wish to consider is provided at the end of the chapter. Each chapter also includes at least one case study and research example to provide the reader with examples of application and encourage a focus on topics. Further questions at the end of each chapter encourage readers to reflect on their practice, values and experience, and to debate the issues. To reflect the huge changes in information management since this book was first published in 1994, website addresses are given for resources and further reading where possible.

The book is targeted at a range of students, including those in basic and post-basic training and qualified professionals. By combining an academic critique with a readable and accessible style, this book will inform, stimulate and encourage readers to engage in ongoing enquiry and reflection regarding their health promotion practice. The intention, as always, is to encourage readers to develop their practice through considering its foundation in theory, policy and clear principles.

Jennie Naidoo
Jane Wills
Bristol and London

References

Naidoo, J., Wills, J., 2010. Public Health and Health Promotion: Developing Practice, third ed. Baillière Tindall, London.
World Health Organization, 1986. Ottawa Charter for Health Promotion. WHO, Geneva.

Acknowledgements

It is 21 years since the publication of the first edition of this book, which was initially prompted by our teaching on the first postgraduate specialist courses in health promotion. Students and colleagues at the University of the West of England and London South Bank University have, as always, contributed to this edition through their ideas, debates and practice examples. We continue to be committed to the development of health promotion as a discipline.

We dedicate this fourth edition to our children, Declan, Jessica, Kate and Alice.

Part One

The theory of health promotion

Part One explores the concepts of health, health education and health promotion. Health promotion draws upon many different disciplines, ranging from the scientific (e.g. epidemiology) and the social sciences (e.g. sociology and psychology) to the humanities (e.g. ethics). This provides a wealth of theoretical underpinnings for health promotion, ranging from the scientific to the moralistic. This in turn means that health promotion in practice may range from a scientific medical exercise (e.g. vaccination) or an educational exercise (e.g. sex and relationships education in schools) to a moral query (e.g. end-of-life options). An important first step for health promoters is to clarify for themselves where they stand in relation to these various different strategies and goals. Are they educators, politicians or scientists? In part this will be determined by their background and initial education, but health promotion is an umbrella which encompasses all these activities and more. Working together, practitioners can bring their varied bodies of knowledge and skills to focus on promoting the health of the population, and achieve more

significant and sustainable results than if they were operating on their own.

This first part of the book explores different understandings of the concept of health and well-being, and the ways in which health can be enhanced or promoted. The effect on health of structural factors such as income, gender, sexuality and ethnicity and the way in which social factors are important predictors of health status are explored in Chapter 2. The different ways in which health is measured reflect different views on health, from the absence of disease to holistic concepts of well-being, and these are discussed in Chapter 3. Chapters 4 and 5 debate what health promotion is, adopting an ecological model in which change in health is said to be influenced by the interaction of individual, social and physical environmental variables. Chapters 6 and 7 will help those who promote health to be clear about their intentions and how they perceive the purpose of health promotion. Is it to encourage healthy lifestyles? Or is it to redress health inequalities and empower people to take control over their lives?

Concepts of health

By the end of this chapter you will be able to:

- define the concepts of health, well-being, disease, illness and ill health, and understand the differences between them
- discuss the nature of health and well-being, and how culture and populism influence our definitions
- understand the elements of the medical model of health and how it influences healthcare practice.

Key Concepts and Definitions

Biomedicine Focuses on the causes of ill health and disease within the physical body. It is associated with the practice of medicine, and contrasts with a social model of health.

Disease Is the medical term for a disorder, illness or condition that prevents an individual from achieving the full functioning of all his or her bodily parts.

Health Is the state of complete mental and physical well-being of an individual, not merely the absence of disease or illness.

Ill health Is a state of poor health when there is some disease or impairment, but not usually serious enough to curtail all activities.

Illness Is a disease or period of sickness that affects an individual's body or mind and prevents the individual achieving his or her optimal outputs.

Well-being Is the positive feeling that accompanies a lack of ill health and illness, and is associated with the achievement of personal goals and a sense of being well and feeling good.

Everyone engaged in the task of promoting health starts with a view of what health is. However, these views, or concepts, of health vary widely. It is important at the outset to be clear about the concepts of health to which you personally adhere, and recognize where these differ from those of your colleagues and clients. Otherwise, you may find yourself drawn into conflicts about appropriate strategies and advice that are actually due to different ideas concerning the end goal of health. This chapter introduces different concepts of health and traces the origin of these views. The Western scientific medical model of health is dominant, but is challenged by social and holistic models. Working your way through this chapter will enable you to clarify your own views on the definition of health and locate these views within a conceptual framework.

Defining health, well-being, disease, illness and ill health

Health

Health is a broad concept which can embody a huge range of meanings, from the narrowly technical to the all-embracing moral or philosophical. The word 'health' is derived from the Old English word for heal (*hael*) which means 'whole', signalling that health concerns the whole person and his or her integrity, soundness or well-being. There are 'common-sense' views of health which are passed through generations as part of a common cultural heritage. These are termed 'lay' concepts of health, and everyone acquires a knowledge of them through socialization into society. Different societies and different groups within one society have different views on what constitutes their 'common-sense' notions about health.

 Learning Activity 1.1 What does health mean to you?

What are your answers to the following?
- I feel healthy when…
- I am healthy because…
- To stay healthy I need…
- I become unhealthy when…
- My health improves when…
- (An event) affected my health by…
- (A situation) affected my health by…
- …is responsible for my health.

Health has two common meanings in everyday use, one negative and one positive. The negative definition is the absence of disease or illness. This is the meaning of health within the Western scientific medical model, which is explored in greater detail later in this chapter. The positive definition of health is a state of well-being, interpreted by the World Health Organization in its constitution as 'a state of complete physical, mental and social well-being, not merely the absence of disease or infirmity' (World Health Organization, 1946).

Health is holistic and includes different dimensions, each of which needs to be considered. Holistic health means taking account of the separate influences and interaction of these dimensions.

Figure 1.1 shows a diagrammatic representation of the dimensions of health.

The inner circle represents individual dimensions of health.
- Physical health concerns the body, e.g. fitness, not being ill.
- Mental health refers to a positive sense of purpose and an underlying belief in one's own worth, e.g. feeling good, feeling able to cope.
- Emotional health concerns the ability to feel, recognize and give a voice to feelings, and to develop and sustain relationships, e.g. feeling loved.
- Social health concerns the sense of having support available from family and friends, e.g. having friends to talk to, being involved in activities with other people.
- Spiritual health is the recognition and ability to put into practice moral or religious principles or beliefs, and the feeling of having a 'higher' purpose in life.
- Sexual health is the acceptance and ability to achieve a satisfactory expression of one's sexuality.

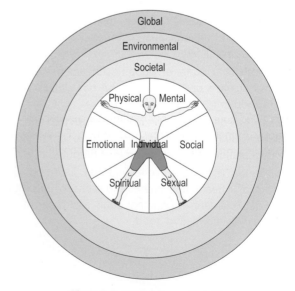

Fig 1.1 ● Dimensions of health.

The three outer circles are broader dimensions of health which affect the individual. Societal health refers to the link between health and the way a society is structured. This includes the basic infrastructure necessary for health (such as shelter, peace, food, income), and the degree of integration or division within society. We shall see in Chapter 2 how the existence of patterned inequalities between groups of people harms the health of everyone. Environmental health refers to the physical environment in which people live, and the importance of good-quality housing, transport, sanitation and pure-water facilities. Global health involves caring for the planet and ensuring its sustainability for the future.

Learning Activity 1.2 Holistic model of health

What are the implications of a holistic model of health for the professional practice of health workers?

Well-being

'Well-being' is a term widely used to describe 'what makes a good life'. It is also used in healthcare discourse to broaden views on what health means beyond the absence of illness. Feeling good and functioning well are seen as important components of mental well-being. This, in turn, leads to better physical health, improved productivity, less crime and more participation in community life (DH, 2010). The New Economics Foundation has developed the Happy Planet Index (New Economics Foundation, 2012) as a headline indicator of how nations compare in enabling long and happy lives for their citizens. In 2012:

- eight of the nine countries that are achieving high and sustainable well-being are in Latin America and the Caribbean
- the highest-ranking Western European nation is Norway in 29th place, just behind New Zealand in 28th place.
- the USA is in 105th position out of 151 countries.

Similarly, the UNICEF index of child well-being (UNICEF, 2013) shows that well-being is greater in more egalitarian countries, such as Norway and other Scandinavian countries.

Evidence (Government Office for Science, 2008) suggests that there are five methods or steps that individuals can take to enable themselves to achieve well-being:

- connect
- be active
- take notice
- give
- keep learning.

More recently, 'Care (about the planet)' has been added to this list.

Learning Activity 1.3 Five steps to well-being

What evidence is there for each of the steps to well-being?

Disease, illness and ill health

Disease, illness and ill health are often used interchangeably, although they have very different meanings. Disease derives from *desaise*, meaning uneasiness or discomfort. Nowadays, disease implies an objective state of ill health, which may be verified by accepted canons of proof. In our modern society these accepted canons are couched in the language of scientific medicine. For example, microscopic analysis may yield evidence of changes in cell structure, which may in turn lead to a diagnosis of cancer. Disease is the existence of some pathology or abnormality of the body which is capable of detection. Disease can be due to exogenous (outside the body, e.g. viral infection) or endogenous (inside the body, e.g. inadequate thyroid function) factors.

Illness is the subjective experience of loss of health. This is couched in terms of symptoms, for example the reporting of aches or pains, or loss of function. One way that illness is given meaning is through the narratives we construct about how we fall sick. The process of making sense of illness is a task most sick people engage in to answer the question 'why me?' Illness and disease are not the same, although there is a large degree of coexistence. For example, a person may be diagnosed as having cancer through screening, even when there have been no reported symptoms; thus a disease may be diagnosed in someone who has not reported any illness. When someone reports symptoms, and further investigations such as blood tests prove a disease process, the two concepts of disease and illness coincide. In these instances, the term ill health is used. Ill health is therefore an umbrella term used to refer to the experience of disease plus illness. Health is the normal functioning of the body as a biological entity. Health is both not being ill and the absence of symptoms.

Social scientists view health and disease as socially constructed entities. Health and disease are not states of objective reality waiting to be uncovered and investigated by scientific medicine; rather, they are actively produced and negotiated by ordinary people. Cornwell's (1984) study of London's Eastenders used three categories of health problems.
1. Normal illness, e.g. childhood infections.
2. Real illness, e.g. cancer.
3. Health problems, e.g. ageing, allergies.

Illness has often been conceptualized as deviance – as a different state from the healthy norm and a source of stigma. Goffman (1968) identified three sources of stigma.
1. Abominations of the body, e.g. psoriasis.
2. Blemishes of character, e.g. human immunodeficiency virus (HIV)/acquired immunodeficiency syndrome (AIDS).
3. Tribal stigma of race, nation or religion, e.g. apartheid.

The subjective experience of feeling ill is not always corroborated by an objective diagnosis of disease. When this lack of corroboration happens, doctors and health workers may label sufferers 'malingerers', denying the validity of subjective illness. This can have important consequences. For example, a sick certificate, and therefore sick pay, may be withheld if a doctor is not convinced that someone's reported illness is genuine. The acceptance of reported symptoms as signs of an illness leads to a debate about how to manage the illness. Several conditions, such as chronic fatigue syndrome and repetitive strain injury, have taken a long time to be recognized as legitimate illnesses.

> **Learning Activity 1.4 The medicalization of health**
>
> What examples are there of a condition or behaviour where its medicalization has led to its acceptance or otherwise?

It is also possible for an individual to experience no symptoms or signs of disease, but to be labelled sick as a result of medical examination or screening. Hypertension and pre-cancerous changes to cell structures are two examples where screening may identify a disease even though the person concerned may feel perfectly healthy.

Figure 1.2 gives a visual representation of these discrepancies. The central point is that subjective perceptions cannot be overruled, or invalidated, by scientific medicine.

The Western scientific medical model of health

In modern Western societies, and in many other societies as well, the dominant professional view of health adopted by most healthcare workers during their training and practice is labelled Western scientific medicine. Western scientific medicine operates within a medical model using a narrow view of health,

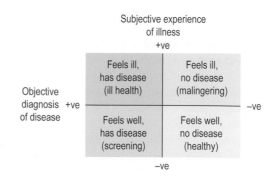

Fig 1.2 ● The relationship between disease and illness.

which is often taken to mean the absence of disease and/or illness. In this sense, health is a negative term, defined more by what it is not than by what it is.

This view of health is extremely influential, as it underpins much of the training and ethos of a wide variety of health workers. Its definitions become powerful because they are used in a variety of contexts, not just in professional circles. For example, the media often present this view of health, disease and illness in dramas set in hospitals or documentaries about health issues. By these means, professional definitions become known and accepted in society at large.

The scientific medical model arose in Western Europe at the time of the Enlightenment, with the rise of rationality and science as forms of knowledge. In earlier times, religion provided a way of knowing and understanding the world. The Enlightenment changed the old order, and substituted science for religion as the dominant means of knowledge and understanding. This was accompanied by a proliferation of equipment and techniques for studying the world. The invention of the microscope and telescope revealed whole worlds which had previously been invisible. Observation, calculation and classification became the means of increasing knowledge. Such knowledge was put to practical purposes, and applied science was one of the forces which accompanied the Industrial Revolution. In an atmosphere when everything was deemed knowable through the proper application of scientific method, the human body became a key object for the pursuit of scientific knowledge. What could be seen, and measured and catalogued was 'true' in an objective and universal sense.

This view of health is characterized as:

- *biomedical* – health is assumed to be a property of biological beings
- *reductionist* – states of being such as health and disease may be reduced to smaller and smaller constitutive components of the biological body
- *mechanistic* – this conceptualizes the body as if it were a machine, in which all the parts are interconnected but capable of being separated and treated separately
- *allopathic* – this works by a system of opposites; if something is wrong with a body, treatment consists of applying an opposite force to correct

the sickness, e.g. pharmacological drugs which combat the sickness

- *pathogenic* – this focuses on why people become ill
- *dualistic* – the mind and the body can be treated as separate entities.

Health is predominantly viewed as the absence of disease. This view sees health and disease as linked, as if on a continuum, so that the more disease a person has, the further away he or she is from health and 'normality'.

The pathogenic focus on finding the causes for ill health has led to an emphasis on risk factors, whether these are health behaviours or social circumstances. Antonovsky (1993) called for a *salutogenic* approach which looks instead at why some people remain healthy. He identifies coping mechanisms which enable some people to remain healthy despite adverse circumstances, change and stress. An important factor for health, which Antonovsky labels a 'sense of coherence', involves the three aspects of understanding, managing and making sense of change. These are human abilities which are in turn nurtured or obstructed by the wider environment.

The medical model focuses on etiology, and the belief that disease originates from specific and identifiable causes. The causes of contemporary long-term chronic diseases in developed countries are often 'social'. Medicine and medical practice thus recognize that disease and the diseased body must be placed in a social context. Nevertheless, the professional training of many healthcare workers provides an exaggerated view of the benefits of treatment and pays little attention to prevention. In part this is due to the dominant concern of the biomedical model with the organic appearance of disease and malfunction as the causes of ill health.

 Research Example 1.1 Carers' health

An ageing population means that caring for the elderly will become a more common experience for younger adults or even children. This has significant implications for the health of the population as a whole. Research studies have reported a clear association between caring and

Continued

care givers' poor mental and physical health, emotional distress and increased mortality. A more intense caring role (e.g. having to provide 24-hour cover, or caring for someone with both mental and physical ill health) is associated with poorer health outcomes on the part of the carer. Yet evidence also shows that not all carers report poor health. Indeed, caring has the opposite effect on some carers, conferring positive benefits through feelings of altruism, fulfilment of familial obligations and personal growth. It is likely that the impact of caring on the health of carers will be to some extent dependent on the existence, or lack, of a supportive environment, including, for example, community activities and respite opportunities. It also seems likely that the existence of personal religious and faith beliefs is associated with improved health and caring, as religion provides an overarching rationale for existence, even if this is compromised by poor health. Religious centres often provide supportive and caring activities for members of their faith, enabling carers to cope better with their burden of care, and providing some respite care for people with disabilities.
See for example Awad et al., 2008; Rigby et al., 2009; Vellone et al., 2008.

Table 1.1 contrasts the traditional views of a medical model with those of a social model of health.

A critique of the medical model

The role of medicine in determining health

The view that health is the absence of disease and illness, and that medical treatment can restore the body to good health, has been criticized. The distribution of health and ill health has been analysed from a historical and social science perspective. It has been argued that medicine is not as effective as is often claimed. The medical writer Thomas McKeown (McKeown, 1976) showed that most of the fatal diseases of the nineteenth century had disappeared before the arrival of antibiotics or immunization programmes. McKeown concluded that social advances in general living conditions, such as improved sanitation and better nutrition made available by rising real wages, have

Table 1.1 The medical and social model of health

Medical model	Social model
• Health is the absence of disease	• Health is a product of social, biological and environmental factors
• Health services are geared towards treating the sick and disabled	• Services emphasize all stages of prevention and treatment
• High value is placed on specialist medical services	• Less emphasis is placed on the role of specialists – there is more attention to self-help and community activity
• Health workers diagnose and treat, and sanction 'the sick role'	• Health workers enable people to take greater control over their own health
• The pathogenic focus emphasizes finding biological causes for illness	• A salutogenic focus emphasizes understanding why people are healthy

been responsible for most of the reduction in mortality achieved during the last century. Although his thesis has been disputed, there is little disagreement that the contribution of medicine to reduced mortality has been minor when compared with the major impact of improved environmental conditions.

 Learning Activity 1.5 The impact of medicine

- What effects do medical advances in knowledge have on death rates?
- What other reasons could account for declining death rates?

The rise of the evidence-based practice movement (see Chapter 20) is attributed to Archie Cochrane (1972). His concern was that medical interventions were not trialled to demonstrate effectiveness prior to their widespread adoption. Instead, many procedures rest on habit, custom and tradition rather than rationality. Cochrane advocated greater use of the randomized controlled trial as a means to gain scientific knowledge and the key to progress.

The role of social factors in determining health

Most countries are characterized by profound inequalities in income and wealth, and these in turn are associated with persistent inequalities in health (see www.who.int/social_determinants/sdh_definition/en/). The impact of scientific medicine on health is marginal when compared to major structural features such as the distribution of wealth, income, housing and employment. Tarlov (1996) claimed that medical services contributed only 17 percent to the gain in life expectancy in the twentieth century. As Chapter 2 shows, the distribution of health mirrors the distribution of material resources within society. In general, the more equal a society is in its distribution of resources, the more equal, and better, is the health status of its citizens (Wilkinson and Pickett, 2009).

Medicine as a means of social control

Social scientists argue that medicine is a social enterprise closely linked with the exercise of professional power. Foucault (1977) argues that power is embedded in social organizations, expressed through hierarchies and determined through discourses. Medical power derives from its role in legitimizing health and illness in society, and the socially exclusive and autonomous nature of the profession. The medical profession has long been regarded as an institution for securing occupational and social authority. Access to such power is controlled by professional associations that have their own vested interests to protect (Freidson, 1986). The 1858 Medical Act established the General Medical Council, which was authorized to regulate doctors, oversee medical education and keep a register of qualified practitioners. The Faculty of Public Health Medicine opened membership to non-medically qualified specialists in 2003, becoming the Faculty of Public Health.

Medicine is a powerful means of social control, whereby the categories of disease, illness, madness and deviancy are used to maintain a status quo in society. Doctors who make the diagnoses are in a powerful position. The role of the patient during sickness as conceptualized by Parsons (1951) is illustrated

Table 1.2 The sick role

Rights	Responsibilities
• Patient is relieved of normal responsibilities and tasks • Patient is given sympathy and support • Patient has the right to a diagnosis, examination and treatment	• Patient must want to recover as soon as possible and only then can he or she be seen as 'sick' • Patient must seek professional advice and comply with treatment

in Table 1.2. Increasingly, too, doctors are involved in decisions relating to the beginning and ending of life (terminations, assisted reproduction, neonatal care, euthanasia). The encroachment of medical decisions into these stages of life subverts human autonomy and, it is argued, gives to medicine an authority beyond its legitimate area of operation (Illich, 1975).

Medicine as surveillance

Public health medicine has been concerned with the regulation and control of disease. Historically this included the containment of bodies, such as those infected with the plague, tuberculosis or venereal disease. Mass-screening programmes have given rise to what has been called medical surveillance. The wish to identify the 'abnormal' few with 'invisible' disease justifies monitoring the entire target population. Another critique of the pervasive power of medicine suggests the mapping of disease and identification of risk have subtly handed responsibility of health to individuals. This may invite new forms of control in the name of health, e.g. random drug testing or linking deservingness for surgery to lifestyle factors. The ability to identify risk also means there can be a moral discourse in which reducing one's risk factors, e.g. eating 'sensibly' and living 'well', is seen as a good thing.

Medicine as harm

According to Illich (1975), doctors and health workers contribute to ill health and create harm (iatrogenesis).
• Clinical iatrogenesis is ill health caused by medical intervention, for example

Case Study 1.1 Reducing antibiotic dependence

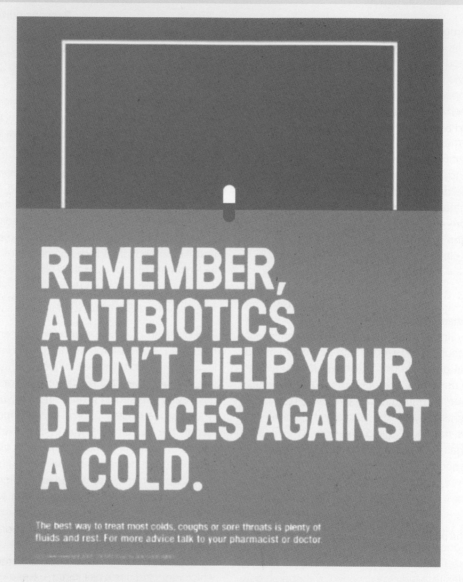

European Antibiotic Awareness Day on 18 November 2013 supported a campaign to reduce people's dependence on antibiotics, as their overuse is leading to resistance. Running noses and green phlegm do not mean patients need antibiotics. Such symptoms are often caused by viruses, and the use of antibiotics is leading to viral resistance. Public Health England (https://www.gov.uk/government/news/ green-phlegm-and-snot-not-always-a-sign-of-an-infection-needing-antibiotics) said its own research showed that 40 percent of people thought antibiotics would help a cough if the phlegm was green, while very few thought it would make a difference to clear-coloured phlegm. (This is from a Department of Health campaign 2008 [Crown copyright 2008. 290981/Goal 1p 40k Oct08 (MRP)].)

side-effects caused by prescribed medicine, dependence on prescribed drugs and cross-infection in medical settings such as hospitals.

- Social iatrogenesis is the loss of coping and the right to self-care which have resulted from the medicalization of everyday life.
- Cultural iatrogenesis is the loss of the means whereby people cope with pain and suffering, which results from the unrealistic expectations generated by medicine.

Challenges to medicine

The dominance of medicine has been challenged in recent years by:

- managerialism and challenges to clinical autonomy
- a rise in complementary therapies
- consumerism and a rise in the number of informed patients who are using the internet
- social movements and advocacy, e.g. the home birth movement
- patient-centred care and shared decision-making.
  These trends are related to wider forces that challenge the expertise of professionals. The response of most professions, including medicine, has been to introduce democratic decision-making, giving far more credence to lay knowledge. This has led to new concepts such as the 'expert patient'.

Learning Activity 1.6 The changing practice of medicine

In your lifetime as a patient, what changes have you noticed in the practice of medicine and healthcare?

Case Study 1.2 The active birth movement

A cultural concern with safety, science, professionalism and technology has ensured the medical domination of midwifery. At the same time the alternative birth movement has resisted hegemonic understandings about childbirth as a medicalized issue. The active

birth movement, initiated by Janet Balaskas in the early 1980s, challenged the medicalization of birth, whereby women were placed in stirrups or the lithotomy position with their feet above or at the same level as their hips, rendering them passive recipients of medical care and attention. The active birth movement campaigns for women to give birth in whatever position feels most comfortable and natural, thereby taking control of their bodies and their childbirth. Balaskas had researched birthing positions across different cultures, and found the Western preferred position (flat on the back) reduced the diameter of the pelvic outlet, rendering the birth process longer and more painful. The active birth movement is a challenge to the increasing medicalization of childbirth. Current statistics show that 25 percent of current births are caesareans, with large local variations. NHS Information Centre statistics show that a third of babies born at London's Chelsea and Westminster NHS Trust are delivered by caesarean section, a figure more than double that in Nottingham (http://www.hscic.gov.uk/catalogue/PUB12744).

Lay concepts of health

For people concerned with the promotion of health, there is another problem with the dominance of scientific medicine: the focus within medicine on illness and disease, and the neglect of health as a positive concept in its own right. Many researchers have studied the general public's beliefs about health or lay concepts of health. The findings present an interesting picture, where there are continuities in definitions but also differences attributable to age, sex and class.

Blaxter (1990) identified five common concepts of health.

1. 'Health as not-ill' – health is the absence of symptoms or medical input; widely used by all groups.
2. 'Health as physical fitness' – health as having energy and strength; mostly used by younger men.
3. 'Health as social relationships'; mostly used by women.
4. 'Health as function' – health as the ability to carry out tasks and activities; mostly used by older people of both sexes.

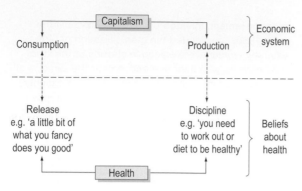

Fig 1.3 • Cultural views about health in capitalist society. Adapted from Crawford (2000).

5. 'Health as psychosocial well-being'; less used by young men, most used by higher socioeconomic groups.

The concepts of 'control' and 'release' are also commonly found in lay accounts. Release is the taking of known risks (e.g. binge drinking), whereas control is the management of health.

As illustrated in Figure 1.3, Crawford (2000) suggests that capitalism also requires individuals to be healthy consumers, having fun and seeking immediate gratification. Adherence to a healthy lifestyle has to be offset by pleasure or release. In capitalist societies we are encouraged to be disciplined and controlled about pleasures such as alcohol. This is couched as being balanced and moderate.

Researchers have found these issues of control and release in many accounts of health, together with a moral view about taking risks. The following extract is from a study of laymen's views:

I eat healthy food generally and I cheat now and again. Alcohol is bad for you, but we all drink. Mostly everyone I know likes a drink 'cause its good for you, it actually cheers you up… we've got like this throwaway society and I think people's perceptions are changing, everybody wants everything yesterday… and that's it, get fit one day, get drunk the next

Robertson (2006), p. 179.

Learning Activity 1.7 Moral identities and health

How do morality and moral identities influence the ways in which people experience health and ill health?

There is often a difference between lay and professional concepts of health. The gap between the two has been identified by health workers as a problem, giving rise to concern. The concern centres around two issues.

1. The perceived lack of communication or poor communication between health worker and client.
2. Clients' lack of compliance with prescribed treatment regimens.

However, there is also a crossover between lay and professional beliefs about health. Health workers acquire their professional view of health during training. These beliefs overlie their original views of health adopted at an early age from family and society, so professionals are familiar with both. The general public is also aware of, and operates with, both sets of beliefs. In searching for meaning, lay patients frequently adopt professionals' explanations and interpretations about health and illness. So the two sets of beliefs, scientific medicine and lay public, are not discrete entities but overlap each other and exist in tandem.

Cornwell (1984) describes how people operate with both official and lay beliefs about health. Her study of London's Eastenders found that accounts of health were either public or private. Public accounts are couched in terms of scientific medicine and reflect these dominant beliefs. Health and illness are related to medical diagnosis and treatment, and medical terms and events are used to explain health status. These public accounts were offered first in Cornwell's interviews. What she terms 'private accounts' reflect lay views of health, which typically use more holistic and social concepts to explain health and illness. For example, private accounts related health to general life experiences, such as employment, housing and perceived stress. Private accounts were offered in subsequent interviews, when a relationship had been established between Cornwell and the women she was interviewing. Cornwell suggests that people are therefore aware of both systems of beliefs and can use either when asked to talk about health. In encounters with strangers who are perceived as professionals, people use public accounts; but in more informal settings they use private accounts.

Cultural views of health

We are able to think about health using the language of scientific medicine because that is part of our cultural heritage. We do so as a matter of course, and think it is self-evident or common sense. However, other societies and cultures have their own common-sense ways of talking about health which are very different. Many cultures view disease as the outcome of malign human or supernatural agencies, and diagnosis is a matter of determining who has been offended. Treatment includes ceremonies to propitiate these spirits as an integral part of the process. Ways of thinking about health and disease reflect the basic preoccupations of a society, and dominant views of the society and the world. Anthropologists refer to this phenomenon as the cultural specificity of notions of health and disease.

In any multicultural society, a variety of cultural views coexist at any one time. For example, traditional Chinese medicine is based on the dichotomy of yin and yang, female and male, hot and cold, which is applied to symptoms, diet and treatments, such as acupuncture and Chinese herbal medicine. Complementary therapists offer therapies based on these cultural views of health and disease alongside (or increasingly within) the National Health Service, which is based on scientific medicine.

 Learning Activity 1.8 Understanding health beliefs

People's explanations for their health and illness are complex. Why is it important for health promoters to understand the health beliefs of those with whom they work? How might they do this?

A unified view of health

Is there any unifying concept of health which can reconcile these different views and beliefs? Attempts at such a synthesis have come from philosophers such as Seedhouse (1986) and from organizations concerned with health, such as the World Health Organization.

1. *Health as an ideal state* provides a holistic and positive definition of health. It is important in showing the interrelationship of different dimensions of health. A medical diagnosis of ill health does not necessarily coincide with a sense of personal illness or feeling unwell. Equally, a person free from disease may be isolated and lonely.
2. *Health as mental and physical fitness* is a perspective developed by Talcott Parsons (1951), a functional sociologist. It suggests that health is when people can fulfil the everyday tasks and roles expected of them.
3. *Health as a commodity* leads to unrealistic expectations of health as something which can be purchased. Health cannot be guaranteed by paying a higher price for healthcare.
4. *Health as a personal strength* is a view which derives from humanistic psychology, and suggests that an individual can become healthy through self-actualization and discovery (Maslow, 1970).

 Learning Activity 1.9 Theories of health

Figure 1.4 shows four theories of health.
1. Health as an ideal state.
2. Health as mental and physical fitness.
3. Health as a commodity.
4. Health as a personal strength.
What problems can you identify with each of these four views of health?

Seedhouse (1986) suggests that these four views can be combined in a unified theory of health as the foundation for human achievement. Health is thus a means to an end rather than a fixed state to which a person should aspire.

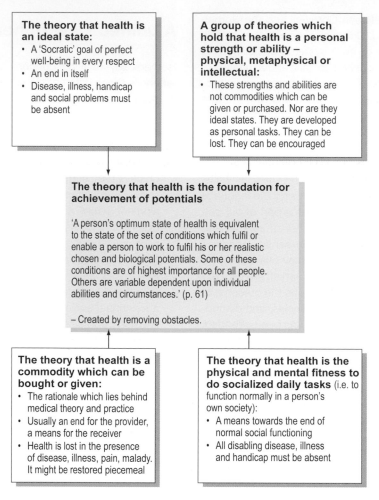

The theory that health is an ideal state:
- A 'Socratic' goal of perfect well-being in every respect
- An end in itself
- Disease, illness, handicap and social problems must be absent

A group of theories which hold that health is a personal strength or ability – physical, metaphysical or intellectual:
- These strengths and abilities are not commodities which can be given or purchased. Nor are they ideal states. They are developed as personal tasks. They can be lost. They can be encouraged

The theory that health is the foundation for achievement of potentials

'A person's optimum state of health is equivalent to the state of the set of conditions which fulfil or enable a person to work to fulfil his or her realistic chosen and biological potentials. Some of these conditions are of highest importance for all people. Others are variable dependent upon individual abilities and circumstances.' (p. 61)

– Created by removing obstacles.

The theory that health is a commodity which can be bought or given:
- The rationale which lies behind medical theory and practice
- Usually an end for the provider, a means for the receiver
- Health is lost in the presence of disease, illness, pain, malady. It might be restored piecemeal

The theory that health is the physical and mental fitness to do socialized daily tasks (i.e. to function normally in a person's own society):
- A means towards the end of normal social functioning
- All disabling disease, illness and handicap must be absent

Fig 1.4 ● A summary of theories of health. Adapted from Seedhouse (1986).

[Health is] the extent to which an individual or group is able, on the one hand, to realize aspirations and satisfy needs; and, on the other hand, to change or cope with the environment. Health is, therefore, seen as a resource for everyday life, not an object of living; it is a positive concept emphasizing social and personal resources, as well as physical capacities.

World Health Organization (1984)

Provided certain central conditions are met, people can be enabled to achieve their potential. The task of practitioners working for health is to create these conditions for people to achieve health:

- basic needs of food, drink, shelter and warmth
- access to information about the factors influencing health
- skills and confidence to use that information.

This definition acknowledges that people have different starting points which set limits for their potential for health. It encompasses a positive notion of health which is applicable to everyone, whatever their circumstances. However, it could be argued that this definition does not acknowledge the social construction of health sufficiently. People as individuals have little scope to determine optimum conditions for realizing their potential.

By health I mean the power to live a full, adult, living, breathing life in close contact with what I love… I want to be all that I am capable of becoming.

Mansfield (1977), p. 278.

The view of health as personal potential is attractive because it is so flexible, but this very flexibility causes problems. It leads to relativism (health may mean a thousand different things to a thousand different people), which makes it impracticable as a working definition for health promoters.

Health is regarded by the World Health Organization as a fundamental human right, and there are certain prerequisites for health, which include peace, adequate food and shelter and sustainable resource use.

Looking at health this way establishes it as a social as well as an individual product, and it emphasizes its dynamic and positive nature. Health is viewed as both a fundamental human right and a sound social investment. This view was publicly affirmed by the Jakarta Declaration, which linked health to social and economic development (World Health Organization, 1997). This definition provides a variety of reasons for supporting health which are likely to meet the concerns of a range of groups. It establishes a broad consensus for prioritizing health, and legitimizes a range of activities designed to promote it. For example, in addition to the more acceptable strategies of primary healthcare and personal skills development, the World Health Organization also identified in the Ottawa Charter the more radical strategies of community participation and healthy public policy as essential to the promotion of health (World Health Organization, 1986). However, it could still be argued that such a broad definition makes it difficult to identify practical priorities for health promotion activities.

There is no agreement on what is meant by health. Health is used in many different contexts to refer to many different aspects of life. Given this complexity of meanings, it is unlikely that a unified concept of health which includes all its meanings will be formulated.

Conclusion

There are no rights and wrongs regarding concepts of health. Different people are likely to hold different views of health and may operate with several conflicting views simultaneously. Where people are located socially, in terms of social class, gender, ethnic origin and occupation, will affect their concept of health. The medical model has dominated Western thinking about health, yet its value for health promotion is limited.

- It relies on a concept of normality that is not widely accepted.
- It ignores broader societal and environmental dimensions of health.
- It ignores people's subjective perceptions of their own health.
- The focus on pathology and malfunction leads to practitioners responding to ill health rather than being proactive in promoting health.

There is such a range of meaning attached to the notion of health that in any particular situation it is important to find out what views are in operation. Clarifying what you understand about health, and what other people mean when they talk about health, is an essential first step for the health promoter.

Questions for further discussion

- How would you describe your own concept of health? What have been the most important influences on your views?

Summary

Definitions of health arise from many different perspectives. While scientific medicine is the most powerful ideology in the West, it is not all-embracing. Social sciences' perspectives on health produce a powerful critique of scientific medicine, and point to the importance of social factors in the construction and meaning of health. Lay concepts of health derived from different cultures coexist alongside scientific medicine. Attempts to produce a unified concept of health appear to founder through over-generalization and vagueness.

Further reading and resources

Barry, A., Yuill, C., 2012. Understanding the Sociology of Health: An Introduction, third ed. Sage, London. *An accessible introduction to the sociology of health and illness exploring key concepts and the social structures that shape and pattern health.*

Lupton, D., 2012. Medicine as Culture: Illness, Disease and the Body in Western Societies, third ed. Sage, London. *An interesting account of the dependence on, and disillusionment with, medicine.*

Naidoo, J., Wills, J., 2015. Health Studies: An Introduction, third ed. Palgrave Macmillan, Basingstoke. *An accessible introduction to different disciplinary perspectives on health including sociology, culture and anthropology and biology.*

 ## Feedback to learning activities

1.1 Health is a complex concept that encompasses different dimensions, including physical, mental, social and emotional health. Some theorists suggest there is a hierarchy of health, whereby physical health needs are the most basic, and it is only once these needs have been met that people can move on to identify and meet mental, social and emotional health needs. Maslow (1943) identified a hierarchy of needs (often represented as a pyramid), with the most basic need (the base of the pyramid) being physiological, moving through safety, belonging and esteem to self-actualization (the tip of the pyramid).

1.2 A holistic model of health implies that professional health workers can only address some aspects or causes of health or ill health (and not necessarily the most basic or important causes). Many of the most important factors affecting health, such as social equality or environmental quality, are beyond the remit of health workers. A holistic model of health also implies that health workers need to work collaboratively with others (e.g. social workers or environmental health officers) in order to achieve optimum results.

1.3 Evidence suggests that a small improvement in well-being can help to decrease some mental health problems and also help people to flourish. The New Economics Foundation, on behalf of Foresight, presented a document which sets out five actions to improve personal well-being based on this evidence (www.neweconomics.org).

- Connect: Having social support and relationships is beneficial to well-being and acts as a buffer against mental ill health.
- Be active: Regular physical activity is associated with a greater sense of well-being and possibly delays cognitive decline.

- Take notice: Being aware of sensations, thoughts and feelings enhances well-being. Being in a state of mindfulness (being attentive to, and aware of, what is taking place in the present) is positive.
- Give: Mutual cooperation is associated with feelings of regard. Active participation in social and community life is associated with positive affect.
- Keep learning: Learning is important in social and cognitive development, enhances self-esteem and encourages interaction.

1.4 According to Hart and Wellings (2002), homosexuals, formerly considered to be sinners, were labelled as ill up to the late 1970s in the USA. Commitments to mental institutions, hormonal treatments and castrations were used to deal with their unwanted sexual behaviour. In 1973 the American Psychiatric Association redesignated homosexuality as non-pathological.

1.5 There were few effective medicines or therapies available to combat infectious diseases before the mid-1930s, so medical care did not play an important role during this period. Historical epidemiologists, such as McKeown (1976), observed that a large share of the decline in infectious disease mortality during the twentieth century preceded the advent of medical treatments, and concluded that rising living standards, better nutrition and public health measures that improved water supplies, sanitation systems and household hygiene were responsible for the drop in mortality rates. Since the late twentieth century the principal causes of mortality have been attributed to 'lifestyles', and medical advances such as the treatment of hypertension and diabetes and the medical and surgical treatment of coronary artery disease have contributed to increased life expectancy.

1.6 You may have mentioned receiving more lifestyle advice; less willingness of GPs to prescribe medication; and more attempts to find out your wishes. If you have a chronic condition, you may use tele-healthcare and have the condition monitored electronically at home. Healthcare has become more patient-centred and consumer-driven, pushed by three fundamental forces: availability of information, choice and control.

1.7 Moral identity, such as strength of character and personal control, is frequently cited in lay accounts of health. In a survey of disadvantaged areas, Popay et al. (2003) found that some respondents suggested that stress mediated the relationship between the experience of disadvantage and poor health. As you will find in Chapter 2, psychosocial pathways provide an important conceptual link within lay understandings to the moral framework within which explanations for health and illness are 'constructed'. Individual resilience and strength of character are seen as the means to avoid ill health.

1.8 There is often a gulf between healthcare professionals' and patients' knowledge, expectations and values regarding illness and healthcare. Healthcare professionals often assume their prioritization of Western scientific medicine and associated values is universal and shared by all their patients. However, this is not the case. Patients' cultural values vary widely and have a significant impact on their understanding of medical diagnoses and prescribed care, as well as their ability to manage illness, disability and death. Gender and position within the family may also impact on patients' ability to understand and cope with ill health. Cultural values impact on all stages of ill health, from receiving and understanding a diagnosis, through management of illness and treatment, to coping with death and bereavement.

1.9 Definitions of health.
- The definition of health as a complete state of well-being is unrealistic and does not help health professionals or lay people set practical or achievable goals. The requirement for complete health means that most people are unhealthy most of the time. This view therefore supports the tendencies of the medical technology and drug industries, in association with professional organizations, to redefine diseases, detect more and more abnormalities through screening, and thus expand the scope of the healthcare system (see Huber et al., 2011).
- The definition of health as normal social functioning ignores the fact that people can be contented and healthy but unable to fulfil social roles (e.g. employee) due to factors such as chronic illness or disability.
- The definition of health as something that can be acquired (e.g. through medicine) suggests health can be slotted into different activities which have a price. However, this is not how people experience health and illness.
- The definition of health as individually defined strength ignores the fact that health and ill health are created within a social context. It is this social context, as much as the individual, which determines what is perceived and recognized to be health and ill health.

References

Antonovsky, A., 1993. The sense of coherence as a determinant of health. In: Beattie, A., Gott, M., Jones, L., et al. (Eds.), Health and Wellbeing: A Reader. Macmillan/Open University, Basingstoke, pp. 202–214.

Awad, A.G., Voruganti, L.N., 2008. The burden of schizophrenia on caregivers: a review. Pharmacoeconomics 26, 149–162.

Blaxter, M., 1990. Health and Lifestyles. Tavistock/Routledge, London.

Cochrane, A.L., 1972. Effectiveness and Efficiency. Nuffield Provincial Hospitals Trust, London.

Cornwell, J., 1984. Hard-Earned Lives. Tavistock, London.

Crawford, R., 2000. The ritual of health promotion. In: Williams, S.J., Gabe, J., Calnan, M. (Eds.), Health, Medicine and Society: Key Theories, Future Agendas. Routledge, London, pp. 219–235.

Department of Health, 2010. Healthy Lives Healthy People: Our Strategy for Public Health in England. Available online at: https://www.gov.uk/government/uploads/system/uploads/attachment_data/file/216096/dh_127424.pdf [accessed 14.09.15].

Freidson, F., 1986. Professional Powers: A Study of the Institutionalization of Formal Knowledge. University of Chicago Press, Chicago.

Foucault, M., 1977. Discipline and Punish: The birth of the prison. Vintage Books, New York.

Goffman, E., 1968. Stigma: Notes on the Management of a Spoiled Identity. Penguin, Harmondsworth.

Government Office for Science, 2008. Foresight Report: Mental Capital and Wellbeing. Government Office for Science, London. Available online at: https://www.gov.uk/government/uploads/system/uploads/attachment_data/file/292450/mental-capital-wellbeing-report.pdf [accessed 14.09.15].

Hart, G., Wellings, K., 2002. Sexual behaviour and its medicalisation: in sickness and in health. British Medical Journal 324, 896–900.

Huber, M.1, Knottnerus, J.A., Green, L., van der Horst, H., Jadad, A.R., Kromhout, D., Leonard, B., Lorig, K., Loureiro, M.I., van der Meer, J.W., Schnabel, P., Smith, R., van Weel, C., Smid, H., 2011. How should we define health? British Medical Journal 343 (4163), 235–237.

Illich, I., 1975. Medical Nemesis, Part One. Calder and Boyers, London.

McKeown, T., 1976. The role of medicine. Dream, mirage or nemesis? The Nuffield Provincial Hospitals Trust, Oxford. Available online at: http://www.nuffieldtrust.org.uk/sites/files/nuffiled/publication/The_Role_of_Medicine.pdf [accessed 14.09.15].

Mansfield, K., 1977. In: Stead, C.K. (Ed.), The Letters and Journals of Katherine Mansfield: A Selection. Penguin, Harmondsworth.

Maslow, A.H., 1943. A theory of human motivation. Psychological Review 50 (4), 370–396.

Maslow, A.H., 1970. Motivation and Personality, second ed. Harper and Row, New York.

New Economics Foundation, 2012. Happy Planet Index. www.happyplanetindex.org.

Parsons, T., 1951. The Social System. Free Press, Glencoe, IL, USA.

Popay, J., Bennett, S., Thomas, C., Williams, G., Gatrell, A., Bostock, L., 2003. Beyond 'beer, fags, egg and chips'? Exploring lay understandings of social inequalities in health. Sociology of Health & Illness 25 (No. 1), 1–23.

Rigby, H., Gubitz, G., Phillips, S., 2009. A systematic review of caregiver burden following stroke. International Journal of Stroke 4, 285–292.

Robertson, S., 2006. Not living life in too much excess: lay men understanding health and well-being. Health 10, 175–189.

Seedhouse, D., 1986. Health: Foundations for Achievement. John Wiley, Chichester.

Tarlov, A.R., 1996. Social determinants of health: the sociobiological translation. In: Blane, D., Brunner, E., Wilkinson, R. (Eds.), Health and Social Organisation: Towards a Health Policy for the 21st Century. Routledge, London.

UNICEF, 2013. Report Card 11 Child Well-Being in Rich Countries. www.unicef.org.uk.

Vellone, E., Piras, G., Talucci, C., Cohen, M., 2008. Quality of life of caregivers of people with Alzheimer's disease. Journal of Advanced Nursing 61, 222–231.

Wilkinson, R., Pickett, K., 2009. The Spirit Level: Why Equality is Better for Everyone. Penguin, London.

World Health Organization, 1946. Constitution. World Health Organization, Geneva. Available online at: http://www.who.int/governance/eb/who_constitution_en.pdf [accessed 14.09.15].

World Health Organization, 1984. Health Promotion: A Discussion Document on the Concept and Principles. World Health Organization Regional Office for Europe, Copenhagen. Available online at: http://apps.who.int/iris/bitstream/10665/107835/1/E90607.pdf [accessed 14.09.15].

World Health Organization, 1986. Ottawa Charter for Health Promotion. Journal of Health Promotion 1, 1–4. Available online at: http://www.euro.who.int/en/publications/policy-documents/ottawa-charter-for-health-promotion,-1986 [accessed 19.03.15].

World Health Organization, 1997. 4th International Conference on Health Promotion. New Players for a New Era – Leading Health Promotion into the 21st Century. World Health Organization, Jakarta. Available online at: http://www.who.int/healthpromotion/conferences/previous/jakarta/declaration/en/index1.html [accessed 19.03.15].

Chapter Two

Influences on health

By the end of this chapter you will be able to:
- identify and critically discuss the social factors influencing health and the mechanisms by which they do so
- understand the associations between social class and health; gender and health; and ethnicity and health
- have a critical understanding of theories of social determinants of health and explanations for health inequalities
- describe the range of policy interventions to address health inequalities aimed at individuals and populations.

Key Concepts and Definitions

Health inequalities The avoidable and unfair differences in health status between groups of people who are united by their shared socio-economic status or gender rather than by any health-related attributes, e.g. medical conditions such as diabetes.

Inequity is a lack of equity or fairness.

Social class describes a group of people united through having the same educational, social or economic status, e.g. working-class.

Social determinants are economic and social factors (e.g. income, social class, gender) that have a profound effect on health. These differences are not natural, but are created and maintained by social and economic policies and legislation.

Importance of the Topic

Chapter 1 showed that there is a wide range of meanings attached to the concept of health, and different perspectives are offered by the scientific medical model and social science. It emphasized the importance of social factors in the construction and meaning of health. This chapter shows how the major influences on mortality and morbidity are social and environmental factors. It summarizes the considerable body of research suggesting that the existence of inequalities in health status between groups of people reflects structural inequalities linked to social class, gender and ethnicity.

Determinants of health

Since the decline in infectious diseases in the nineteenth and early twentieth centuries, the major causes of sickness and death are now cancers (30%), circulatory disease, including coronary heart disease (CHD) and stroke (29%) and respiratory disease (14%) (Office for National Statistics, 2013a; Fig. 2.1).

In the last 20 years cancers have become the leading cause of mortality in both men and women. This is a considerable change from 100 years ago, when bronchitis was the leading cause of death, killing more than 39,000 people, and tuberculosis and pneumonia were among the 10 leading causes. Alzheimer's disease and dementia currently account for 5.1% of deaths in men and 10.3% of deaths in women. Nearly 40% of deaths occur in people over the age of 85 and 0.6% of deaths in those under the age of one.

In the UK increased longevity and the current average lifespan of women of 82 years and men of 79 years account for the increase in degenerative diseases in the population as a whole. Despite the increase in life expectancy, epidemiologists who study the pattern of diseases in society have found that not all groups have the same opportunities to achieve good health, and that there are population patterns which make it possible to predict the likelihood of people from different groups dying prematurely (Case Study 2.1).

As well as differences within countries, there are also differences across countries.

- In South Africa the death rate from HIV/AIDS per 100,000 is 555.7. In Finland it is 0.1 per 100,000.
- In Afghanistan the death rate from birth trauma is 30.8 per 100,000, while in Ireland it is 0.2 per 100,000.
- In India the death rate from lung disease is 142.1 per 100,000, while in Japan it is 4.0 per 100,000 (www.healthdata.org/gbd).

In trying to determine what affects health, social scientists and epidemiologists seek to compare at least two variables: firstly, a measure of health, or rather ill health, such as mortality or morbidity; and secondly, a factor such as gender or occupation that could account for the differences in health. Of course, effects on health can be due to several variables interacting together. For example, research into CHD has linked the disease with a large number of factors, including high levels of blood cholesterol, high blood pressure, obesity, cigarette smoking and low levels of physical activity. Other research indicates there may be links between CHD and psychosocial factors, such as stress and lack of social support, depression and anger (Marmot and Wilkinson, 2006). Many studies have tried to establish whether there is a coronary-prone personality that is competitive, impatient and hostile (known as type A). We also know that mortality from CHD is higher among lower socio-economic groups, among men rather than women and among South Asians (British Heart Foundation, 2012). Figure 2.2 illustrates in a simple form how health status can be accounted for not by one variable, but by many factors interacting together. It shows that some factors have an independent effect on health while others may be mediated by intervening variables. While physical inactivity, smoking and raised blood cholesterol are the major risk factors for CHD, it is important to look 'upstream' and understand the causes of these risk factors and their roots in the social context of people's lives.

What is clear is that ill health does not happen by chance or through bad luck. A report by Lalonde (1974), published in Canada, was influential in identifying four fields in which health could be promoted.

1. Genetic and biological factors which determine an individual's predisposition to disease.
2. Lifestyle factors and health behaviours, such as smoking, which contribute to disease.
3. Environmental factors, such as housing and pollution.
4. The extent and nature of health services.

Genetic factors remain largely unalterable, and what limited scope there is for intervention lies in the medical field. Chapter 1 outlined McKeown and Lowe's (1974) work showing that medical interventions in the form of vaccination had remarkably little impact on mortality rates. This suggests that factors other than the purely biological determine health and well-being, and that probably the greatest opportunities to improve health lie in the environment and individual lifestyles.

THE DISTRIBUTION OF CAUSES OF MORTALITY IN ENGLAND IN THE 21st CENTURY

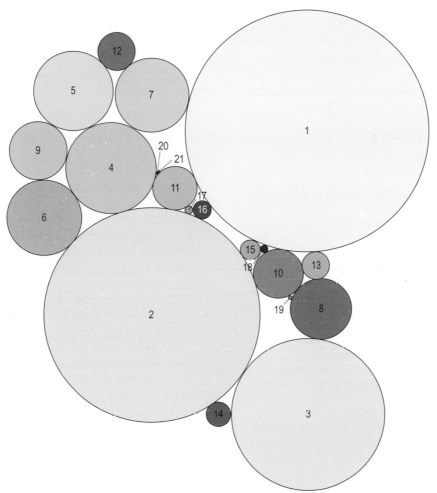

1	Circulatory diseases	2,114,550
2	Cancer and neoplasms	1,686,133
3	Respiratory diseases	836,894
4	Digestive diseases	300,225
5	Mental and behavioural disorders**	227,377
6	External causes of morbidity and mortality	207,576
7	Diseases of the nervous system	199,409
8	Other causes	135,516
9	Genitourinary diseases	122,446
10	Endocrine, nutritional and metabolic diseases	87,890
11	Certain infectious and parasitic diseases	68,123
12	Musculoskeletal system and connective tissue	52,438
13	Neonatal (no cause registered)	26,620
14	Skin	20,468
15	Congenital malformations, deformations and chromosomal abnormalities	14,695
16	Blood diseases	12,230
17	Babies dying before, during or after childbirth	2,446
18	Drug-resistant tuberculosis*	2,275
19	Pregnancy and childbirth	539
20	Diseases of the ear and mastoid process	269
21	Diseases of the eye and adnexa	158

*Drug-resistant tuberculosis was given its own special code but could be considered with the certain infectious disease grouping.

**The number of deaths registered as being due to mental and behavioural disorders was particularly affected by the switch between volumes due to vascular dementia being pushed into this category.

Fig. 2.1 ● The distribution of causes of mortality in England in the twenty-first century. (Adapted from The Office for National Statistics, 2013a. Licenced under the Open Government Licence v.3.0. Available online at: http://www.theguardian.com/news/datablog/interactive/2013/oct/24/how-people-died-21st-century.)

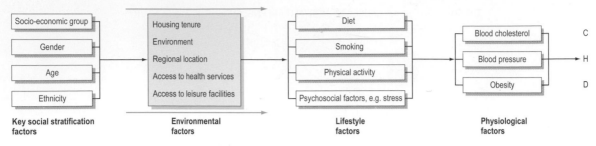

Fig. 2.2 ● Factors influencing the development of coronary heart disease (CHD).

Case Study 2.1 Differences in health in the UK

- Women live around four years longer than men, but the gap has been shrinking and is expected to shrink further over time.
- Black African women who are asylum seekers are estimated to have a mortality rate seven times higher than white women.
- Black Caribbean and Pakistani babies are twice as likely to die in their first year compared to Bangladeshi or white British babies.
- Three times as many men as women commit suicide, and rates are particularly high for younger men aged 25 to 44.
- Evidence suggests that lesbian, gay, bisexual and transgender people may have an increased risk of attempted suicide.
- Children from ethnic minorities are up to twice as likely as white British children to be involved in road traffic accidents while walking or playing.
- The risk of mental health problems is nearly twice as likely for Bangladeshi men as for white men.

Equality and Human Rights Commission (2011).

Learning Activity 2.1 Influences on health

Lifestyles are frequently the focus of health promotion interventions. Figure 2.3 shows a whole range of factors that may influence behaviour. Take one of the lifestyle factors implicated in CHD, e.g. physical activity, and identify the influences on that health behaviour.

Dahlgren and Whitehead (1991) thus talk of 'layers of influence on health' that can be modified (Fig. 2.3):

- personal behaviour and lifestyles, and the knowledge, awareness and skills that can enable change in relation to, for example, diet or physical activity
- support and influence within communities which can sustain or damage health
- living and working conditions, and access to facilities and services
- economic, cultural and environmental conditions, such as standards of living or the labour market.

In all societies, health behaviours and physical and mental health vary between social groups. The main axes of variation include socio-economic status, gender, ethnicity and place of residence. The specific features and pathways by which societal conditions affect health are termed the social determinants. The social determinants of health refer to factors determined by social policies which affect health, e.g. working conditions, housing and the physical environment. These social policies in turn are determined by political beliefs and economics (see Chapters 7 and 11). The medical model of health tends to focus on individuals and their biological bodies rather than socially patterned behaviours. For example, poor diet is linked to many causes of ill health and premature mortality, and most medical advice is focused on trying to persuade individuals to change their dietary behaviour. Yet the social forces implicated in unhealthy dietary choices (advertising, pricing and availability of products) remain untouched, because they are viewed as economic or political factors beyond the remit of the health services.

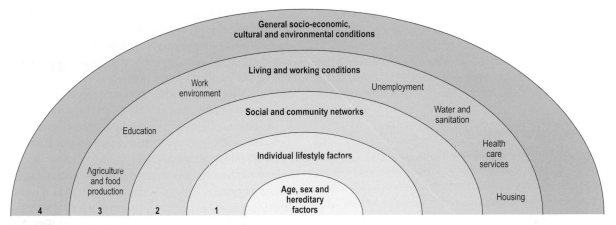

Fig. 2.3 ● The main determinants of health. (From Dahlgren, Whitehead, M., 1991. Policies and Strategies to Promote Social Equity in Health. Institute for Future Studies, Stockholm.)

There is a large body of research supporting the link between socio-economic status and health in all countries (CSOH, 2008). This research shows there is an undisputed link between lower socio-economic status and poorer health. While describing and documenting health inequalities are now a key part of research and policy, addressing such inequalities requires a distinction between inequality and inequity. Inequalities refer to differences between groups which are largely avoidable. If these differences are deemed inequitable, this implies a judgement that they are not only avoidable but also unfair and unjust.

There are three types of health inequalities.

1. Inequalities in the determinants of health, e.g. education, employment and housing, which can all have an influence on health status.
2. Inequalities in health outcomes, e.g. there is a 6-year difference in life expectancy at birth across different boroughs in London (see http://life.mappinglondon.co.uk).
3. Inequalities in access to healthcare, e.g. refugees and homeless people often have difficulty in obtaining access to primary healthcare services, such as registering with a general practitioner (GP).

It is important to understand social stratification in order to analyse and assess how inequalities are created and perpetuated, how different groups are perceived and understood, and the impact of this on policy.

Social class and health

Most research in the UK which has sought to identify the major determinants of health and ill health has focused on the links between social class and health. A report was published of a Department of Health and Social Security working group on inequalities in health (Townsend and Davidson, 1982). Known as the Black Report after the group's chairman, Sir Douglas Black, it provided a detailed study of the relationship between mortality and morbidity and social class.

The terms social class, social disadvantage, socio-economic status and occupation are often used interchangeably. The classification of social class derives from the Registrar General's scale of five occupational classes, ranging from professionals in class I to unskilled manual workers in class V. This was largely unchanged from 1921 (although class III was divided into manual and non-manual work in 1971). From 2001 the National Statistics Socio-Economic Classification (NS-SEC) has been used for all official statistics and surveys (Table 2.1).

Although social class classification is not a perfect tool, it does serve as an indicator of the way of life and living standards experienced by different groups. It correlates with other aspects of social position, such as income, housing, education and working and living environments.

The Black Report and a later report commissioned by the Health Education Authority, *The Health Divide* (Whitehead, 1988), found significant differences in death rates between socio-economic classes. More recently, another government inquiry (Marmot, 2010) drew together data which show that, far from ill health

Table 2.1 Social class classification
1. Higher managerial and professional
1.1 e.g. company directors, bank managers, senior civil servants
1.2 e.g. doctors, barristers and solicitors, teachers, social workers
2. Lower managerial and professional, e.g. nurses, actors and musicians, police, soldiers
3. Intermediate, e.g. secretaries, clerks
4. Small employers and own-account workers, e.g. publicans, playgroup leaders, farmers, taxi drivers
5. Lower supervisory, craft and related occupations, e.g. printers, plumbers, butchers, train drivers
6. Semi-routine occupations, e.g. shop assistants, traffic wardens, hairdressers
7. Routine occupations, e.g. waiters, road sweepers, cleaners, couriers
8. Never worked and long-term unemployed

Source: NS-SEC.

being a matter of bad luck, health and disease are socially patterned, with the more affluent members of society living longer and enjoying better health than disadvantaged social groups. Although the health of the whole population has steadily improved, there is still a strong relationship between socio-economic group and health status.

A wealth of research has shown the relationship between socio-economic status and health status in most Western countries. People from lower socio-economic groups have much poorer health than those in higher groups. This is evident in relation to disease prevalence, life expectancy and infant mortality.

Figure 2.4 shows the step-wise social gradient in health whereby the poorest have the worst health and the richest enjoy the best health. In general, and in all countries, the lower an individual's socio-economic position, the worse is his or her health. This health gradient is evident in death rates as well as in reports of ill health.

Although infant deaths are declining, children from manual backgrounds are more likely to die in the first year of life or from accidental injury. Low birth weight is probably the most important predictor of death in the first month of life and this is clearly

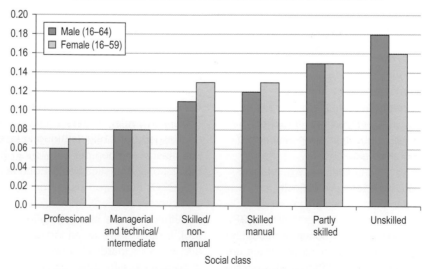

PROPORTION OF DEVIATION FROM PERFECT HEALTH BY SOCIAL CLASS

Note: Based on QALY measure of self-reported health. Does not cover Scotland and Wales.

Fig. 2.4 ● Self-reported health and social class. (Open government licence/Crown copyright.)

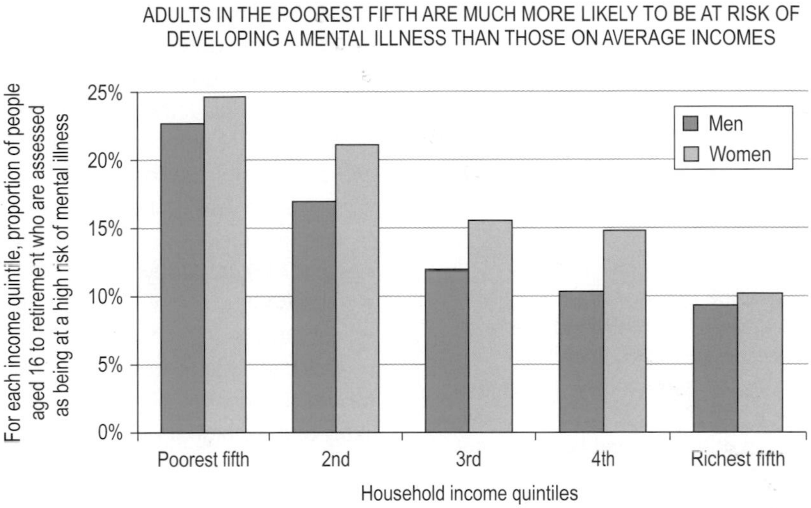

ADULTS IN THE POOREST FIFTH ARE MUCH MORE LIKELY TO BE AT RISK OF DEVELOPING A MENTAL ILLNESS THAN THOSE ON AVERAGE INCOMES

Fig. 2.5 ● The social gradient of mental ill health. (Open government licence/Crown copyright.)

class-related, with two-thirds of babies weighing under 2.5 kg being born to mothers in social class V (Office for National Statistics, 2013a). Although it is common to talk of 'diseases of affluence', such as CHD, being the major killers in contemporary Europe, most disease categories are more common among lower socio-economic groups. Particularly large differentials have developed for respiratory disease, lung cancer, accidents and suicide. An exception to this is the death rate from breast cancer, which is evenly distributed across all social groups. People from lower socio-economic groups experience more sickness and ill health, and measures of mental health and well-being also reflect a social gradient, as shown in Figure 2.5.

In our companion book *Public Health and Health Promotion: Developing Practice* (Naidoo and Wills, 2010) we discuss the determinants of health in more detail. The most immediate causes of socio-economic inequalities in health were summarized by Macintyre (2007) as:

- exposures, e.g. damp housing, hazardous work, adverse life events
- behaviours, e.g. smoking, diet, exercise
- personal strengths and capabilities (see Chapter 1).

The pathways by which members of different socio-economic status groups are at risk of such exposures and vulnerabilities are often due to political and economic forces and social stratifications in society. Some of these pathways are discussed in the next section.

Income and health

Better health is strongly associated with income. The UK is the world's sixth-largest economy, yet one in five of the UK population live below the official poverty line, meaning that they experience life as a daily struggle (see www.poverty.org.uk). Those most likely to be in this category are the unemployed, pensioners, lone parents, families with three or more children and the low paid.

Poverty can affect health directly by, for example, children not having enough to eat, eating a high-processed diet and having limited access to food outlets. Across the UK dietary initiatives such as breakfast clubs, cookery clubs and community cafés promote healthy eating in low-income communities (e.g. see www.communityfoodandhealth.org.uk in Scotland).

In low-income countries, infectious diseases such as diarrhoeal illness and malaria are associated with lack of income resulting in lack of access to clean water, food and medical services. Disease then further impoverishes the poor, preventing people from working and incurring high medical costs.

 ### Research Example 2.1 Children, poverty and health

A systematic review of 34 studies, mainly from America but including some British research, found a strong causal link between household income and children's achievements in education, their well-being and positive behavioural outcomes. Children in richer households were more likely to do better in all spheres of life, including education and health. The link between household income and childhood well-being appears to be due to money rather than any other confounding factors such as parental expectations. While a parent's level of education, attitude towards bringing up children and other parental factors have a bearing, research shows that having more money has a direct positive impact on children's social and behavioural development and educational achievement. The evidence is strongest for a link between income and educational outcomes. Conversely, reductions in family income, including benefit cuts, are likely to have wide-ranging negative effects. Money seems to have more of an effect among low-income families.

Research evidence supports two theories as to why income matters so much. The family stress model focuses on the stress and anxiety caused by low income, while the investment model focuses on parental ability to invest in services and goods that support child development. Research findings are more supportive of the family stress model than the investment model.

Cooper and Stewart (2013).

Housing and health

Frank Dobson, briefly health minister in 1997, remarked: 'everyone with a grain of sense knows that it's bad for your health if you don't have anywhere to live'. The issues of housing stock, dampness, inadequate heating and energy efficiency are recognized as key determinants of health (Parliamentary Office of Science and Technology, 2011).

For example, there are 40,000 excess winter deaths (deaths which would not be expected if the average death rate for the rest of the year applied in winter) each year in the UK. These are attributable to:

* energy efficiency
* level of occupancy
* income
* cost of fuel.

Cold and damp housing has been shown to contribute to illness. Children living in damp houses are likely to have higher rates of respiratory illness, symptoms of infection and stress. These will be exacerbated by overcrowding. The high accident rates to children in social class V are associated with high-density housing where there is a lack of play space and opportunities for parental supervision. Psychological and practical difficulties accompany living in high-rise flats and isolated housing estates, which may adversely affect the health of women at home and older people.

Employment and health

Work is important to consider as a social determinant of health because:

* it determines income levels
* it affects self-esteem
* the type of employment may itself directly affect health.

The traditional focus of occupational health has been to consider how particular types of employment carry high occupational health risks. This may be because of the risk of accidents (e.g. in mining), exposure to hazardous substances or stress. Some occupations encourage lifestyles which may be damaging to health. Publicans, for example, are at high risk of developing cirrhosis.

There has been considerable interest in how the psychosocial environment of work can affect health (Marmot et al., 2006). Most research has identified high demands and low control over work decisions as contributing to job stress and cardiovascular risk. These factors, together with the amount of social support people get at work, have been confirmed in workplace studies in many developed countries (see Chapter 14 for further discussion). There is also a considerable body of evidence, mostly gathered in the 1980s, that unemployment can damage health (McLean et al., 2005). It is, however, uncertain whether unemployment itself can lead to a deterioration in health or whether it is the poverty associated with unemployment which contributes to the poor health of the unemployed.

Research Example 2.2 The Whitehall studies

The Whitehall studies are important because they have followed employees of the British Civil Service over a number of years, and have shed light on the causation of ill health among employees. The original Whitehall study began in 1967 and studied the careers and health of 18,000 men. The study found that premature death was more prevalent among men in the lowest employment grades. Furthermore, it appeared to be the lower employment status rather than any other confounding factors (such as smoking) that was responsible for the increased mortality rate. The second Whitehall study, started in 1985, recruited over 10,000 employees, including women, and has collected data from 10 cohorts of civil servants. The study sought to clarify risk factors for ill health and premature mortality. Consistent findings are that psychosocial factors (e.g. work-related stress and conflict, unfairness at work, domestic conflict) make a significant contribution to poor health outcomes. The study also found that environmental changes were more effective than targeting individuals in getting employees to change their behaviour, e.g. to quit smoking. The Whitehall studies support the view that social hierarchy is an important factor impacting on health, and that the more subordinate individuals lower down in the hierarchy suffer increased ill health and premature death due to their low status. The impact of social position is greater than that of individual risk behaviours such as smoking.

More details available at http://www.ucl.ac.uk/whitehallII/history.

Learning Activity 2.2 Unemployment and health

Consider the following evidence concerning the effects of unemployment on health. What could account for this relationship?

1. The unemployed report higher rates of mental ill health, including depression, anxiety and sleep disturbance.
2. Suicide and parasuicide rates are twice as high among the unemployed as among the employed.
3. The death rates among the unemployed are at least 20% higher than expected after adjustment for social class and age.
4. The unemployed have higher rates of bronchitis and ischaemic heart disease than the employed.
5. Over 60% of unemployed people smoke, compared to 30% of employed people.

Moller (2012).

Gender and health

Gender refers to the social categorization of people as men or women, and the social meaning and beliefs about sexual difference. Some of the sex differences in morbidity have been viewed as an artefact of measurement of the use of health services. Women are more likely to report illness, as they are less likely to be in full-time employment and have easier access to primary care, or because they are more inclined to take care of their health, resulting in increased consultation rates. However, this does not explain the sex difference in mortality. Nor is there a consistent tendency for women's greater willingness to consult: women are no more likely than men to visit their GPs for musculoskeletal, respiratory or digestive problems.

The biological explanation suggests that women are more resistant to infection and benefit from a protective effect of oestrogen, accounting for their lower mortality rates. Paradoxically, female hormones and the female reproductive system are claimed to render women more liable to physical and mental ill health. But biological explanations are unable to account for the social class difference in women's health, whereby women in professional and managerial social classes experience better health than women in lower socio-economic groups. It is also important to note that greater female longevity only arose in the twentieth century, and is mostly attributable to the dramatic decline in infectious disease mortality and a decline in the number of births. It is not evident in low-income countries.

Lifestyle explanations argue that women are socialized to be passive, dependent and sick. Women readily adopt the sick role because it fits with preconceived notions of feminine behaviour. Men, by contrast, are encouraged to be aggressive and risk-taking, both at work and in their leisure time. The higher rates for accidents and alcoholism among men are cited as evidence for this. Men are far less likely to take part in weight-management programmes and the national bowel cancer screening programme, or to set quit dates for smoking cessation (see https://www.menshealthforum.org.uk/professionals/search?f%5B0%5D=im_field_pro_content_type%3A30).

Learning Activity 2.3 Men's health

What could account for why men under the age of 45 visit their GPs only half as often as women (www.menshealthforum.org.uk)?

More recently, the focus has been on the distinct roles and behaviours of men and women in a given culture, dictated by that culture's gender norms and values, and how these give rise to gender differences. Globally, there is considerable concern about how women, because of gender norms, are disempowered from, for example, receiving healthcare because they cannot travel alone to a clinic, or protecting themselves against HIV because of their male partners' promiscuity or refusal to use a condom.

In most societies, when compared with men, women tend to have:

- lower status
- lower income
- lower power
- limited access to financial and other assets

- lower educational status
- lower levels of participation in legal and political institutions, and hence less influence on decision-making
- limited access to work
- increased likelihood of being victims of domestic violence.

Yet women often have greater health needs (e.g. pregnancy and child-related care). In most cases women take the leading role in caring for children and dependants, and are also expected to look after the house and work in the fields producing food.

Case Study 2.2 Gender-based interventions: football fans in training

The prevalence of obesity in men in the UK is among the highest in Europe, but men are less likely than women to use existing weight-loss programmes. Developing weight-management programmes which are appealing and acceptable to men is a public health priority. Football Fans in Training (FFIT), a men-only weight-management programme delivered to groups of men at top professional football clubs, encourages men to lose weight by working with, not against, cultural ideals of masculinity. The setting enabled men to join a weight-management programme in circumstances that felt 'right' rather than threatening to them as men. FFIT is an example of how to facilitate health promotion activities in a way that is consistent with, rather than challenging, common ideals of masculinity.

More details from http://www.ffit.org.uk, including the results of a randomized controlled trial published in *The Lancet*.

Health of ethnic minorities

Race commonly refers to a biological marker of difference assigned to a group of people who are recognized as sharing common physical or physiognomic characteristics and/or a common lineage of descent, such as 'Asian' or 'Chinese'. Essentialist racism emphasizes race difference in hierarchical terms of biologic inequality, and 'scientific' categories such as the Aryan superiority assumed by the Nazis over the Jews. A racial logic becomes a system of differentiation based upon the ascription of people to specific categories on the basis of assumed biological, physiognomic or cultural differences, usually bestowing privilege to one group. It becomes a means of exclusion and subordination, and a way of making a group of people inferior within society. In extreme cases this is demonstrated by extermination, e.g. in Rwanda and Nazi Germany.

Contemporary sociological and political theory focuses rather on 'race' as a social construct, and specifically on the ways in which racial concepts, categories and divisions structure and become embedded in areas of social life and national states. Ethnicity is a complex concept that is used to refer to those with a shared culture, social background, language or religion.

The Fourth National Survey of Ethnic Minorities in England and Wales (Nazroo, 1997) notes:

- two-fifths of Caribbeans, Pakistanis and Bangladeshis have poor general health
- Pakistanis and Bangladeshis have a greater risk of heart disease than white people
- one in 18 people from an ethnic minority group is diagnosed as diabetic
- 50% of Bangladeshi men smoke.

That particular diseases, poor perceived health or premature deaths are more common in ethnic minority groups is a complex issue. In the past, explanations tended to focus on simple differences in culture.

The factors influencing ethnic health inequalities were summarized by Bhopal (2014) as:

- culture, e.g. taboos on alcohol
- social education and economic status, e.g. knowledge of biology and health influences, languages spoken and read
- environmental, e.g. before and after migration
- lifestyle, e.g. behaviours in relation to diet, alcohol and tobacco
- access to and concordance with healthcare advice, willingness to seek health and social services, and use of complementary/alternative methods of care or treatment
- genetic and biological factors, e.g. birth weight, body composition.

Socio-economic factors have a profound impact, but it is important not to put all members of ethnic minorities into one disadvantaged category. More data would enable us to find out how many people from ethnic minority groups are disadvantaged, and in what way. It would also then be possible to determine whether the poor health of black and ethnic minority groups is associated with the low-income, poor working conditions or unemployment and poor housing shared by those in lower social classes, or whether there is, in addition, ill health resulting from other factors. Racism in service delivery, either directly or through the ethnocentrism of services which are based on the needs of the majority, is often invoked as the explanation for inequalities.

 Learning Activity 2.4 Healthcare and ethnicity

In your experience, do you think that healthcare differs according to the ethnicity of the patient?

Place and health

In the 1980s mortality rates were shown to increase steadily in the UK, moving from the south-east to the north-west, with a north–south divide present for most diseases. This seemed to be associated with poverty and disadvantage. Glasgow's Shettleston, for example, has twice the national average mortality rate. In the UK, Danny Dorling has written extensively on the impact of place on health (see http://www. dannydorling.org/?page_id=70). One obvious explanation for the geographic differences in death rates might be differences in social class distribution – those areas with high mortality rates being areas with a greater proportion of people in lower socio-economic groups. Increasingly, the effect of place on health has been seen as more complex, including not only the socio-economic characteristics of individuals concentrated in particular places but also the local physical and social environment and the shared norms and traditions that might promote or inhibit health.

Explaining health inequalities

Inequality means a lack of uniformity, or difference. In this chapter we note differences in health outcomes according to gender and ethnicity. In the context of health and healthcare, the term 'inequalities' is mainly used to refer to differences that arise from socio-economic factors, including income, work, housing and location of residence. Our companion volume *Public Health and Health Promotion: Developing Practice* (Naidoo and Wills, 2010) explores these social determinants of health in more detail.

You may believe that people in the lower socio-economic groups choose more unhealthy ways of living, or you may believe they have low incomes which prevent them from adopting a healthy lifestyle and cause them to live in unhealthy conditions. There is a continuing debate over this question, and no simple answer. Explanations for health inequalities focus on cultural/behavioural, materialist/structural and psychosocial explanations which suggest that adverse environmental conditions at different points in the life course can lead to ill health.

Health inequalities as a consequence of lifestyles

This argument suggests that the social distribution of ill health is linked with differences in the prevalence of risk behaviours. These behaviours – smoking, high alcohol consumption, lack of exercise, high-fat and high-sugar diets – are more common among lower socio-economic groups.

For example, although smoking has decreased in all social classes over the last 20 years, there are still major differences in the proportion of smokers in each socio-economic group: data from the General Lifestyle Survey show that in 2010, 28% of smokers were from manual occupations, whereas 13% were from managerial and professional backgrounds. Smokers from manual backgrounds started smoking early in their lives: 48% of men and 40% of women were smoking by the age of 16,

compared to 33% of men and 28% of women from managerial and professional backgrounds (Office for National Statistics, 2013b).

Behaviour cannot, however, be separated from the social context in which it takes place. Graham (1992), in many studies on smoking, has shown how the decision to smoke by many working-class women is a coping strategy to deal with the stress associated with poverty and isolation. The decision to smoke *is* a choice, but it is not taken through recklessness or ignorance; it is rather a choice between 'health evils' – stress versus smoking.

 Learning Activity 2.5 Attitudes to lifestyle inequalities

Smoking is the biggest single cause of the differences in death rates between rich and poor people. Which of the following views comes closest to your own?

'Poor people bring ill health upon themselves. They don't care about their health. If they are so poor, how can they afford to smoke and drink and eat junk food?'

'People's use of tobacco and alcohol is to a large extent determined by their social relations and networks, which in turn affect their self-esteem and levels of stress. Tobacco offers a prop of sorts'.

Some writers claim that there are cultural differences between social groups in their attitudes towards health and protecting their health for the future. Thus giving up cigarettes, as a form of deferred gratification, is more likely to appeal to middle-class people who, as we saw in Chapter 1, may have a stronger locus of control and are more likely to believe that they determine the course of their lives. Working-class people, who may have to struggle to get by each day, do not make long-term plans and have a fatalistic view of health, believing it to be a matter of luck. These attitudes are passed on from generation to generation. This phenomenon is referred to as the 'culture of poverty' or 'cycle of deprivation'. According to such views, ill health can be explained in terms of the characteristics of poor people themselves and their inadequacy and incompetence. In 1986 Edwina

Currie, a newly appointed health minister, caused a storm of controversy by suggesting that the high levels of premature death, permanent sickness and low birth weights in the northern regions were due to ignorance and people failing to realize that they had some control over their lives.

A behavioural explanation, which sees lifestyles and cultural influences determining health, has considerable appeal to any government that wants to reduce public expenditure. If individuals are seen as responsible for their own health, government inactivity is legitimized. Such viewpoints, which are particularly associated with neoliberal governments (see Chapter 7), have been widely criticized as victim-blaming, in that people are seen as being responsible for factors which disadvantage them but over which they have no control.

Health inequalities as a consequence of the life course

This explanation for health inequalities suggests that early life circumstances predict future morbidity and mortality rates. There are cumulative effects of both material and psychosocial hazards over the life course of an individual that explain observed differences in health and life expectancy, as shown in Figure 2.6.

1. The early life environment has a significant impact on the later health of the adult, regardless of other health-related factors. For example, fetal exposure to passive smoking (due to maternal smoking or maternal exposure to passive smoking) may impact on fetal health and result in low birth weight. Low birth weight is linked to poorer health outcomes (e.g. greater mortality from CHD, stroke and respiratory disease) in adult life.
2. The early life environment of an individual is linked to later lifestyle factors which have a direct impact on health. For example a lower socio-economic family background is associated with poorer educational attainment and poorer housing, job security and work opportunities. Early interventions can change this association. Interventions in the early years can help individuals achieve better educational, work and social outcomes (e.g. home ownership, higher incomes), which in turn are associated with better health outcomes.

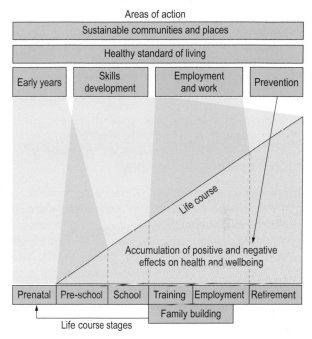

THE MARMOT REVIEW (2010): ACTION ACROSS THE LIFE COURSE MODEL

Fig. 2.6 ● The social gradient of health across the life course. (Marmot, M., 2010. Fair Society, Healthy Lives. DH, London. © The Marmot Review, Marmot Review Secretariat, Department for Epidemiology & Public Health. University College, London, 1-19 Torrington Place, London WC1E 7HB, Email: P.Hallam@ucl.ac.uk.)

3. The environment to which individuals are exposed is also an important factor in determining their health status. Exposure to a health-damaging environment, e.g. smoky indoor areas, will have a cumulative effect on an individual's health. The intensity and duration of the exposure are directly linked to later outcomes, e.g. mortality from cancer, CHD, strokes or respiratory illness.

The 1958 birth cohort study, which follows a group of individuals from childhood to adulthood, demonstrates that socio-economic status is linked to factors such as low birth weight and height. Childhood development in all spheres (physical, psychological, social and intellectual) is sensitive to the wider environment and is an important determinant of health status in later life (Graham and Power, 2004).

Learning Activity 2.6 The life course and health

Chart your own life course in relation to health.
- Are there any external factors which influenced your and your family's health?
  - Were there any personal events which affected your physical and psychological well-being?

Learning Activity 2.7 Characteristics of a healthy society

The quality of the social life of a society is one of the most powerful determinants of health (and this, in turn, is very closely related to the degree of income equality)

Wilkinson (1996), p. 5.

Which of the following, in your view, reflects the characteristics of life in a healthy society?
1. High level of civic activities.
2. High gross national product.
3. Low crime rates.
4. High percentage of adults receiving a university education.
5. High levels of employment.
6. Narrow differences in income.
7. Sense of social solidarity and cohesion.

Health inequalities as a consequence of psychosocial factors

There is a growing body of evidence demonstrating that it is *relative* inequalities in income and material resources, coupled with the resulting social exclusion and marginalization, which are linked to poor health (Wilkinson, 1996; Wilkinson and Pickett, 2010). The key evidence on this comes from international data on income distribution and national mortality rates. In high-income countries it is not the richest nations which have the best health, but the most egalitarian, such as Sweden. While the exact mechanisms linking social inequality to ill health are uncertain, it is likely that social cohesion – as measured by levels of trust – provides the causal link between the two. The most plausible explanation for income inequality's apparent effect on health and social problems is 'status anxiety'. This suggests that income inequality is harmful because it places people in a hierarchy which increases status competition and causes stress, leading to poor health and other negative outcomes (Wilkinson and Pickett, 2010). Healthy egalitarian societies are more socially cohesive and have a stronger community life with greater social capital.

The degree to which an individual is integrated into society and has a social support network has been shown to have a significant impact on health. Wilkinson and Pickett (2010) demonstrate that people with stronger social relationships are half as likely to die as those with weaker social ties. Indicators of social relationships and networking, such as marital status, feeling lonely, size of social network and participation in social activities, are as important to health as smoking, and much more important to survival than heavy drinking, physical activity or obesity.

The negative emotional experience that arises from living in an unequal society is illustrated in the Whitehall II study (Marmot et al., 2006), a longitudinal study of civil servants and their experience of ill health (described in Research Example 2.2). Irrespective of health behaviour, those in control of their working lives (those in higher grades) are less likely to suffer from CHD, diabetes and metabolic syndrome.

Health inequalities as a consequence of material disadvantage

This explanation argues that the distribution of health and ill health in the population reflects a profoundly unequal distribution of resources in society. Thus those who experience ill health are those who are lower in the social hierarchy, are least educated and have least money and fewest resources. Low income may be the result of unemployment or ill-paid hazardous occupations. It can lead to poor housing in polluted and unsafe environments with few opportunities to build social support networks; and in turn such conditions lead to poor health. Lack of money can make it difficult for households to implement what they may know to be healthy choices.
- People on low incomes eat more processed foods, which are much higher in saturated fats and salt.

- They also eat a smaller variety of foods, due to the need to buy cheaper in bulk and from fear of potential waste.
- People living on state benefits eat less fruit and vegetables, which are less widely available and relatively expensive (Darmon and Drewnowski, 2008).

Absolute poverty is the inability to meet basic human needs such as access to food, shelter, warmth and safety. More than a billion people worldwide live in such extreme poverty. Relative poverty is determined by the standards of the rest of the society in which the individual lives. Although a person's basic needs may be met, relative poverty means he or she may be unable to afford any social participation and is then more likely to suffer from a range of physical health problems, e.g. CHD, as well as social and emotional health problems such as stress and depression, marital breakdown and addiction to drugs or alcohol.

Poverty is just one aspect of socio-economic disadvantage, and is associated with other factors:

- having a family to provide for
- being unable to work due to incapacity or illness
- being geographically isolated from services or supports
- being a young person leaving the care system
- being a single parent
- living in substandard housing or experiencing homelessness
- lacking skills.

 Case Study 2.3 Food banks

Across Europe there has been a huge rise in the number of people relying on food banks for emergency supplies. Over a million people, including nearly 400,000 children, received at least three days' emergency food from the Trussell Trust's 400 food banks in 2014/15 (http://www.trusselltrust.org/resources/documents/Press/Trussell-Trust-foodbank-use-tops-one-million.pdf). In 2014 German food banks provided more than 1.5 million people (from children to senior citizens) with food (http://blogs.lse.ac.uk/europpblog/2013/07/11/germany-foodbanks/). The reliance on emergency food is said to be triggered by low wages and limited welfare with no crisis payments.

http://www.trusselltrust.org/mid-year-stats-2014.

Health inequalities as a consequence of limited healthcare

A common response to the evidence of health inequalities is to see these as a consequence of restricted access to services. The intention of the National Health Service – to provide a universal service freely available to all – might have been expected to reduce inequalities in health status. Yet in the early 1970s a GP writing in *The Lancet* put forward the radical view that good healthcare tends to vary inversely with the needs of the population (Tudor Hart, 1971):

> *In areas with most sickness and death, GPs have more work, larger lists, less hospital support and inherit more clinically ineffective traditions of consultation than in the healthiest areas; and the hospital doctors shoulder heavier caseloads with less staff and equipment, more obsolete buildings and suffer recurrent crises in the availability of beds and replacement of staff. These trends can be summed up as the Inverse Care Law: that the availability of good medical care tends to vary inversely with the needs of the population served.*
> Tudor Hart (1971).

Equality of access requires that, for different communities:

- travel distance to facilities is equal
- transport and communication services are equal
- waiting times are equal
- patients are equally informed about the availability and effectiveness of treatments
- charges are equal (with equal ability to pay)
- the quality of services offered does not vary between groups or locations.

 Learning Activity 2.8 Equality of access to healthcare services

Even in the UK, where services are universally available and not dependent on the ability to pay, some groups are more able to access services than others. Why is this?

There is evidence of variation in the quality and quantity of care available to people in different social groups, and between regions and different ethnic groups (House of Commons Health Committee, 2009). However, since medical care has had little impact on the overall death rate from heart disease or cancers, and probably only about 5% of deaths are preventable through medical treatment, it must be concluded that differences in health status are not wholly attributable to variations in the amount and type of care received.

Tackling inequalities in health

Life expectancy, health and health-related behaviours have shown a steady improvement over the last 50 years, but there are gross inequalities in health between countries. Life expectancy at birth, for example, ranges from 34 years in Sierra Leone to 81.9 years in Japan (World Health Organization, 2004). Within countries, too, there are inequalities. In the USA Native Americans from South Dakota can expect to live only 58 years while Asian-American women from New Jersey have the highest national life expectancy at 91 years (Murray et al., 2005). Mortality statistics can reveal a social gradient in disease in *all* countries. As we have seen in this chapter, such inequalities are linked to chronic non-communicable diseases related principally to tobacco, alcohol, diet and obesity; to poverty; to violence; to access to health services; and to the circumstances in which people live and work.

In England, the Marmot Review, *Fair Society, Healthy Lives* (Marmot, 2010), emphasizes the 'causes of the causes' of health inequalities, and the need to address these wider determinants. To tackle inequalities and reduce the steepness of the social gradient, the Marmot Review recommends actions of sufficient scale and intensity to be universal but also proportionately targeted. Strategies need to target those at the lower end of the gradient as well as throughout the whole of society, according to the level of disadvantage.

The report specifically proposes action on six policy objectives.
- Give every child the best start in life.
- Enable all children, young people and adults to maximize their capabilities and have control over their lives.

- Create fair employment and good work for all.
- Ensure a healthy standard of living for all.
- Create and develop healthy and sustainable places and communities.
- Strengthen the role and impact of ill-health prevention.

 Learning Activity 2.9 Indicators for tackling health inequalities

Give an indicator for the successful tackling of each of the following.
Education.
Economic stability.
Social and community context.
Health and healthcare.
Neighbourhood and the built environment.

For example, interventions to reduce inequalities in health, e.g. in relation to diet, could address:
- the structural level, e.g. trade policy, food-labelling regulations, food fortification
- the local/community level, e.g. food gardens, free fruit and vegetables in school, food outlets
- the individual/family level, e.g. nutrition education in school or during pregnancy; mass-media campaigns, e.g. to reduce salt, weight-loss programmes.

Although many health promoters may feel powerless to effect change at a macro-structural level, it is possible to address health inequalities in planning health promotion interventions, as these examples illustrate. One of the central tasks for health promoters is to acknowledge socio-economic factors as crucial in determining individual and population health (Naidoo and Wills, 2010).

 Learning Activity 2.10 What improves health?

In your experience, what long-term social policy initiatives would be most effective in bringing about an improvement in the health of your clients or patients, or people you know?

Conclusion

Health promotion is not a purely technical activity. As we have seen, even identifying the causes of ill health will lead to political judgements being made. In any area of work or discipline, there will always be debate about what constitutes good practice. It is important to clarify your thinking and where you stand, because it will affect your views on the purpose of health promotion and what would be appropriate health promotion activities. It is also important that you share these thoughts with colleagues and clients to reach a common understanding of the ideals upon which health promotion activities are based.

In practice, behavioural and structural explanations are often aligned to the right or left of the political spectrum, and have become linked with very different policies and approaches to health promotion. The behavioural approach, which focuses on individual lifestyles, has informed much of health education because it suggests that information, advice or mass-media messages can change behaviours such as smoking or sexual activity. A structural approach, which sees health as determined by social and economic conditions, and reflecting the unequal distribution of power and resources in society, requires the health promoter to become involved in political activity.

Summary

This chapter has reviewed the evidence concerning health differences in the population and the physical, social and environmental variables that are implicated in ill health: poverty, unemployment, inadequate housing, stressful and dangerous working conditions, lack of social support, and air and water pollution. It goes on to consider the ways in which risk factors associated with personal behaviour – smoking, nutrition, exercise – are influenced by the social environment.

Several explanations for inequalities in health have been discussed. None offers a complete explanation, but the chapter concludes that there is sufficient evidence to point to social and economic factors determining health. It argues that disadvantage can give rise to, or exacerbate, health-damaging behaviours such as smoking or poor nutrition, and so health behaviours should not be separated from their social context.

Further reading and resources

Commission on Social Determinants of Health CSDH, 2008. Closing the Gap in a Generation: Health Equity through Action on the Social Determinants of Health. Final Report of the Commission on Social Determinants of Health. World Health Organization, Geneva. Available online at: http://apps.who.int/iris/bitstream/10665/43943/1/9789241563703_eng.pdf [accessed 16.09.15].

Marmot, M., Wilkinson, R.G. (Eds.), 2006. Social Determinants of Health, second ed. Oxford University Press, Oxford.

An overview of the factors known to affect health including unemployment, work and social support.

Useful websites include: the Institute of Health Equity at: http://www.instituteofhealthequity.org.

The Black Report can be downloaded from: http://www.sochealth.co.uk/history/black.htm.

The Marmot Review 2010 Fair Society Healthy Lives. Available online at: http://www.instituteofhealthequity.org/projects/fair-society-healthy-lives-the-marmot-review.

 Feedback to learning activities

2.1 Lifestyle behaviours are often viewed as being individual choices. While on one level this is true, many other factors influence individual behaviours. Taking the example of physical activity, it can be argued that individual motivation and willpower are all that is necessary. However, many factors will impact on the likelihood and ease of taking more physical activity, e.g. availability of suitable facilities, access to facilities and social norms depicted in the mass media.

2.2 It seems that unemployment has a profound effect on mental health, damaging a person's self-esteem and social structure. Employment, as well as providing wages which provide for people's material needs, is also often part of someone's self-identity. The higher incidence of smoking among unemployed people appears paradoxical given the cost involved, but smoking is often used as a psychological prop. Unemployment also means lower income and material disadvantage, as well as social isolation (McLean et al., 2005).

2.3 There are several reasons why men under the age of 45 do not visit their GPs as often as women. The obvious reason is that they suffer less ill health and disease than women, but this is not corroborated by medical statistics. Some issues, e.g. contraception, are seen as being women's responsibility. Pregnancy and childbirth will also contribute significantly to women's use of GPs. The sick role and its associated features, e.g. dependency, are typically viewed as more feminine than masculine, and therefore women may feel more at ease reporting ill health and using their GPs than men. There are therefore both medical and social reasons why women visit their GPs more frequently than men.

2.4 Healthcare is a cultural as well as a medical activity and is based on various premises, e.g. that the doctor knows best, and that the patient should be passive and should cooperate with medical advice and treatment. Sometimes patients from minority ethnic groups may have different expectations about their role and treatment. If there is a disparity between the expectations and role behaviours of health staff and patients, healthcare may suffer.

2.5 The first comment suggests that individuals must take full responsibility for their health-related behaviour. The second comment recognizes that behaviours take place in social contexts, and that many factors impact on individual behaviours. While behaviour is an individual attribute, its causes, meanings and significance are all socially determined. While it is logical to think poor people should smoke less, because of the cost of cigarettes, the social reality is that smoking is often used for social bonding and as a marker of individual identity, which are both rendered precarious by poverty.

2.6 Reflecting on your own life course to date in this way will illuminate the variety of factors that have

impacted on your health. These factors will probably include both external factors, e.g. the impact of economic recession or growth, and personal events, e.g. unemployment, migration or sickness. While we are encouraged to believe that we forge our own destinies, many other familial, social and societal factors and events have a profound impact on our lives.

2.7 It could be argued that all the above factors reflect a healthy society. Several factors (1, 6 and 7) are characteristic of egalitarian societies with a high level of social capital or networking, which is arguably a bedrock of good health. Other factors (2 and 5) are indicative of a thriving economy which, while it does not guarantee good health for all, provides a supportive backdrop. Factors 3 and 4 suggest a society investing in education and the next generation.

2.8 Accessing services, even when they are free and universally available, requires some initiative and confidence on the part of the user. To access NHS services, people need to negotiate with medical staff and make their needs known. This requires a degree of confidence, and such communication is much easier if the service user and service provider share a common cultural background, i.e. the user comes from the same social class as the medical staff.

2.9 There is a wide variety of indicators that could be used, including government statistics, e.g. increasing number of young people in higher education or increasing percentage of students achieving pass grades in exams; lay people's feedback and views, e.g. the percentage of people who feel their neighbourhood is safe; and service users' views, e.g. the percentage of patients who report feeling well cared for by the NHS.

2.10 Effective long-term social policy initiatives are varied, and include extending educational and business opportunities for young people (e.g. through apprenticeships), provision for older people with chronic ill health (e.g. nursing homes) and ensuring that everyone has sufficient income to meet their needs (e.g. welfare benefits).

References

Bhopal, R.S., 2014. Migration, Ethnicity, Race and Health in Multicultural Societies. Oxford University Press, Oxford.

British Heart Foundation, 2012. Coronary Heart Disease Statistics 2012. British Heart Foundation. Available online at: http://www.bhf.org.uk/publications/view-publication.aspx?ps=1002097 (accessed 01.08.14).

Cooper, K., Stewart, K., 2013. Does Money Affect Children's Outcomes? Joseph Rowntree Foundation. Available online at: https://www.jrf.org.uk/report/does-money-affect-children's-outcomes (accessed 16.09.15).

CSDH, 2008. Closing the gap in a generation: health equity through action on the social determinants of health. Final Report of the Commission on Social Determinants of Health. Geneva, World Health Organization. Available online at: http://apps.who.int/iris/bitstream/10665/43943/1/9789241563703_eng.pdf (accessed 16.09.15).

Dahlgren, G., Whitehead, M., 1991. Policies and Strategies to Promote Social Equity in Health. Institute for Future Studies, Stockholm.

Darmon, N., Drewnowski, A., 2008. Does social class predict diet quality? American Journal of Clinical Nutrition. Available online at: http://bvs.per.paho.org/texcom/nutricion/1107cn.pdf (accessed 06.03.15).

Dobson, F., 1997. Healthy Houses for Healthy Lives: Address to National Housing Federation 16/10/97. Department of Health Press Release 97/282.

Equality and Human Rights Commission, 2011. How Fair Is Britain? Equality, Human Rights and Good Relations in 2010. EHRC, London. Available online at: http://www.equalityhumanrights.com/sites/default/files/documents/triennial_review/how_fair_is_britain_-_complete_report.pdf (accessed 06.03.15).

Graham, H., 1992. Smoking Among Working Class Mothers with Children. Department of Applied Social Studies, University of Warwick, Warwick.

Graham, H., Power, C., 2004. Childhood Disadvantage and Adult Health: A Life Course Framework. Health Development Agency, London.

House of Commons Health Committee, 2009. Health Inequalities: Third Report of Session 2008–2009. Stationery Office, London.

Lalonde, M., 1974. A New Perspective on the Health of Canadians. Ministry of Supply and Services, Ottawa, Canada.

Macintyre, S., 2007. Inequalities in Health in Scotland: What Are They and What Can We Do about Them? Occasional paper 17. MRC Social and Public Health Sciences Unit, Glasgow. Available online at: http://www.google.com/url?sa=t&rct=j&q=&esrc=s&source=web&cd=1&ved=0CB0QFjAAahUKEwiGhIHMiPzHAhUD7RQKHWZvDAM&url=http%3A%2F%2Fwww.sphsu.mrc.ac.uk%2Freports%2FOP017.pdf&usg=AFQjCNGfBh5wGNpVoRKknyRQnRyWCEFt2g (accessed 16.09.15).

Marmot, M., 2010. Fair Society, Healthy Lives. DH, London. Available online at: http://www.instituteofhealthequity.org/projects/fair-society-healthy-lives-the-marmot-review (accessed 06.03.15).

Marmot, M., Siegrist, J., Theorell, T., 2006. Health and the psychosocial environment at work. In: Marmot, M., Wilkinson, R. (Eds.), The Social Determinants of Health, second ed. Oxford University Press, Oxford, pp 97-131.

Marmot, M., Wilkinson, R. (Eds.), 2006. The Social Determinants of Health, second ed. Oxford University Press, Oxford.

McKeown, T., Lowe, C.R., 1974. An Introduction to Social Medicine. Blackwell Science, Oxford.

McLean, C., Carmona, C., France, C., et al., 2005. Worklessness and Health: What Do We Know about the Causal Relationship? Health Development Agency, London. Available online at: http://www.employabilityinscotland.com/media/83147/worklessness-and-health-what-do-we-know-about-the-relationship.pdf (accessed 04.08.14).

Moller, H., 2012. Health Effects of Unemployment. Wirral Performance & Public Health Intelligence Team. Available online at: http://info.wirral.nhs.uk/document_uploads/Short-Reports/Unemployment-2%20Sept%2012.pdf (accessed 06.03.11).

Murray, C., Kulkarni, S., Ezzati, M., 2005. Eight Americas: new perspectives on US health disparities. American Journal of Preventive Medicine 29, 4–10.

Naidoo, J., Wills, J., 2010. Public Health and Health Promotion: Developing Practice, third ed. Baillière Tindall, London.

Nazroo, J., 1997. The Health of Britain's Ethnic Minorities. Policy Studies Institute, London.

Office for National Statistics, 2007. Childhood, Infant and Perinatal Mortality Statistics. HD3. ONS, London.

Office for National Statistics, 2013a. The 21st Century Mortality Files. ONS, London. Available online at: http://www.ons.gov.uk/ons/publications/re-reference-tables.html?edition=tcm%3A77-325379 (accessed 01.08.14).

Office for National Statistics, 2013b. General Lifestyle Survey Overview: A Report on the 2011 General Lifestyle Survey. Available online at: http://www.ons.gov.uk/ons/rel/ghs/general-lifestyle-survey/2011/rpt-chapter-1.html (accessed 20.01.16).

Parliamentary Office of Science and Technology, 2011. Post Note: Housing and Health. Available online at: http://www.parliament.uk/documents/post/postpn_371-housing_health_h.pdf (accessed 01.08.14).

The Marmot Review, 2010. Fair Society Healthy Lives. is available online at: http://www.instituteofhealthequity.org/projects/fair-society-healthy-lives-the-marmot-review (accessed 20.01.16).

Townsend, P., Davidson, N., 1982. Inequalities in Health: The Black Report. Penguin, Harmondsworth.

Tudor Hart, J., 1971. The inverse care law. Lancet 1, 405–412. Available online at: http://www.thelancet.com/journals/lancet/article/P11SO140-6736(71)92410-X/abstract (accessed 16.09.15).

Whitehead, M., 1988. The Health Divide. HEC, London.

Wilkinson, R., 1996. Unhealthy Societies: The Afflictions of Inequality. Routledge, London.

Wilkinson, R., Pickett, K., 2010. The Spirit Level: Why Equality Is Better for Everyone. Penguin, London.

World Health Organization, 1986. Ottawa Charter for Health Promotion. Journal of Health Promotion 1, 1–4.

Chapter Three

3

Measuring health

Learning Outcomes

By the end of this chapter you will be able to:
- identify sources of health information
- understand and use some frequently used epidemiological terms
- use available health information to describe health needs.

Key Concepts and Definitions

Epidemiology The scientific study of the distribution and causes of health and disease in defined populations. Epidemiology is used in public health to inform policy and practice through the identification of risk factors for disease and the application of this knowledge to control health problems.

Morbidity The incidence of disease or illness in a specified population.

Mortality The number of deaths at a given time and location. The mortality or death rate is typically expressed as the number of deaths per 1000 individuals per year.

Indicator The health indicators are quantifiable characteristics of a population (e.g. life expectancy) which may be used to justify public health interventions.

Rate A measure, quantity, or frequency, typically one measured against another quantity or measure.

Importance of the Topic

We saw in Chapter 1 how people define health in different ways, and in Chapter 2 how there are different determinants of health. This would suggest that measuring health is not a simple task. This appears to be borne out by the existence of a number of ways of measuring health, and a lack of clear agreement about which are the best ways to do this and which sources of information are most useful. This chapter looks first at why we might want to measure health. It goes on to investigate the different means of measuring health currently in use, and unpacks some of the assumptions underlying their use. Finally, the uses of the different kinds of measures are explored. The practical uses of measuring health are discussed further in Chapters 18 and 19 on needs assessment and programme planning, and in Chapter 20 on evaluation.

Why measure health?

Finding a means to measure health is an important practical task for health promoters. There are several reasons why this is so.

1. *To establish priorities.* Collecting and evaluating information about the health status and health problems of a community are important ways of identifying needs.
2. *To assist planning.* Health promoters need information to assist the planning and evaluation of health promotion programmes. It is important to establish baseline data in order to plan priorities and have a standard against which health promotion interventions can be evaluated.
3. *To justify resources.* Health promotion is often in competition with other activities for scarce resources. To make a claim for resources and prove that their activities are effective, health promoters need information on the health status of populations.
4. *To assist the development of the profession.* Measurements of health gain are important to the professional development of health promoters. Unless there is a means of measuring the effect of our actions, health promotion work will remain invisible, underfunded and low priority. By demonstrating the efficacy of health promotion interventions, it is possible to argue for resources, credibility and funding.

Ways of measuring health

Depending on the purpose, different measures of health may be used or developed. The means of measuring health depend primarily on the view of health which is held. If health is basically about physical functioning, then measures of physical fitness will be an adequate measure of health. If health is defined as having no disease, then measures of the extent of disease may be used (in reverse) as measures of health. However, if health is defined as including social and mental aspects, and meaning something other than being not ill, specific measurements of health will need to be developed.

Learning Activity 3.1 Describing the health of populations

If you wanted to describe the health of the people where you live or work, what information would you need?

Community health workers who profile their communities have many different ways of building a picture of their area. Some of these are described in Chapter 18 on needs assessment. In this chapter we look at sources of information available to describe a community's health. A great deal of information is available online. For example, in the UK you can find out about your local area by visiting http://neighbourhood. statistics.gov.uk, and, for those living in Scotland, www.groscotland.gov.uk/statistics.

Case Study 3.1 outlines a profile of the borough of Tower Hamlets in London and, using a variety of indicators, paints a picture of an area of disadvantage.

Case Study 3.1 Describing Tower Hamlets in London

At the last census conducted in 2011 the population size of Tower Hamlets was 254,096. Thirty-two percent of the population classified themselves as Bangladeshi, making this the largest ethnic group in the borough (2012-12 Census 2011 Second Release - Headline Analysis FINAL VI.pdf). Tower Hamlets ranks as the seventh most deprived local authority out of 326 in England on the Index of Multiple Deprivation (Tower Hamlets Indices of Deprivation 2011 Research Briefing 2011-03). Seventy-two percent of its lower super output areas (LSOAs) are in the 20% of the most deprived LSOAs nationally; 39.6% of the population live in social housing compared to 24.1% of the population in London; 6% of males aged 16 to 74 have never worked, compared to an average in England of 4.7%; and 7.9% of the population cannot speak English well or at all, while 18% say Bengali is their preferred language.

We look next at the contribution of epidemiology in the measurement of health as a negative variable, and move on to consider the measurement of health as a positive variable. Measuring health as a negative variable means measuring the opposite to health (e.g. disease or death) and using these results to infer the degree of health. Health is therefore being defined as a negative (health is not being ill or dead), not as a positive (health as positive well-being).

Measuring health as a negative variable (e.g. health is not being diseased or ill)

Epidemiology is the study of the occurrence and spread of diseases in the population. It is concerned with the health status (or, more usually, the ill-health status) of populations. Health promoters use epidemiological evidence to identify health problems, at-risk groups and the effectiveness of preventive measures. Figure 3.1 shows the key functions of epidemiology and Table 3.1 illustrates some of the key questions it answers.

The most common means of assessing a population's health are mortality and morbidity rates. This reflects the reductionist model of health, which sees health as a simple matter of illness or its absence. Thus data on deaths and illnesses are often used as surrogate measures of health. There are clearly shortcomings to this approach. Measuring conditions which limit health, such as illness, is not the same as measuring health itself. Measuring mortality rates does not reflect the extent of illness in the population, nor does it say anything about the quality of health experienced by people when they were alive. Conditions such as arthritis or schizophrenia cause considerable suffering and pain, but do not lead to premature death and so are not reflected in mortality rates.

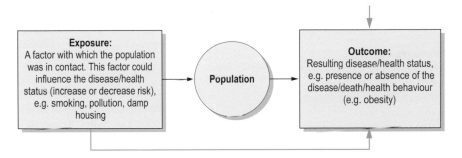

Fig. 3.1 ● The key functions of epidemiology.

Table 3.1 The application of epidemiology to public health

Distribution	Determinants
How many diseases are there?	Why do diseases happen?
How often do diseases happen (frequency)?	What determines/causes diseases/health-related events?
Where do they happen (places)?	What works to reduce the burden or risk of the disease? What is effective?
When do they happen or how do they change over time?	Is there a relationship between the disease and factors surrounding
Who has them and who does not (which population groups are at higher risk)?	people's lives? Which factors are associated with a higher risk of getting the disease? How much higher is the risk associated with these factors? What kind of factors (e.g. genetic or lifestyle) determine which populations are at risk and which populations are relatively immune?

Statistics concerning mortality are readily obtainable in developed countries. A death certificate is taken to the registrar of births, deaths and marriages and the director of public health in every health authority, and the total number of deaths, the geographic and population variations and the causes of death are all collated in each district's annual public health report. The statistics can also be used in international comparisons because most countries hold some form of database on deaths and disease rates.

All countries have systems of collecting data on the health status of the population and the use of services. Although these statistics are often presented as if they were objective facts, it is important to remember that statistics are devised by people in a social context, and are subject to assumptions, bias and error. At every stage of the data-collecting process, decisions are taken which help shape the ultimate form of information presented.

 Learning Activity 3.2 Mortality rates and food hygiene as an indicator of health status

If you wished to develop a health promotion intervention to improve food hygiene, why would mortality rates be a poor indicator of its priority?
- How else could you find out about the extent of poor food hygiene in your area?
- Why might mortality statistics be a good indicator of the necessity of health promotion around food hygiene in a low-income country?

Mortality statistics

There are several different ways of expressing death rates. The crude death rate is the number of deaths per 1000 people per year. However, this figure is affected by the age structure of the population, which may vary over time and regions. An area with a high proportion of older people, such as an English south-coast retirement town, would have consistently higher death rates than a more deprived area with a higher percentage of premature deaths but a younger population, such as an inner-city area. The standardized mortality ratio (SMR) measures the death rate, taking into account

differences in age structure. It is the number of deaths experienced within a population group (which may be defined by geographic or socio-economic factors) compared to what would be expected for this group if national averages applied, taking age differences into account. The overall average for England and Wales is 100, so SMRs of below 100 indicate a lower than average mortality rate, whereas SMRs of more than 100 indicate higher than average mortality rates.

 Learning Activity 3.3 The International Classification of Diseases

The *International Classification of Diseases, Injuries and Causes of Death* (ICD) (World Health Organization, 2010) (http://apps.who.int/classifications/icd10/browse/2015/en) classifies death according to diagnosed diseases which cause death, for example lung cancer. Death certificates which use the ICD thus give no information about contributory risk factors, such as smoking or diet.
- What impact do you think this has on our perception of risk factors and causes of disease, and on suitable strategies for prevention and treatment?
- Is it likely to foster understanding of social, environmental or biological causes of disease?

The infant mortality rate (IMR) is another commonly used statistic: it is the number of deaths in the first year of life per 1000 live births. The IMR is strongly associated with adult mortality rates. It reflects maternal health, particularly nutrition, and the provision of social care and child welfare. The IMR is therefore capable of being used as an indicator of the general health of the population, particularly when comparisons between countries are being drawn. The perinatal mortality rate is the number of stillbirths and deaths in the first 7 days after birth per 1000 births. The neonatal death rate is the number of deaths occurring in the first 28 days after birth per 1000 live births. Both the SMR and the IMR are readily available statistics, and therefore easy to use as surrogate measures of health.

Table 3.2 illustrates the marked inequalities across countries as shown by health indicators. For example, reducing infant mortality was one of the UN Millennium Development Goals, with a target reduction of two-thirds. There has been some progress: for example,

Table 3.2 Key health indicators worldwide (2012)

Country	Life expectancy (years)		Adult mortality rate (probability of dying aged 15 to 60) per 1000 population		Infant mortality rate (per 1000 live births), MDG 4
	Men	Women	Men	Women	
Belgium	78	83	102	59	4
Canada	80	84	84	53	5
UK	79	82	91	57	4
USA	76	81	131	77	6
Zimbabwe	53	55	501	473	43
China	74	77	112	81	13
Argentina	72	79	154	85	13
Sweden	80	84	71	44	2
India	64	67	247	159	47
Australia	80	84	80	46	4

Institute for Health Metrics and Evaluation Seattle. www.healthmetricsandevaluation.org. Contact data@healthdata.org to clarify conditions for commercial publication.

since 2000 measles vaccines have averted over 14 million deaths. But four out of every five deaths of under-5-year-olds occur in sub-Saharan Africa or Southern Asia. Improving education for girls and women is a priority, as children of educated mothers – even mothers with only primary schooling – are more likely to survive than children of mothers with no education.

Learning Activity 3.4 Key health indicators worldwide

Table 3.2 compares key health indicators for different countries worldwide in 2012.
- Which country has the highest life expectancy for women and men?
- Which country has the lowest life expectancy for women and men?
- Which country has the highest IMR?
- What reasons can you give to explain these findings?

Death rates are also available broken down by gender and cause (and, in the UK, by social class and occupation). People in the lower socio-economic groups have higher than average death rates at all ages and for virtually all causes. These differences show no sign of diminishing. Indeed, inequalities in

IMRs and life expectancy continue to grow, although there are some signs of progress, for example in child poverty and housing indicators. It may well take some time for any strategies currently being implemented to have an impact on mortality indicators. Reductions in mortality for selected causes among targeted groups in the population constitute the majority of targets in public health strategies.

Learning Activity 3.5 Data collection in low-income countries

In low-income countries mortality statistics may not be complete. Can you think of reasons why this might be the case?

Morbidity statistics

Statistics measuring illness and disease are more difficult to obtain. This is due in part to the difficulty in establishing a hard-and-fast line between health and disease. There is no one source of data for the whole population concerning disease and illness; instead, there are a number of different sources of relevant information. These are summarized below.

Case Study 3.2 Sources of health information in the UK

These sources of data may be accessed from public health departments, hospital-based datasets, the Health Protection Agency, primary care consultation rates, local delivery plans, local surveys and the Office for National Statistics. Useful websites include www.statistics.gov.uk (Office for National Statistics) for local information and health trends; www.hpa.org.uk (Health Protection Agency, which is now part of Public Health England) for communicable disease information; www.apho.org.uk (Association of Public Health Observatories) for neighbourhood profiles; and www.rcgp.org.uk (Royal College of General Practitioners) and www.hse.gov.uk (Health and Safety Executive). Child health information is available from www.chimat.org.uk.

Mortality

- Death by cause, age, sex and area of residence.
- Infant deaths (in children under one year).
- Perinatal deaths (after 28th week of pregnancy and in the first 7 days after birth).
- Neonatal deaths (within the first 28 days of birth).

Morbidity

- General Household Survey (annual survey of health behaviour and experience of illness).
- Health service records on consultation and treatment episodes in hospital and general practice, for example hospital episodes and statistics available from the Health and Social Care Information Centre (http://www.hscic.gov.uk).
- Registers for specific conditions such as cancers, disability, blindness and partial sight, people at risk of harm and drug addiction.
- Notification systems for infectious (communicable) diseases from the Health Protection Agency and the Communicable Diseases Surveillance Centre (Wales).
- National General Practice Morbidity Survey, conducted by the Office for National Statistics and the Royal College of General Practitioners.
- Surveys on mental health and psychiatric morbidity (for England, Scotland and Wales), since 1993.

Reporting of Injuries, Diseases and Dangerous Occurrences Regulations (RIDDOR) data, available from the Health and Safety Executive (HSE)

- Data regarding incidence of disease obtained from screening programmes, for example for cervical cancer.
- Notifiable congenital malformations.

Information on health status and behaviour

GP records on diagnoses, and communicable and respiratory disease monitoring, for example PRIMIS+ (primary care information services)

- Dental health records.
- Child health surveillance records.
  - Child measurement (of obesity) from 5 to 11.
- National surveys for the Office for National Statistics, for example the annual Health Survey for England, the Living Costs and Food Survey, Smoking, Drinking and Drug Use Among Young People in England, the Infant Feeding Survey and occasional surveys, for example Active People Survey (Sport England). The HSCIC has links to the major national surveys at http://www.hscic.gov.uk/public-health.

Demographic data

- Census information on the whole population is collected every 10 years (information includes numbers in household by age, sex, marital status, place of birth, occupation, ethnicity (since 1991), educational level, house type and tenure, accommodation and facilities). Information on self-reported health is collected.
- Register of births, including birth weight and mother's occupation.
- Claimants of unemployment benefit, free school meals, housing benefit and income support.

Environmental indicators and deprivation indices

- Services available.
- Levels of pollution: air, water and noise.
- Crime statistics.
- Type of housing.
- Leisure facilities.
- Road traffic accidents.
- Education, skills and training.
- Employment.

The health services collect routine data on the use of their services and activity rates. These data can be used to express the disease experience of different populations, but there are several problems with adopting this approach. The main problem with using many of the health authority measurements is that they were developed primarily for administrative, planning or management tasks, and reflect available services and their use rather than health itself. Health authority data are primarily collected as a management tool. To some extent, this determines what data are collected. Routinely available morbidity data represent only the tip of the illness iceberg. Many people who are ill do not seek help from primary care services or hospitals. However, the advantage of using data of this kind is that they are routinely collected, consistent across regions and easily accessed.

 Learning Activity 3.6 Hospital Episode Statistics as an indicator of health status

Hospital Episode Statistics (HES) is a patient-based dataset that contains all finished episodes of hospital care by diagnosis and treatment (http://www.hscic.gov.uk/hes).
- What will these data tell you about the health status of the local population?
- What do these data not tell you?
- Why do you think data are collected in this way?

The General Household Survey (GHS) is a continuous government survey of a sample of the population. The GHS includes questions on people's experience of illness, both long term (chronic) and within the last fortnight (acute). GHS data are difficult to use comparatively over time, as the wording of the questions changes occasionally. The following are examples of questions used in the GHS.
- Over the last 12 months would you say your health has on the whole been good, fairly good or not good?
- Do you have any long-standing illness, disability or infirmity? By long-standing I mean anything that has troubled you over a period of time or that is likely to affect you over a period of time.

- Now I'd like you to think about the two weeks ending yesterday. During those two weeks, did you have to cut down on any of the things you usually do (about the house, at work or in your free time) because of (any chronic condition cited earlier in the interview) or some other illness or injury?

The GHS is useful in providing information on people's subjective experience of illness, because it relies on self-reported illness rather than use of services. It also collects information on people's health-related behaviour, such as smoking, drinking and exercise. For example, one question asks: 'Do you smoke cigarettes at all nowadays?'

A number of proxy measures of health are used, such as the number of days at work lost due to sickness. However, such data are only available for people in paid employment. The large section of the population who are not in paid employment, and their experience of illness, is therefore invisible.

 Learning Activity 3.7 Indicators of health

The following are used to describe the health of populations. Which are good indicators of health?
- Standardized mortality rates.
- Infant mortality rates.
- Life expectancy.
- General Certificate of Secondary Education (GCSE) rates.
- Childhood obesity.
- Smoking prevalence.
- Depression rates.
- Happiness.

These measures of mortality and morbidity are inadequate for assessing people who are not ill but have some limited function which affects their everyday life. Different health indicators or health outcome measures have been developed to assist in the analysis of the consequences of disease. The concept of morbidity has been extended to incorporate the personal and social consequences of diseases as well as quality of life measures.

The various measures of health outcome are presented from a historical perspective.

In particular, the combined indicator of mortality and non-fatal outcomes, the DALY (disability adjusted life year), is examined in some detail and compared to other related measures.

- Years of healthy days of life lost (YHLLs). This composite indicator combines morbidity and mortality to provide quantitative measures of losses from particular diseases and gains from particular interventions.
- Quality-adjusted life years (QALYs). The QALY measures years of survival weighted for the quality of life, which people may be expected to have in the context of different states of illness.
- Disability adjusted life years (DALYs). The DALY combines years of healthy life lost from disability with those lost from premature death. DALYs were calculated for over 100 specific diseases for eight demographic regions worldwide. The measure is based on the incidence and duration of conditions resulting in non-fatal outcomes and weighted according to the severity of the disability and its impact.

Measuring health and disease in populations

The Global Burden of Disease (GBD) study is a comprehensive regional and global assessment of mortality and disability from major diseases, injuries and risk factors. It measures the burden of disease using the disability adjusted life year (DALY). The GBD for the UK from the latest study (Murray et al., 2013) shows an increase over the past 20 years in the contributions to premature mortality of Alzheimer's disease, cirrhosis and drug-use disorders. Compared with Europe, the UK had significantly lower rates of road injury, diabetes, liver cancer and chronic kidney disease, but significantly higher rates for ischaemic heart disease, chronic obstructive pulmonary disease, lower respiratory-tract infections, breast cancer, other cardiovascular and circulatory disorders, oesophageal cancer, pre-term birth complications, congenital anomalies and aortic aneurysm. The leading risk factor in the UK was tobacco, followed by increased blood pressure and high body-mass index.

Diet and physical inactivity accounted for 14.3% of UK DALYs in 2010.

Epidemiological studies examine the distribution and patterns of health and disease in populations. Epidemiological data help to build up a picture in the following ways.

1. Showing the scale of the problem.
2. Showing the natural history and aetiology of the condition.
3. Showing causation and association.
4. Identifying risk.

Scale of the problem

- *Incidence.* The number of people developing a disease over a specified period, for example in 2012 there were 1300 cases of breast cancer diagnosed in women aged 35 to 39 in the UK (www.info.cancerresearchuk.org).
- *Prevalence.* The number of people with a condition or characteristic at a specified time, for example in 2014 in Great Britain 22% of adult men and 19% of adult women were smokers (www.ash.org.uk)
- How the condition is distributed by gender, age, socio-economic status, ethnicity, etc., for example data from the National Child Measurement Programme show that obesity is more common in young children aged 5 years from Black African and Black Other ethnic groups, and in boys from the Bangladeshi ethnic group (http://www.noo.org.uk/uploads/doc/vid_9444_Obesity_and_ethnicity_270111.pdf).

Natural history and aetiology of the condition

- Indicate if primary prevention is possible.
- Show severity of the problem and ways in which individuals, families or communities may be affected.

Causation and association

- Show if there is evidence that exposure to a particular environmental, lifestyle or socio-economic factor contributes to ill health. There is a difference between causation (without which the ill health would not have occurred) and association (which links a socio-economic factor with ill health).

Identifying risk

- Assessing the chance or probability of a disease or condition occurring.
- Assessing how much illness is due to a particular factor (the *attributable risk*).

Epidemiologists assess risk in terms of the statistical probability of adverse events or death occurring. The link between these events and identified contributory factors varies from negligible to high. Lay people, by contrast, assess risk in the light of their personal experience. This difference in focus (whole populations vs specific individuals at a specific time) is problematic for health promoters. Rose (1981) called this the 'prevention paradox': for one person to benefit, many people have to change their behaviour, even though they will not benefit from so doing. Public awareness of this paradox can become a barrier to behaviour change.

Epidemiological studies of mortality, illness, disease and disability are often used to talk about health. Such usage reinforces, albeit in an indirect way, the definition of health as 'not disease'. But the advantage of such statistics is that they are already collected, relatively consistent and readily available. Recognizing the limitations of such measures has prompted health promoters to develop new means of measuring health as an independent phenomenon distinct from illness or disease. These measures may be conveniently divided into those describing health as an objective quality which is an attribute of people or environments, and those describing health as a subjective reality which is socially produced.

Measures of health as an objective attribute

There are a number of ways of measuring health as an objective factor, including:
- health measures
- health behaviour indicators

- socio-economic or deprivation indicators
- environmental indicators.

Health measures

There are various measures of the health status of people, including vital statistics such as height, weight and dental health (the decayed, missing and filled teeth, or DMF, index). Floud (1989) argues that the average height of a population may be taken as a measure of health, as it represents a proxy for nutritional status and therefore welfare. The *Health Survey for England 2012* (Health and Social Care Information Centre, 2013) includes height and weight measurements for this reason. In the same way, the percentage of low-birth-weight babies is used as an indicator of health status as it indicates whether a child has a 'healthy start' – and also serves as a health outcome related to maternal health risk.

Health behaviour indicators

Measurements of people's behaviour are used as a measure of health. For example, the number of people smoking, the proportion of children who are overweight or obese, the percentage of the population who do more than 150 minutes of exercise a week as per the government guidelines and the average daily consumption of fruit and vegetables may all be used to describe different populations and make comparisons between them regarding relative health status. This information may be routinely collected, such as smoking prevalence in young people, or it may be obtained from commissioned surveys. For example, sun protection surveys are carried out annually in Victoria, Australia. These lifestyle measures are sometimes narrowed down to more specific behaviour in relation to the health services. For example, the percentage of children immunized against childhood illnesses, or the percentage of women screened for cervical and breast cancer, may be used to describe the health status of a population.

Socio-economic indicators

Socio-economic status (SES), including educational attainment, occupational status and income, is related to health in developed countries, with higher SES being associated with better health. Other factors that are strongly associated with health include well-developed primary healthcare systems (Macinko et al., 2003), redistributive and egalitarian policies (Navarro et al., 2006) and more equal income distribution, high levels of female education and reduced ethnic fragmentation and conflict (Filmer and Pritchett, 1999).

The socio-economic environment shapes resources, opportunities and exposures, and can directly and indirectly influence health. Characteristics of the socio-economic environment can be measured through specific data and provide a picture of health in a neighbourhood or population.

- Wealth and income: financial stress, older age provision.
- Housing: supply and affordability.
- Transport and infrastructure: travel time to work, access to public transport, internet access.
- Productivity and employment: innovation and new businesses, jobs available, rates of pay.

The social environment may also be measured in terms of its 'healthiness'. One of the measures most commonly used to assess the social environment is wealth. The gross domestic product (GDP – the value of all goods and services produced within a nation in a given year) measures economic well-being, but this forms only part of social well-being (also called quality of life or social welfare). Happiness and life satisfaction are only weakly related to GDP for the developed Organisation for Economic Co-operation and Development (OECD) countries. The OECD issues an annual report on levels of happiness in 140 countries. For the last decade, European countries and Australia, New Zealand and Canada have ranked in the top countries but the USA has not made the top 10. Norway has the highest GDP per capita, but ranks behind Denmark in population happiness.

 Learning Activity 3.8 Measuring happiness

What might account for the high scores for happiness in north-west European countries and the low score for the USA?

The UN Development Programme has introduced a new way of measuring development that incorporates health. The human development index is a single statistic that combines indicators of life expectancy, educational attainment and income, and was first used in 1990 (http://hdr.undp.org/en/humandev/hdi/). Since then, gender inequalities have also been added, leading to the gender-related development index.

Environmental indicators

The same method may be applied to physical environments. Measurements of the physical environment include air and water quality, and housing type and density. These measures are routinely collected by the environmental health departments of local authorities. The European Happy Planet Index is a global index of sustainable well-being, combining measures of carbon footprints, life expectancy and life satisfaction (Thompson et al., 2007).

Many countries now have sustainability indicators that may measure a variety of factors pertaining to social capital, economic capital and natural capital. The latter includes:
- climate and atmosphere
- land
- ecosystems
- wildlife
- natural resources
- water
- waste disposal and recycling
- the origins of food consumed.

Combining a number of discrete elements to measure health is attractive, because it gives a more rounded picture of health and provides a clear basis and direction for health promoters.

Measuring deprivation

Much of the evidence which finds that people who are most disadvantaged experience more illness and premature death has derived from the link between occupational class and health status. Occupational class is still the main measure of socio-economic status (SES), although other factors such as gender, age and ethnicity are also recognized as having an important impact on SES. The limitations of using occupational categories are discussed in Chapter 2. The classification of socio-economic classes is derived from census information on type of employment. Since 2001 eight socio-economic classes have been used (see Chapter 2 for further details).

The income deprivation domain combines discrete domains of deprivation at a local area level to form a single score. The eight domains of deprivation are income; employment; health and disability; education, skills and training; access to services; barriers to housing and other services; living environment; and crime (Department of Communities and Local Government, 2011). Each domain includes several different indicators. For example, the income domain includes:

- adults and children in income support households
- adults and children in income-based job seeker's allowance households
- adults and children in working families' tax credit households whose equivalized income (excluding housing benefits) is below 60% of median before housing costs
- adults and children in disabled person's tax credit households whose equivalized income (excluding housing benefits) is below 60% of the median before housing costs
- adults and children in pension credit (guarantee) families
- asylum seekers in England in receipt of subsistence or accommodation support, or both.

In addition, indices for income deprivation affecting children and older people have been developed. The indices of deprivation measure relative levels in small areas of England called super output areas (SOAs). Lower-layered SOAs include about 1500 people and enable smaller area analysis.

Subjective health measures

The previous section outlined means of measuring health as if it were an objective property of beings, societies or environments, capable of scientific scrutiny. However, it is apparent that health is not such a simple or uncontested attribute. Chapter 1 highlighted the importance of subjective interpretations of health and the multiple meanings health may have in different contexts. This has led some researchers to attempt to devise measurements of health which incorporate subjective reporting. Herzlich (1973) identified three different aspects to people's accounts of health.

1. Health as a vacuum (not being ill).
2. Health as a reserve (of strength and resilience).
3. Health as equilibrium (balance and well-being).

Bowling (2005) identifies five dimensions of subjective health.

1. Functional ability.
2. Health status.
3. Psychological well-being.
4. Social networks and social support.
5. Life satisfaction and morale.

This is very similar to Blaxter's (1990) classification, with the one difference being the last category, where Blaxter identified physical fitness and vitality instead of life satisfaction and morale.

Physical well-being, functional ability and health status

Most measures of functional ability use people's self-reports of physical activity, such as the degree of mobility and the ability to perform everyday tasks like personal care and domestic activities. A widely used tool to measure health is the short-form 36-item (SF-36) health survey (Ware and Sherbourne, 1992). The SF-36 is a multi-item scale that assesses eight health concepts.

1. Limitations in physical activities because of health problems.
2. Limitations in social activities because of physical or emotional problems.
3. Limitations in usual role activities because of physical health problems.
4. Bodily pain.
5. General mental health.
6. Limitations in usual role activities because of emotional problems.

7. Vitality.

8. General health perceptions.

A short version is the SF-12 health survey, which is published in both standard (4-week) and acute (1-week) recall versions for self-administration.

 Learning Activity 3.9 Using the Short Form (SF-36) health survey

What are the advantages and disadvantages of the SF-36 health survey?

Psychological well-being

Several questionnaires have been developed to measure psychological well-being, including Goldberg's general health questionnaire (GHQ) (Goldberg and Hillier, 1997). Goldberg's GHQ, which measures minor psychological distress and social dysfunction, has been validated for use worldwide and includes items such as:

- ability to concentrate
- enjoyment of normal activities
- capability to make decisions
- feeling unhappy and depressed
- losing much sleep.

Well-being is commonly assessed using the Warwick–Edinburgh Mental Well-Being Scale (WEMWBS), which is a 14-item scale of subjective well-being covering psychological functioning and well-being in the past 2 weeks. It is worded positively and addresses aspects of positive mental health. As WEMWBS scores show a roughly normal distribution, WEMWBS can be expected to capture the full spectrum of positive mental health without floor or ceiling effects, and is suitable for both monitoring trends over time and evaluating the effect of mental health promotion programmes or interventions.

Social capital and social cohesion

Health includes the dimension of social health, which may be defined as the degree to which people function adequately as members of the community. A key characteristic of social health is social support, incorporating both the extent of a person's social networks and their perceived adequacy (Antonovsky, 1987). The concept of 'social capital' is now widely used to describe these networks and the trust which links people together in a community (Wilkinson, 1996). This is discussed in Chapter 10. Higher levels of social capital are associated with better health, less violent crime, better schooling, more tolerance and more economic and civic equality (Putnam, 2001; Rocco and Suhrcke, 2012). Attempts to measure social capital have used data regarding membership of voluntary organizations, clubs and committees as well as data on informal networks and questions about trust to assess the degree of civic participation (see the Office for National Statistics guide to social capital at http://www.ons.gov.uk/ons/guide-method/user-guidance/social-capital-guide/the-social-capital-project/guide-to-social-capital.html). It has been argued that a reduction or disinvestment in social capital, triggered by increased income inequality, leads to increased mortality (Kawachi et al., 1997).

 Learning Activity 3.10 Measuring social capital

Why and in what contexts might it be important to measure social capital, social cohesion or social connectedness?

Quality of life

Because health is multidimensional and includes physical, social and mental domains, composite measures have been developed, known as health-related quality of life measures. The desire to include a measurement of health in evaluating healthcare outcomes has led to the development of QALYs. QALYs are an explicit attempt to include not just years of life saved but also the quality of life when making resource allocation decisions regarding different medical procedures. The quality of life includes things such as freedom from pain and discomfort, and the ability to live independently. The assessment of quality of life is made by both health professionals and lay people. The QALY is the arithmetic product of life expectancy and an adjustment for the quality of the remaining life years gained (Baldwin et al., 1990). These two components are quite separate. QALYs are an important tool in making decisions about how to ration health-care resources.

There is much theoretical and methodological confusion in attempts to measure different aspects of positive health, and a lack of consensus in how this may best be achieved. It is an area which is currently being refined and researched, and is undoubtedly important to any adequate conceptualization and measurement of health.

 ### Research Example 3.1 The Framingham Heart Study

The Framingham Heart Study started in 1948, enrolling 5209 people in the town of Framingham in Massachusetts, USA. Their offspring cohort of 5124 started to be followed in the 1970s, and their offspring, a third generation of 4095 people, started in 2002 (see https://www.framinghamheartstudy.org/about-fhs/history.php). The original intention was to uncover the risk factors for cardiovascular disease. For 20 years from 1983 to 2003 the participants completed a happiness assessment. Clusters of happy and unhappy people are visible in the network of participants, and people's happiness extends up to three degrees of separation (for example, to the friends of one's friends' friends). People who are surrounded by many happy people and those who are central in the network are more likely to be happy in the present and in the future.

Fowler and Christakis (2008).

Conclusion

Indicators used to describe health will depend on what they are being used for and the extent to which stakeholders such as local people are involved. But, as with all measurement, indicators need to be:
- measurable
- understandable
- comparable
- available
- targetable
- geographic and temporal.

Measuring health is an important activity for health promoters, and is integral to the planning and evaluation of health promotion programmes. Yet there is no consensus on the best means to measure health, and a wide variety of methods have been used. Some are opportunistic, relying on data already collected and available, such as the annual Health Survey for England and QALYs. The drawback of using these methods is that they use data which have been collected for specific reasons, often managerial or administrative. Other methods, such as the SF-36, have arisen from research which has addressed the issue of how to measure health. The concept 'health' can have many different meanings, as outlined in Chapter 1, and this also contributes to the variety of different methods used. Some methods focus on one dimension of health, whereas others try to span different dimensions. Different measures may suit different purposes. It is unlikely that any one method will ever prove to be a comprehensive measure of health, even if it combines different measurements within a weighted index. What is important, first, is to be specific about *why* you wish to measure health, and then to go on to select the most appropriate means of doing so, bearing in mind constraints on the time and money you have at your disposal.

 ### Learning Activity 3.11 Health records

Susan is a 27-year-old mother of one child, 7-year-old Stephen. She collapses while out shopping with her son, and is taken by ambulance to her local accident and emergency department. The staff are keen to treat Susan as effectively as possible, which will entail checking her medical records to identify any pre-existing conditions or sensitivities to particular drugs. The staff are also anxious to keep an eye on Stephen and avoid any unnecessary distress to him. What information about Susan and Stephen will staff routinely be able to access?

Summary

This chapter has examined the reasons for attempting to measure health, and demonstrated that the most commonly used measures of health are in fact measures of ill health, disease and premature death. Recently there has been more activity directed towards trying to find ways of measuring health as an independent positive variable in its own right. Different approaches have been taken, including attempts to combine the measurement of health as an objective property of people or environments with the measurement of health as it is subjectively experienced and interpreted by people. These different approaches have been identified and described.

Questions for further discussion

- Thinking of your own work or practice you have seen, how is health conceptualized and measured? Are you more likely to use positive (e.g. well-being) or negative (e.g. absence/presence of disease) indicators?

Further reading and resources

There are many accessible textbooks providing introductions to epidemiology. The following provide short overviews and examples of how health and social care professionals can use health information.

Bowling, A., 2005. Measuring Health: A Review of Quality of Life Measurement Scales, third ed. Open University Press, Milton Keynes. *A detailed and comprehensive account of the different ways of measuring health and their comparative validity and reliability. Health measures include subjective measures of function, health status and psychological health as well as social health, life satisfaction and quality of life.*

Carr, S., Unwin, N., Pless-Mulloli, T., 2007. An Introduction to Public Health and Epidemiology, second ed. Open University, Buckingham. *A basic introduction to epidemiology which explains core concepts in a simple and readable form.*

Crichton, N., 2015. Epidemiology. In: Naidoo, J., Wills, J. (Eds.), Health Studies: An Introduction, third ed. Palgrave Macmillan, Basingstoke. *A concise and readable introduction to epidemiological theories and methods, including features designed to help readers reflect on the material and relate it to their own concerns.*

Harvey, J., Taylor, V. (Eds.), 2013. Measuring Health and Wellbeing. Sage, London. *This very useful book provides an introduction to the health surveillance competencies for public health practitioners.*

Jones, L., Douglas, J. (Eds.), 2012. Public Health: Building Innovative Practice. Sage, London. *This book contains a useful section on techniques in statistics and epidemiology that allows the student to use data with confidence, and shows how to use research techniques to identify needs and set priorities.*

Feedback to learning activities

3.1 It is likely that you included:
- information about the health status of the community (e.g. the number of deaths and the main causes of death; the number of episodes of illness and the main types of illness)
- information on the determinants of health (e.g. people's lifestyles; the quality of housing; levels of employment; the adequacy and accessibility of health services)
- information about the community itself (e.g. the age, gender, ethnic and socio-economic breakdown of the population).

3.2 Poor food hygiene in developed countries is likely to lead to illness but unlikely to lead to death. Mortality rates are therefore unlikely to flag up poor food hygiene as a priority. Poor food hygiene may be linked to ill health and loss of income, and therefore may be a priority for health promotion even though it does not figure in mortality data. In developing countries poor food hygiene may be linked with life-threatening illnesses (e.g. *Salmonella*, *Shigella*, *Campylobacter*), but mortality rates may still be inappropriate when trying to gauge the extent and impact of poor food hygiene.

3.3 The use of medical conditions, illnesses and diseases in classifying causes of death tends to obscure the significance of lifestyle behaviours in causing ill health and premature death. This in turn impacts on the funding of health promotion, which is perceived as being of less importance than clinical medicine in reducing ill health and premature deaths. This has a knock-on effect on public awareness and knowledge of risk factors for ill health and premature death.
The net result of the medicalization of classification of causes of death and ill health is less priority to,

funding for and awareness of health promotion, and of the enormous benefits it could bring.

3.4 In 2011 Sierra Leone had the lowest life expectancy for both sexes (47 years), closely followed by the Central African Republic at 48 years and the Democratic Republic of the Congo at 49 years. Japan, San Marino and Switzerland had the highest life expectancy for both sexes (83 years). Many factors contribute to life expectancy, for example economic factors; whether or not a country is at war; the state of its infrastructure, for example is clean water universally available; and the availability of medical help against disease and illness.

In 2011 Sierra Leone had the highest IMR of 119. The Democratic Republic of the Congo had an IMR of 111. These very high rates are due to many factors, including lack of basic sanitation and clean water; lack of medical care and facilities; and lack of social stability. Both countries also had volatile mining sectors.

In 2011 several countries shared the lowest IMR, or probability of dying by the age of 1 per 1000 live births. Finland, Iceland, San Marino, Singapore, Slovenia, Sweden, Luxembourg and Japan all had an IMR of 2. Again, this is due to several different factors, including economic infrastructure, stability of the country and the availability of medical help when required – http://www.who.int/gho/publications/world_health_statistics/EN_WHS2013_Part3.pdf.

3.5 There are several reasons why mortality statistics may not be complete.
- In rural areas the infrastructure for recording may not exist.
- Particular causes of mortality may be easier to recognize or be less stigmatized than others.
- People in higher socio-economic groups are more likely to have sought medical care prior to death and thus have a detailed cause of death recorded.

3.6 Hospital Episode Statistics (HES) is a secure data repository established in 1987 that collects monthly data on all hospital admissions, outpatient appointments and accident and emergency attendances at NHS hospitals in England. The data enable hospitals to be paid for the services they provide, and are also used by providers, researchers and service users for a range of other purposes, including healthcare analysis, monitoring and regulation, and research. HES enables activities such as monitoring of NHS hospital activity, supporting local service planning, enhancing patient choice and public accountability, and revealing health trends.

HES will reveal local use of NHS hospital services, but does not provide details of the health status of local populations or their use of primary healthcare facilities, for example GPs or community nurses. The dataset is primarily administrative, and designed to enable NHS planning and payment for services provided.

3.7 A good indicator is one that accurately and reliably describes an aspect of health of the population. Most available indicators measure ill health or death rather than health. The SMR is the ratio of observed deaths in the study group to expected deaths in the general population. A ratio of 1.0 means the number of observed deaths is equal to that of expected deaths. If the SMR is greater than 1.0 there is a higher number of deaths than expected. IMRs and life expectancy are used to compare populations internationally, and were both used to set targets to reduce inequalities in England. GCSE rates are used in the Marmot Review (2010) as an indicator of social disadvantage. Childhood obesity is measured through the National Child Measurement Programme. Smoking prevalence rates are estimates based on national surveys. Depression rates depend on the condition being identified as such and recorded by the clinician. Factors that are strongly associated with health include well-developed primary healthcare systems (Macinko et al., 2003), redistributive and egalitarian policies (Navarro et al., 2006), more equal income distribution (Wilkinson, 1996), high levels of female education and reduced ethnic fragmentation and conflict (Filmer and Pritchett, 1999).

3.8 Happy life expectancy (HLE) is calculated by multiplying life expectancy by a happiness index. Happiness is a subjective concept, but it is associated with various factors such as security and good health. Seventy percent of the statistical variance in HLE scores is explained by four characteristics: affluence, freedom, education and tolerance. Happiness is being measured as part of the National Wellbeing measurement in the UK that includes indicators on relationships, job satisfaction, economic security, education and environmental conditions, as well as individuals' assessment of their own well-being.

3.9 The SF-36 measures people's subjective assessment of their physical, mental and social health.

Continued

It does not measure physical health in an objective manner, for example screening for markers of disease. The main criticism of such measures is that people may become accustomed to limitations of bodily function and not perceive them as such.

3.10 Social capital is now measured as a contributor to health status. Higher levels of social capital are associated with better health, higher educational achievement, better employment outcomes and lower crime rates. There are a number of different aspects to social capital, which makes its measurement in communities complex. Generally, social capital focuses on:

- levels of trust – for example, whether individuals trust their neighbours and consider their neighbourhood to be a place where people help each other
- membership – for example, to how many clubs, societies or social groups do individuals belong
- networks and how much social contact individuals have in their lives – for example, how often individuals see family and friends.

The Office for National Statistics outlines how it measures social capital at http://www.ons.gov.uk/ons/guide-method/user-guidance/social-capital-guide/the-social-capital-project/guide-to-social-capital.html (accessed 01.03.15).

3.11 Susan will have been monitored throughout her pregnancy, with the following information about her being routinely recorded:

- height and weight
- blood pressure
- whether or not she smokes, drinks alcohol (and if so, how much per week) and takes, or has ever taken, any illegal drugs

- results of tests for HIV, hepatitis B and C, syphilis, rubella, sickle cell, thalassaemia, fetal anomaly and blood glucose.

Susan's records will also include demographic information about her socio-economic status:

- postcode, which gives an indication of her socio-economic status
- ethnicity
- employment status (of Susan and any partner)
- marital status.

Staff will be able to access a wealth of information about Stephen. All children are given an NHS number and registered on local child health and GP systems after they have been registered (civil registration) by their parent/s. Information on newborn babies includes medical conditions identified from a blood sample and recorded at birth (e.g. sickle cell disease, cystic fibrosis), and additional information recorded on the Child Health Information System (CHIS). Information held on CHIS includes whether or not Stephen was breastfed, measurements of his head circumference and body length, hearing and sight test results and all his vaccinations. Any medical conditions will be recorded in Stephen's medical records. At school Stephen's weight will be recorded as part of the National Child Measurement Programme.

Everyone has data held on them by different agencies, including health authorities. Linking up all the data held on someone by different agencies (health, education, housing, social services) can provide an overview of the person's health and living conditions and socio-economic status, but it is a time-consuming task. There is also concern about the levels of information held about individuals in relation to intrusion of privacy.

References

Antonovsky, A., 1987. Unravelling the Mystery of Health: How People Manage Stress and Stay Well. Jossey-Bass, San Francisco.

Baldwin, S., Godfrey, C., Propper, C., 1990. Quality of Life: Perspectives and Policies. Routledge, London.

Blaxter, M., 1990. Health and Lifestyles. Routledge, London.

Bowling, A., 2005. Measuring Health: A Review of Quality of Life Measurement Scales, third ed. Open University Press, Buckinghamshire.

Crichton, N., 2015. Epidemiology. In: Naidoo, J., Wills, J. (Eds.), Health Studies: An Introduction, third ed. Palgrave Macmillan, Basingstoke.

Department of Communities and Local Government, 2011. The English Indices of Deprivation 2010. Available online at: http://www.gov.uk/government/uploads/system/uploads/attachment_data/file/6871/1871208.pdf (accessed 21.09.15).

Filmer, D., Pritchett, L., 1999. The impact of public spending on health: does money matter? Social Science and Medicine 49, 1309–1323.

Floud, R., 1989. Measuring European inequality: the use of height data. In: Fox, J. (Ed.), Health Inequalities in European Countries. Gower, Aldershot, pp. 231–249.

Fowler, J., Christakis, N., 2008. Dynamic spread of happiness in a large social network: longitudinal analysis over 20 years in the Framingham Heart Study. BMJ 337, a2338.

Goldberg, D.P., et al 1997. The validity of two versions of the GHQ in the WHO study of mental illness in general health care. Psychological Medicine 27 (1), 191–197 www.ncbi.nlm.nih.gov/pubmed/9122299.

Health and Social Care Information Centre (HSCIC), 2013. The Health Survey for England, Available online at: http://www.hscic.gov.uk/catalogue/PUB13218 (accessed 21.09.15).

Herzlich, C., 1973. Health and Illness. Academic Press, London.

Kawachi, I., Kennedy, B.P., Lochner, D., et al., 1997. Social capital, income inequality and mortality. American Journal of Public Health 87, 1491–1498.

Macinko, J., Starfield, B., Shi, L., 2003. The contribution of primary care systems to health outcomes within Organization for Economic Cooperation and Development (OECD) countries 1970–1998. Health Services Research 38, 831–865.

Marmot Review, 2010. Healthy Healthy Lives: The Marmot Review. Available online at: http://www.instituteofhealthequity.org/projects/fair-society-healthy-lives-the-marmot-review.

Murray, C.J., Richards, M.A., Newton, J.N., et al., 2013. UK health performance: findings of the Global Burden of Disease Study 2010. The Lancet 381 (9871), 997–1020. Available online at: http://www.thelancet.com/pdfs/journals/lancet/PIIS0140-6736(13)60355-4.pdf (accessed 21.09.15).

Navarro, V., Muntaner, C., Borrell, C., et al., 2006. Politics and health outcomes. Lancet 368, 1033–1037. Available online at: www.thelancet.com/pdfs/journals/lancet/PIIS0140-6736(06)69341-0.pdf(accessed 21.09.15).

Putnam, R., 2001. Social capital: measurement and consequences. Isuma, Canadian Journal of Policy Research 2, 41–51.

Rocco, L., Suhrcke, M., 2012. Is Social Capital Good for Health? A European Perspective. WHO Regional Office for Europe, Copenhagen. Available online at: http://www.euro.who.int/__data/assets/pdf_file/0005/170078/Is-Social-Capital-good-for-your-health.pdf (accessed 06.03.15).

Rose, G., 1981. Strategy of prevention: lessons from cardiovascular disease. British Medical Journal 282, 1847–1851.

Thompson, S., Abdallah, S., Marks, N., et al., 2007. The European Happy Planet Index: An Index of Carbon Efficiency and Well-being in the UK. New Economic Foundation/Friends of the Earth. Available online at: http://www.foe.co.uk/sites/default/files/downloads/euro_happy_planet_index.pdf (accessed 25.02.15).

Ware, J.E., Sherbourne, C.D., 1992. The MOS 36-item short-form health survey (SF-36): 1: conceptual framework and item selection. Medical Care 30, 473–483.

Wilkinson, R.G., 1996. Unhealthy societies: the afflictions of inequality. Routledge, London.

World Health Organization, 2010. The International Classification of Diseases, Injuries and Causes of Death (ICD-10), tenth ed. WHO, Geneva. Available online at: http://apps.who.int/classifications/icd10/browse/2015/en (accessed 25.02.15).

World Health Organization, 2012. World Health Statistics, Part Three: Mortality. Available online at: http://www.who.int/gho/publications/world_health_statistics/EN_WHS2013_Part3.pdf. (accessed 21.09.15).

Chapter **Four**

4

Defining health promotion

Learning Outcomes

By the end of this chapter you will be able to:
- define health promotion, health education and public health, and the differences between them
- describe the historical origins of health promotion
- understand the role and contribution of the World Health Organization (WHO) in the development of health promotion
- evaluate critically the contribution of health promotion to the health of populations
- assess your own practice in relation to advocacy, mediation and enablement.

Key Concepts and Definitions

Health promotion is a range of activities and interventions to enable people to take greater control over their health. Activities may be directed at individuals, families, communities or whole populations.

Health education involves activities to facilitate health-related learning and behaviour change.

Public health involves activities based on a biomedical understanding of health, focused on the identification of health-related needs and population-based actions such as immunization and screening.

Disease prevention includes activities at primary, secondary and tertiary levels to prevent the onset of disease or to reduce or ameliorate its effects.

Importance of the Topic

The process of attempting to promote health may include a whole range of interventions, including those which:
- foster and enable healthy lifestyles
- encourage access to services and involvement in health decisions
- seek to promote an environment in which the healthy choice becomes the easier choice
- educate about the body and keeping healthy.

Until the 1980s most of these interventions were referred to as 'health education', and the practice was almost exclusively located within preventive medicine or, to a lesser extent, education. In recent years the term 'health promotion' has become widely used. There is no agreed consensus on what health promotion is or what health promoters do when they try to promote health, nor what a successful outcome might be. Many professions, including nursing, have found health promotion to be part of an expanding job description. This development reflects the arguments presented in this book – that it is health and not illness or disease which should underpin healthcare work. Yet what practitioners do in the name of health promotion varies enormously. This chapter outlines the historical development of health promotion and considers different views on the purpose, nature and scope of health promotion practice.

Foundations of health promotion

The term health promotion is recent, used for the first time in the mid-1970s (Lalonde, 1974), and the Alma Ata conference (World Health Organization, 1978) is cited as setting the agenda for health promotion. Its foundations are complex and differ between countries and regions, but in general arose from:

- a change in perceptions of the determinants of health and a shift away from the tendency to equate health simply with healthcare services
- the shift from communicable to chronic diseases attributable to people's lifestyles
- an awareness of the potential of primary healthcare as a first line for prevention and treatment.

'Health promotion' is used in a number of different ways, often without any clarification of meaning. In 1985, when the term was becoming widely adopted, Tannahill (1985) described it as a meaningless concept because it was used so differently. Over a decade later, Seedhouse (1997) described the field of health promotion as muddled, poorly articulated and devoid of a clear philosophy. These early understandings reflect the origins of health promotion, and include:

- 'slick salesmanship of health' (Williams, 1984)
- 'attempts to persuade, cajole or otherwise influence individuals to alter their lifestyle' (Gott and O'Brien, 1990)
- 'any combination of education and related legal, fiscal, economic, environmental and organisational interventions designed to facilitate the achievement of health and the prevention of disease' (Tones, 1990)
- 'an approach and philosophy of care which reflects awareness of the multiplicity of factors which affect health and which encourages

everyone to value independence and individual choice' (Wilson-Barnett, 1993).

Health promotion is defined by building on the Ottawa Charter (World Health Organization, 1986) definition, as Nutbeam (1998, pp. 1–2) explains:

Health promotion represents a comprehensive social and political process. It not only embraces actions directed at strengthening the skills and capabilities of individuals, but also actions directed towards changing social, environmental and economic conditions so as to alleviate their impact on public and individual health. Health promotion is the process of enabling people to take control over the determinants of their health and thereby improve their health.

 Learning Activity 4.1 Distinguishing health promotion from health education

- What do you consider to be the main features of health education?
- And what do you consider to be the main features of health promotion?
- Is your work mostly health education or health promotion?

A shared understanding of the meaning and purpose of health promotion is elusive. A diversity of disciplinary and ideological perspectives and policy changes has resulted in apparently conflicting conceptualizations. Health promotion as a concept can thus be understood as:

- a discrete discipline that draws from other disciplines (e.g. psychology, education, sociology) to understand a particular problem
- a process or way of working that seeks to empower individuals and groups by enabling them to address their own needs and valuing their experience
- a field of activity that includes supporting people to develop personal health skills, fostering public participation, building partnerships and coordinating policy and strategy.

Origins of health promotion in the UK

The first phase of health promotion development is known as the 'social hygiene period', and had roots in both public health and health education. These origins of health promotion lie in the nineteenth century, when epidemic disease eventually led to pressure for sanitary reform for the overcrowded industrial towns. Alongside the public health movement emerged the idea of educating the public for the good of their health. The medical officers of health appointed to each town under the public health legislation of 1848 frequently disseminated everyday health advice on safeguards against 'contagion'. Voluntary associations were also formed, including the London Statistical Society (1839), the Health of Towns Association (1842) and the Sanitary Institute (1876). The temperance movement held Band of Hope mass meetings, and through schools and churches lectured to young people on the virtue of abstinence from alcohol. By the 1920s health education had become associated with diarrhoea, dirt, spitting and venereal disease! The evidence that 10% to 20% of soldiers in the First World War had contracted venereal disease led to propaganda, one-off lectures and the first 'shock-horror' techniques in which soldiers were shown lurid pictures of diseased genitals to dissuade them from having sex (Blythe, 1986; Welshman, 1997).

The second phase of health promotion development is known as the 'personal services' period. Changing patterns of morbidity and mortality shifted attention away from disease to personal behaviour. The Central Council for Health Education was established in 1927, paid for by local authority public health departments, and public health doctors formed the majority of its members. An extract from some of the tasks it listed as important reflects an emphasis on information and education to bring about change in personal habits and behaviour:

- the provision of better and cheaper posters and leaflets
- the provision of exhibits for exhibition
- the production of a readable monthly bulletin
- the provision of a panel of lecturers who really could lecture and hold an audience.

The Central Council was principally concerned with propaganda and instruction. During the Second World War it delivered 3799 lectures on sex education and venereal disease which were attended by 340,000 people (Amos, 1993).

 Learning Activity 4.2 Comparing health education slogans

The twentieth century saw widespread use of propaganda approaches to health education, using slogans and striking images to persuade the population to adopt healthy living. Compare examples from 1920s' insurance cards with slogans from contemporary Africa.

1920s' England
- 'Have a hot bath at least once a week'.
- 'Moderation in all things: every hour you steal from digestion will be reclaimed by indigestion'.
- 'Do not spit – it dries in the dust and other people breathe it in'.

Contemporary Africa
- 'Arrive alive'.
- 'Say NO to sex. Virgin power'.
- '**SAFE: S**urgery, **A**ntibiotics, **F**acial cleanliness, **E**nvironmental Improvement'.

The Health Education Council (HEC), which was set up in 1968 as a quango – a quasi-autonomous non-governmental organization – reflected the Department of Health and Social Security's (as it then was) medical model of health. The members were drawn from public health and the medical and dental professions, with the inclusion of advertising and consumer affairs representatives. Its brief was to create a 'climate of opinion generally favourable to health education, develop blanket programmes of education and selected priority subjects' (Cohen Committee, 1964). Similar health education agencies were set up in Wales, Scotland and Northern Ireland.

The HEC came to be associated with mass publicity campaigns such as 'Look After Yourself' (LAY), which was launched in 1978. LAY reflected the view that people could be encouraged to adopt lifestyles which would lead to better health. The lead agency for health education in England consistently emphasized such mass campaigns and short-term initiatives. Sutherland, the first director of education and training at the HEC, has vividly described the pressures and lobbying which led the HEC away from confrontation with vested interests, such as agriculture and tobacco, and kept it confined to mass-media campaigns despite evidence of their limited effect (Sutherland, 1987).

By the 1970s there was an increasing recognition that health policy could not continue to be confined to clinical and medical services, which were both proving expensive and not improving the health status of the population. Health education and the prevention of disease represented a means of cutting costs and an ideology which could place the onus of responsibility on the individual.

 Learning Activity 4.3 Changing views on disease prevention

What does this extract from the government document *Prevention and Health: Everybody's Business* (Department of Health and Social Security, 1976) suggest about changing views on prevention, risk and individual behaviour?

To a large extent though, it is clear that the weight of responsibility for his own health lies on the shoulders of the individual himself. The smoking-related diseases, alcoholism and other drug dependencies, obesity and its consequences, and the sexually transmitted diseases are among the preventable problems of our time and, in relation to all of these, the individual must decide for himself.
Department of Health and Social Security (1976)

The view that improving health depends on individuals changing the way they live in order to avoid 'lifestyle' diseases has permeated all UK government white papers (Department of Health, 1987, 1992, 1999, 2004, 2010). The following behavioural priorities have been the focus of these strategies.
- Reducing the numbers who smoke.
- Tackling obesity.
- Improving sexual health.
- Improving mental health and well-being.
- Reducing alcohol-related harm and encouraging sensible drinking.

Alongside this government response, however, was the awareness that poor health was linked to poverty. In 1980 the Black Report, commissioned by the government, showed how those in lower socio-economic groups had a far higher risk of dying prematurely than more advantaged groups (Townsend and Davidson, 1982). The HEC commissioned a further study on inequality, *Inequalities in Health: The Black Report and the Health Divide* (Townsend et al., 1992). The report was published on a national holiday in August, ostensibly to avoid publicity, so damning was its evidence on the extent of poverty and deprivation.

The last three decades have seen a re-emergence of public health measures and a recognition of the need to address the social, economic and environmental determinants of health. The Acheson Report (HM Government, 1998), commissioned by an incoming Labour government, recommended that as part of health impact assessment, all policies likely to have an impact on health should be formulated in such a way as to favour the less well off. More recently the Marmot Review (Marmot, 2010) exposed continuing health inequalities, and the Institute of Health Equity, launched in 2011, seeks to increase health equity through action on the social determinants of health (www.instituteofhealthequity.org). In all countries, making the connection between the social determinants of health and health promotion policy and action is a major task, as discussed by the International Commission on the Social Determinants of Health (http://apps.who.int/iris/bitstream/10665/43943/1/9789241563703_eng.pdf). In many countries, however, much of health promotion remains 'downstream', focusing on the behavioural determinants of ill health such as smoking rather than the material factors and socio-structural conditions outlined in Chapter 2. In addition, most governments are reluctant to challenge or curtail the industries that produce ill health, such as tobacco, alcohol and armaments.

This century has seen challenges to the term 'health promotion'. In England the term 'health development' was used briefly, and currently 'health improvement' has been adopted. In Canada 'population health' replaced 'health promotion' (Raphael, 2008). In the USA 'health education' is more widely used than 'health promotion'. This reflects the neoliberal ideologies (see Chapter 7) of these countries, which seek to equate health promotion to social marketing and individual behaviour change. Likewise, in Africa 'health promotion' is said to reflect neoliberal globalization – Sanders et al. (2008), in analysing African solutions to water sanitation, give the example of using private-sector engineering companies to install water plants rather than investment in the social processes of engaging communities.

Public health

In 1920 the Winslow Professor of Public Health at Yale University described public health as:

The Science and Art of preventing disease, prolonging life, and promoting health and efficiency through organized community effort for:

- *The sanitation of the environment*
- *The control of communicable diseases*
- *The organization of medical and nursing services for the early diagnosis and preventative treatment of disease*
- *The development of social machinery to ensure everyone a standard of living adequate for the maintenance of health, so organizing these benefits so as to enable every citizen to enjoy his birthright of health and longevity.*

(http://www.yale.edu/printer/bulletin/htmlfiles/publichealth/history-of-the-yale-school-of-public-health.html).

In the UK health promotion and public health are terms that are often used interchangeably. Health promotion is sometimes defined as one of the processes in securing public health. In many countries there is understood to be a clear distinction: public health is the practice of public health medicine, with an emphasis on the prevention and control of disease. This distinction is explored in greater detail in our companion volume, *Public Health and Health Promotion: Developing Practice* (Naidoo and Wills, 2010).

Historically, public health has been driven by social policy as much as by medicine. The early UK public health movement in the nineteenth century used a medical scientific model to explain the disease process. The gathering of information and interpretation of quantitative data (epidemiology) were employed to underpin decisions. Social policy interventions were deployed to protect the public and prevent disease (see Chapter 11).

The UK Faculty of Public Health identifies three domains of public health practice: health improvement, service improvement and health protection. The term 'health promotion' is not included. In contrast, in New Zealand the Public Health Clinical Network sees health promotion as one of five core public health functions.

The relationship between public health and health promotion has been much debated and focuses on the multidisciplinary nature of health promotion, embracing environmental, social and individual health dimensions. Our companion volume (Naidoo and Wills, 2010) discusses the similarities and differences between public health and health promotion in more detail. The distinction between a specialist or a mainstream health promotion workforce has also been much debated. Health promotion may be part of the work of practitioners in different settings such as sports centres or workplaces. The mainstreaming of health promotion has frequently resulted in its absorption into a traditional individualized public health discourse. Yet the originators of health promotion viewed it as a moral and political value-based project (Wills and Douglas, 2008).

Case Study 4.1 Midwives' contribution to public health

- Improving the wider determinants of health
  Domestic abuse
  Social connectedness
- Health improvement
  Low birth weight of full-term infants
  Breastfeeding
  Smoking status at time of delivery
  Conceptions among under-18-year-olds
  Diet
  Excess weight in adults
  Proportion of physically active and inactive adults
  Smoking prevalence
  Access to cancer screening programmes
  Self-reported well-being
- Health protection
  Chlamydia diagnoses
  Population vaccination coverage
- Reducing mortality
  Infant mortality
  Mortality from causes considered preventable
  Suicide

Learning Activity 4.4 Critical health promotion

Green et al. (2015, p. 40) refer to health promotion as the critical conscience of public health. What do you think they mean? Do you agree?

The World Health Organization and health promotion

The WHO has played a key part in proposing a broader agenda for health promotion. In 1977 the World Health Assembly at Alma Ata committed all member countries to the principles of *Health for All 2000* (HFA, 2000: World Health Organization, 1977): there 'should be the attainment by all the people of the world by the year 2000 of a level of health that will permit them to lead a socially and economically productive life'. The WHO made explicit five key principles for health promotion in a discussion paper commonly referred to as the Copenhagen document.

1. It involves the population as a whole in the context of their everyday lives, rather than focusing on people at risk of specific diseases.
2. It is directed towards action on the causes or determinants of health to ensure that the total environment which is beyond the control of individuals is conducive to health.
3. It combines diverse, but complementary, methods or approaches, including communication, education, legislation, fiscal measures, organizational change, community development and spontaneous local activities against health hazards.
4. It aims particularly at effective public participation supporting the principle of self-help movements and encouraging people to find their own ways of managing the health of their community.
5. Although health promotion is basically an activity in the health and social fields and not a medical service, health professionals – particularly in primary healthcare – have an important role in nurturing and enabling health promotion (World Health Organization, 1984).

The context for the development of broad-based health strategies thus needs to be based on equity, community participation and intersectoral collaboration. The WHO also noted that improvements in lifestyles, environmental conditions and healthcare will have little effect if certain fundamental conditions are not met. These include:

- peace and freedom from the fear of war
- equal opportunity for all and social justice
- satisfaction of basic needs, including food and income, safe water and sanitation, housing, secure work and a satisfying role in society
- political commitment and public support (World Health Organization, 1985).

The WHO launched a programme for health promotion in 1984, and conferences in Ottawa (1986), Adelaide (1988), Sundsvall (1991), Jakarta (1997), Mexico (2000), Bangkok (2003), Nairobi (2009) and Helsinki (2013) have further outlined areas for action. The practice and principles of health promotion developed in the Ottawa Charter (World Health Organization, 1986) are still widely used to provide a framework for practice.

1. Building a healthy public policy.
2. Creating supportive environments.
3. Developing personal skills, including information and coping strategies.
4. Strengthening community action, including social support and networks.
5. Reorienting health services away from treatment and care, and improving access to health services.

Each of these health promotion actions is the subject of a chapter in Part Two of this book.

Learning Activity 4.5 Implementing the Ottawa Charter action areas

What activities might be included in each of these action areas in relation to diet and nutrition?

Defining health promotion

Disease prevention

In Chapter 1 we saw that there are many different meanings attached to the concept of health, but the notion that health is the 'absence of disease' is dominant. Different perceptions about the nature of health and the factors contributing to it underpin interpretations of health promotion. The shift from infectious and communicable diseases to chronic diseases in the twentieth century highlighted the role of people's lifestyles in disease causation. Prevention therefore became much more important, often through targeting high-risk groups who have an increased likelihood of developing a specific disease.

Health promotion is often categorized as being concerned with primary, secondary or tertiary prevention.

- Primary prevention seeks to avoid the onset of ill health through the detection of high-risk groups and the provision of advice and counselling. Examples of primary prevention include immunization and cervical cytology, as well as health education in schools and workplaces.
- Secondary prevention seeks to change health-damaging behaviour to shorten episodes of illness and prevent the progression of ill health. Examples include education about medication, and advice on healthy eating for diabetics and relaxation for cardiac patients.
- Tertiary prevention seeks to limit disability or complications arising from a chronic or irreversible condition and enhance quality of life. Examples include education about the use of a disability aid and rehabilitation therapy. Medical support and symptom control are important to those living with life-threatening illness, but so too is enhancing their quality of life.

For those working in a clinical setting, this is the usual interpretation of health promotion. It differs little from the education of patients about the condition that brought them to the health service. Its aims are to help patients avoid a recurrence by following a treatment regimen or some change in their lifestyle, and to enhance quality of life when living with a chronic condition. Disease prevention does not, however, look beyond the risk factors or groups to the origins of ill health.

 Learning Activity 4.6 Health promoting palliative care: A contradiction in terms?

What would health promoting palliative care look like?

Health education

Educating people about their health is commonplace, but 'health education' as a formalized activity only emerged in the 1980s. The recognition of the need to diffuse information about the physical and moral 'evils' of squalor and drink can, however, be dated to the mid-nineteenth century. An awareness that individuals make health choices which can contribute to the development of disease led to the view that it was possible to inform people about the prevention of disease and motivate them to change their behaviour through persuasion and mass-communication techniques, and to equip them through education with the skills for a healthy lifestyle.

'Traditional' health education was often criticized for its narrow focus on information provision, based on the assumption of a simple causation relationship between knowledge and behaviour. The emphasis on individual responsibility for health led to accusations of victim blaming. Victim blaming makes individuals feel guilty, although it may be factors beyond their control (poverty, social and environmental factors) that prevent them from making health changes.

 Learning Activity 4.7 Refocusing upstream

McKinlay (1979), in persuading us of the need to refocus upstream, tells a story:

There I am standing by the shore of a swiftly flowing river and I hear the cry of a drowning man. So I jump into the river, put my arms around him, pull him to shore and apply artificial respiration. Just when he begins to breathe, there is another cry for help. So I jump into the river, reach him, pull him to shore, apply artificial respiration, and then just as he begins to breathe, another cry for help. So back in the river again, without end, goes the sequence. You know I am so busy jumping in, pulling them to shore, applying artificial respiration, that I have no time to see who the hell is upstream pushing them all in.

- What examples can you think of in your own work of short-term problem-specific activity?
- What would a reorientation upstream involve?
- Who or what do you think is pushing people in?

Health education may be defined as planned opportunities for people to learn about health and make changes in their behaviour. It includes:

- raising awareness of health issues and factors contributing to ill health
- providing information
- motivating and persuading people to make changes in their lifestyle for their health
- equipping people with the skills and confidence to make those changes.

This might be seen as a limited interpretation of a health promotion role confining activity to information, education and communication, as discussed in Chapter 9.

 Learning Activity 4.8 Is health an individual responsibility?

Is your health in your own hands?

One of the paradoxes of health education and a prevailing professional dilemma is the degree of voluntarism or free choice. Health education is based on an expert-authority model derived from both medicine and education. It is the health educator or doctor who decides if there is a health need and the adequacy of an individual's lifestyle; who decides the nature of the intervention and the most effective means of communication; who tries to ensure compliance; and who will decide if the intervention has 'worked'. When we look at the practice of health education, we might be led to believe that it is the *giving* of information, and success in promoting health is when the client follows the advice. For other health educators, education is a means of *drawing out*. Clients are not 'empty vessels' who will rationally change their behaviour once provided with the relevant information, advice or guidance. After all, information about the risks to health from smoking has been available since 1963 and information about human immunodeficiency virus (HIV) transmission since 1986, yet people continue to smoke and not use condoms. These health educators seek neither to coerce nor to persuade, both because this is unlikely to be effective and also because it is unethical. The health educator is a facilitator and enabler rather than an expert. Rather than telling clients what to do, the health educator works with them to identify their needs and move towards an informed choice, even when this may lead to health-damaging behaviour. The goal is to empower individuals to take health-related decisions by developing health literacy, self-efficacy, self-esteem and coping skills (Nutbeam, 2000; Kickbusch, 2001).

 Learning Activity 4.9 Health literacy

Health literacy may be defined as the capacity of an individual to obtain, interpret and understand basic health information and services in ways that are health enhancing.
US Department of Health and Health Services (2000)

Does this definition help to address inequalities in health?

For many frontline workers there are tensions in health education.

- Should health education be about telling people what is best for them?
- Are health educators failing in their role if they accept their clients' health-damaging behaviour?
- Who should determine what constitutes a healthy life – practitioner or client?
- Should health behaviour and its effects be seen as a matter of individual choice?

 Learning Activity 4.10 Health education approaches

Consider the following case story of a middle-aged manual worker and appropriate health education approaches.

John is a labourer on the roads. He is 47 and single, and his social life revolves around the pub. He drinks a few pints at lunchtime with his sandwiches and usually four pints on the way home. He visits his GP with backache. The GP takes his blood pressure and finds it is dangerously high.

Which of the following do you do?

1. Tell him that the recommended drinking limit for adult males is 28 units per week. Stress the damage to his heart and liver, and that he risks a heart attack.
2. Discuss the reasons for his drinking behaviour and whether he sees it as causing problems.
3. Prescribe medicine to lower his blood pressure, and tell him to visit the practice nurse in 2 weeks to see if his blood pressure has come down.

These issues are discussed further in Chapter 6 on ethical issues and Chapter 11 on developing healthy public policy.

The two strands of voluntarism and authoritarianism reflect the historical development of health education, as educationists and social scientists challenged the mainstream of preventive medicine by contesting the assumption that health education could, or indeed should, seek to bring about behaviour change through information or persuasion. Thus emerged the principle of self-empowerment, which many argue is central to the practice of health education (Green et al., 2015). Empowerment is an approach which enables people to take charge of their lives, including changing their behaviour if they so wish. Tones (1986) argues that an essential element of health education is 'critical consciousness-raising' to increase people's awareness of the fundamental causes of ill health – a notion first espoused by the Brazilian priest Paolo Freire. Only through this process can the structural influences on health be addressed (see Chapter 5 for a discussion of Tones's model of health promotion) and policy change be pursued and accepted.

 Learning Activity 4.11 Health promotion and the informed choice

The aim of health promotion is to enable people to make informed choices about their health. Do you agree?

The range of approaches to health education are outlined and discussed in Chapter 5. They range from the medical model, focusing on health surveillance and achieving behaviour change, to the educational model, which relies on the exploration of attitudes and values. Alongside these are the approaches more closely aligned to health promotion, such as community development, which emphasizes the need to take collective action for health, and a social model which focuses on the need to influence decision-makers at local and national levels.

Figure 4.1 illustrates some specific examples of downstream interventions tackling health behaviours that give rise to problems, and upstream interventions tackling the causes of such behaviours.

Health promotion

The WHO has moved the definition of health promotion away from prevention of specific diseases or the detection of risk groups towards the health and well-being of whole populations. Instead of experts and professionals diagnosing problems, the people themselves define health issues of relevance to them in their local community. Teachers, primary healthcare workers, workplace managers and social and welfare workers can all be involved in promoting health. Instead of health being seen as the responsibility of individuals alone, the social

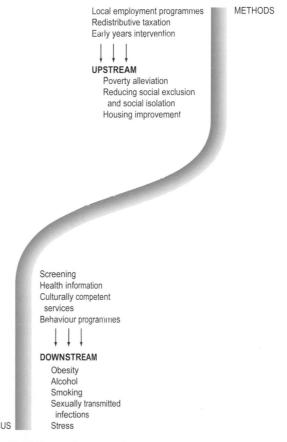

Local employment programmes   METHODS
Redistributive taxation
Early years intervention

UPSTREAM
Poverty alleviation
Reducing social exclusion
and social isolation
Housing improvement

Screening
Health information
Culturally competent
services
Behaviour programmes

DOWNSTREAM
Obesity
Alcohol
Smoking
Sexually transmitted
infections
FOCUS   Stress

Fig. 4.1 ● Downstream and upstream approaches to promoting health. (Ipsos MORI/King's College London: Global trends survey.)

factors determining health are taken into account, and health is viewed as a collective responsibility of society which needs to be prioritized by organizations and governments in their decision-making.

 Learning Activity 4.12 Health promotion approaches

Consider these descriptions of the work of a nurse on an acute medical ward and a community worker with young people. Would you consider them to be practising health education or health promotion? What criteria do you use to make your judgement?

- 'Patient education for coronary care is carried out one to one with information booklets. The overall aim is to alleviate anxiety, promote recovery and educate about the cause of the attack to get the patient back to normal and even healthier. Patients may be given factual information about the working of the heart, be taught relaxation exercises and encouraged to talk about concerns such as sex after a heart attack. They will be educated about their medication, how to eat healthily, keeping their weight down and curbing their cholesterol intake, and ways to increase physical activity.'
- 'Health education on topics such as sexual health passes on knowledge, allows for discussion and leads to understanding. It gives young people the freedom to choose and make health decisions and at the same time it asserts an appreciation and respect for the choices of others. The end result should lead to positive pleasure for the young person while enabling him or her to remain healthy and disease-free'.

The terms health education and health promotion are often used interchangeably, but while health promotion can be seen as an umbrella term incorporating aspects of health education, it is much broader in concept.

Health promotion incorporates all measures deliberately designed to promote health and handle disease... A major feature of health promotion is undoubtedly the importance of 'healthy public policy' with its potential for achieving social change via legislation, fiscal, economic and other forms of 'environmental engineering'

Tones (1990), p. 3.

There are, as we saw in Chapter 2, a range of factors which influence people's health. Some are material–structural and some are behavioural. These need to be addressed other than by education alone. Health promotion thus involves public policy change and community action to enable people to make changes in their lives. A phrase first coined by Milio (1986) has come to encapsulate health promotion – 'making the healthy choice the easier choice' – and was adopted as the strapline for the Public Health Strategy for England (Department of Health, 2004). As we have seen, it is easy for practitioners to confine their health promotion role to offering information and advice on how to adopt a healthier lifestyle. However, for people to make such changes, the factors and situations which led them to adopt 'unhealthy' behaviours need to be addressed. People may smoke because of stress, even though they know it is bad for their health. Others may use an illegal drug because it is widely used by their peer group and is part of their social life. Equally, it is easier for some people to make healthy choices than it is for others. It is easier to eat a diet including fresh fruit and vegetables for people with reasonable incomes who have easy access to supermarkets or high-street shopping. Some factors affecting individual health are outside individual control, for example, inadequate housing, busy roads or lack of childcare.

 Learning Activity 4.13 Making the healthy choice the easier choice

School nurses were concerned that a high proportion of children's packed lunches contained fizzy drinks, jam sandwiches, crisps and a chocolate bar. How can the healthy choice be made an easier choice?

Changing health behaviours without regulation that also then changes social norms will always be difficult. Yet regulation of individual behaviour lays governments open to the charge of being a nanny state. Sparks (2011) refers to a cartoon in the *New Yorker* that depicts a street scene in contemporary Manhattan, with three people in pillories – a medieval form of public humiliation and punishment. Above each person is a word indicative of their offence:

smoking, salt and carbs. The base of the pillory is ironically labelled as the property of the NY Department of Moral Guidance. The UK government has adopted a low-intervention strategy combining 'responsibility deals' with industries such as food manufacturing to reduce salt, sugar and fat in processed foods and 'nudge', which aims to change the 'choice architecture' in which individuals make decisions, for example, removing confectionery counters from supermarket checkout areas.

Research Example 4.1 Does 'nudge' work?

The UK government has adopted a libertarian paternalistic approach to behaviour change, also known as 'nudge' after the book by Thaler and Sunstein (2009). The use of nudge in health is rooted in the idea of influencing behaviour without compulsion, for example, by using subconscious cues to 'nudge' people towards making healthy choices, or manipulating the environment to increase the chances that people act in a healthier way.

A study by Ipsos Mori showed that most people recognize the role of individuals in improving their own health. Some also believe that government has a role to play, even to the extent of citizens being required to improve their health before receiving treatment. Yet they do not want government interference in their personal health choices (Duffy et al., 2010).

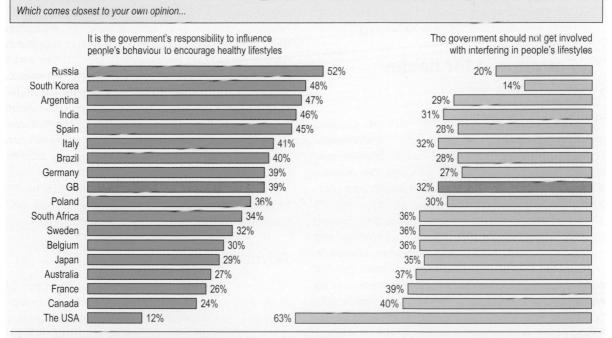

Which comes closest to your own opinion...

It is the government's responsibility to influence people's behaviour to encourage healthy lifestyles | The government should not get involved with interfering in people's lifestyles

Country	Gov responsibility	Gov not involved
Russia	52%	20%
South Korea	48%	14%
Argentina	47%	29%
India	46%	31%
Spain	45%	28%
Italy	41%	32%
Brazil	40%	28%
Germany	39%	27%
GB	39%	32%
Poland	36%	30%
South Africa	34%	36%
Sweden	32%	36%
Belgium	30%	36%
Japan	29%	35%
Australia	27%	37%
France	26%	39%
Canada	24%	40%
The USA	12%	63%

Base: c. 500–1000 adults 15+ in each country (1004 aged 16–75 in GB), 2013/14.

If people are 'nudged', they may believe that they have made a personal choice, but the government is making it easier for them to 'make the right choice'.

There is some evidence to demonstrate that nudging works (Marteau et al., 2011). Incentives have been shown to affect weight loss: people taking part in schemes where they deposited money that is forfeited if they do not attain their goals were successful in weight loss in the short term. In another study, smokers taking part in savings schemes were more likely to give up if, on proving they had quit, they were given access to their savings.

Critiques of health promotion

There are several critiques of health promotion, from different political standpoints. Most common are critiques from right-wing politics of social regulation and the supposed lack of evidence of its effectiveness. Less frequent is a critique from left-wing politics about health promotion's focus on individual behaviour change. Examples include the following.

- Health education is simply advertising admonitions, such as 'don't drink and drive' or 'wear a condom'. These amount to a nanny state.
- Health promotion does not work. Finite resources would be better spent on those who are ill.
- Insufficient attention is paid to the conditions producing ill health. Health promotion fails to address poverty.
- Health promotion is a means of social control that exhorts people to behave in a certain way.

The argument for health promotion

Although health promotion is part of national efforts to improve health, its rejection of a disease-oriented pathogenic model of health differentiates it from medical approaches. Its goals derive from a positive, salutogenic concept of health and well-being (as discussed in Chapter 1). Its methods are empowering, enabling individuals and groups to have a say in how their health is promoted and valuing their perspective, and supporting people to acquire the skills and confidence to take greater control over their health. As such, there are no quick wins.

In practice, health promotion encompasses different political orientations which can be characterized as the individual versus structural approaches. For some, health promotion is a narrow field of activity which seems to explain health status by reference to individual lifestyles, and a process largely determined by an expert who advises on beneficial changes. In its emphasis on personal responsibility it sees a minimal role for the state, and has thus come

to be associated with a conservative viewpoint. For others, including the WHO, health promotion recognizes that health and wealth are inextricably linked, and seeks to address the root causes of ill health and problems of inequity using radical and challenging approaches (www.who.int/social_determinants/en/). It is not helpful to debate whether one form of activity is better or worse than the other: both are necessary. Health promotion may involve lobbying and political advocacy, but it may just as easily involve working with individuals and groups to enhance their knowledge and understanding of the factors affecting their health.

Health education has become equated with persuasive attempts to manipulate behaviour, but this is a narrow interpretation and ignores its importance as a core element of health promotion. Green et al. (2015) propose the term 'new health education' to refocus understanding and activity on education that enables individuals and communities to achieve greater control over their health.

Many practitioners believe that their role in achieving the social changes necessary to eliminate health inequalities or the community change necessary to provide social support is limited. Yet there are ways in which individual practitioners can promote health over and beyond merely informing, advising or listening. The WHO identifies three ways in which practitioners can promote health through their work: advocacy, enablement and mediation.

Advocacy

Advocacy in health promotion is the process of defending or promoting a cause. It may mean representing the interests of disadvantaged groups and speaking on their behalf or lobbying to influence policy. It may also mean action to gain political commitment, policy support, social acceptance and support systems for a particular goal or cause. For example, health promotion networks in Australia, New Zealand, the USA and Canada have long advocated for a focus on the health of indigenous peoples.

Learning Activity 4.14 Advocacy and practice

- To what extent do you work 'on behalf of' clients or the public?
- Do you regard advocacy as part of your health promotion role?

Enablement

Enabling means health promotion practitioners taking action in partnership with others to promote health by identifying needs and developing networks and resources in the community; assisting people to develop knowledge and skills; and helping people identify and address the determinants of their own health. Enablement is an essential core skill for health promoters, since it requires them to act as a catalyst and then stand aside, giving control to the community (see Chapter 10 for further discussion of working with communities).

Mediation

Health promoters mediate between different interests by providing evidence and advice to local groups and influencing local and national policy through lobbying, media campaigns and participation in working groups.

In the definitions of health promotion so far, health promotion has been interpreted as a process of improving the health of individuals or community. It can also be seen as a set of values or principles. The WHO identifies these as empowerment, equity, collaboration and participation. These values should be incorporated in all health and welfare work for it to be health promoting (Naidoo and Wills, 2010).

 Learning Activity 4.15 Enabling engagement in practice

To what extent, and how, do you encourage participation and enable your clients to take more control over their health?

Health promotion is thus an integrating approach to identifying and doing health work. Cribb and Dines (1993) argue that 'the central question is not what is the domain of health promotion but is this being done in a health promoting way? And this is a question that can be asked about any and every example of practice, not merely those which are clearly aimed at disease prevention or health education.' To accept such a definition means there can be no boundaries to health promotion, since any situation or event between client and practitioner has the potential to be health promoting.

 Learning Activity 4.16 Health promoting practice

What would you define as health promoting aspects of your contact with clients?

Conclusion

Many health workers are strongly committed to health education and the promotion of health. However, this has often been manifested in one-to-one programmes limited to providing information. Many may be daunted by the broad definition of health promotion, and feel that this broad approach is beyond their professional remit. Indeed, it would not be possible for any one worker or group to bring about the changes needed for a health promoting society. It is important that we remind ourselves of the WHO's view, which describes the process of promoting health as not only involving political change and interagency collaboration, but also enabling people to take more control over their own health and equipping them with the means for well-being. Health promotion thus includes increasing individual knowledge about the functions of the body and ways of preventing illness, raising competence in using the healthcare system and raising awareness and strengthening community action on the political and environmental factors that influence health.

Summary

This chapter has looked at the origins of health promotion, and shown how different interpretations arise from different origins. It has shown that health promotion is a broad term encompassing interventions which differ in aims and purpose and in the role accorded to the practitioner. It may be seen as a set of activities clearly intended to prevent disease and ill health, to educate people to a healthier lifestyle or to address the wider social and environmental factors which influence people's health. It may also be seen as a set of principles to orient health work towards addressing inequality and promoting collaboration and participation. Health promoters thus need to be clear in their understanding of what health is, what aspect of health is being promoted and the ways in which health is affected by wider influences than individual behaviour.

 Learning Activity 4.17 The aims of teenage pregnancy strategies

The under-18 conception rate in the UK is the lowest since 1969 at 27.9 conceptions per 1000 women aged 15 to 17. Yet it is still the highest in Western Europe: 5432 girls under 16 conceived in 2012, and 60% of these had a legal termination (ONS, 2012). You are responsible for sexual health services in your area. What should be the aim for teenage pregnancy?

1. Reduce teenage pregnancy rates.
2. Educate young people about the risks of under-age sex.
3. Support and advise young mothers.
4. Improve access to services and contraceptive advice.
5. Raise awareness of sexual health among teenagers.
6. Enable young people to make informed and confident choices about their sexual health.

Which of the following activities would you consider a priority for a health promotion intervention? Why?

7. Run a youth counselling drop-in service.
8. Work with teachers to develop a sex education curriculum.
9. Give talks at local schools about the risks of under-age sexual activity.
10. Open a young people's session at the family planning clinic.
11. Write a leaflet for young people on contraception.
12. Research the pattern and trends of teenage pregnancies in the area.
13. Set up a teenage mothers' group.
14. Set up an information stall at the local market.
15. Set up an interagency group with employers and housing, education and leisure services to discuss young people's needs.
16. Lobby the health authority to provide free condoms at all clubs and leisure centres.
17. Run a training course for doctors on counselling young people

Questions for further discussion

- What term do you use to describe your work in improving people's health – health promotion, health education, health improvement, public health or another term? Why do you use this term?
- How do you explain the current emphasis on health promotion in healthcare job remits?

Further reading and resources

Cragg, L., Davies, M., Macdowall, W. (Eds.), 2013. Health Promotion Theory, second ed. McGraw Hill/Open University Press, Maidenhead. *Section 1 contains interesting accounts of the history and development of health promotion.*

Green, J., Tones, K., Cross, R., Woodall, J., 2015. Health Promotion Planning and Strategies, third ed. Sage, London. *A useful textbook which includes thoughtful and provocative discussion on health promotion goals and methods.*

Keleher, H., MacDougall, C., 2010. Understanding Health, second ed. Oxford University Press, Melbourne. *An interesting Australian textbook that applies equity approaches to health promotion.*

Nutbeam, D., 1998. A Health Promotion Glossary. Available at: http://www.who.int/healthpromotion/about/HPR%20 Glossary%201998.pdf (accessed 22.09.15).

Scriven, A., Garman, S. (Eds.), 2005. Promoting Health Global Perspectives. Palgrave Macmillan, Basingstoke. *A collection of views on the challenges facing the promotion of health around the globe.*

Seedhouse, D., 1997. Health Promotion: Philosophy, Prejudice and Practice. Wiley, Chichester. *A stimulating personal analysis of the conceptual roots of health promotion.*

National health promotion agencies or associations can provide useful insights into health promotion work. See for example the following.

Australia: Australian Health Promotion Association at www.health-promotion.org.au and Victorian Health Promotion Foundation at www.vichealth.vic.gov.au.

Canada: Public Health Agency of Canada at http://www.phac-aspc.gc.ca/index-eng.php.

New Zealand: Health Promotion Agency at http://www.hpa.org.nz.

Northern Ireland: Public Health Agency for Northern Ireland at www.publichealth.hscni.net. See health and social well-being improvement.

Scotland: NHS Health Scotland at www.healthscotland.com.

Thai Health and Information at thaihealth.org.

USA: Office of Disease Prevention and Health Promotion at health.gov.

Wales: Health in Wales at www.wales.nhs.uk includes Health Challenge Wales.

Journals can also be helpful. For example, see the following.

American Journal of Health Promotion
Critical Public Health
Health Education Research
Health Promotion International
Health Promotion Journal of Australia
Scandinavian Journal of Health Promotion

The Ottawa Charter can be downloaded from the WHO website at: www.who.int/healthpromotion/conferences/previous/ottawa/en/.

Feedback to learning activities

4.1 There is a large overlap between health education and health promotion, but in general health education is understood to focus on health-related learning (e.g. the effects of tobacco use), whereas health promotion is understood to have a wider remit, focusing on any actions designed to improve health (e.g. legislation outlawing the advertising of tobacco and restrictions on smoking in public places). Most health personnel see their role as including health education but not necessarily health promotion.

4.2 The slogans from 1920s' European insurance companies make some attempt to explain why they are advocating certain actions. The slogans from modern-day West Africa are more didactic and 'snappy', designed to be remembered and to act as a trigger for action.

4.3 In the 1970s health promotion slogans advocated actions which were viewed as being a matter of individual choice. There was no recognition of group or marketing pressure to adopt unhealthy behaviours. Nowadays there is more recognition of the many pressures put upon individuals to adopt unhealthy behaviours, and health promotion is directed at changing these pressures as well as encouraging individual change.

4.4 Critical conscience or consciousness is a concept developed by Freire which focuses on understanding the social and political contradictions that exist in the world, and on taking action against the oppressive forces in one's life. Health promotion as being the critical conscience of public health implies that health promotion takes a broader view of health as a socio-economic concept rather than a medical concept. Health promotion seeks correspondingly broader actions to promote health, such as building a healthier environment, rather than medical interventions such as immunization against diseases.

4.5
- Building a healthy public policy with regard to diet and nutrition might include requirements for healthy school meals (e.g. including fruit and vegetables).
- Creating supportive environments might include ensuring adequate outlets for fresh fruit and vegetables, controlling the number of fast-food outlets and educating schoolchildren regarding the benefits of eating 'five [portions of fruit and vegetables] a day'.
- Developing personal skills might include how to cook fresh vegetables as part of a meal.
- Strengthening community action might include lobbying local councils about limiting the number of fast-food outlets and creating more allotments to allow people to grow their own fruit and vegetables.
- Reorienting health services might include more routine monitoring of people's height and weight when they have contact with health services for any reason, coupled with a fast track to support services to help obese people lose weight.

4.6 Health promoting palliative care might include the fostering of hope and support, prevention of depression, home help and death education (Kellehear and O'Connor, 2008).

4.7 The concept of refocusing upstream is a powerful and persuasive argument for health promotion. It can help us to reorient our thinking away from a belief that medical care can, or will, solve most health problems, and towards prevention.

4.8 Many factors that impact on our health are not in our control (although our actions may have some limited effect), for example, environmental pollution and socio-economic inequalities. Other factors are more directly controllable, for example, exposure to sexually transmitted diseases and eating a healthy diet.

4.9 The concept of health literacy is not new or radical, and can be identified in many of the definitions of empowerment. However, it contains a central message that although knowledge alone is insufficient to achieve change, not understanding the conditions that determine health or knowing how to change them is disempowering (Abel, 2007). We are faced with a society in which there is more choice of foods and other products, more health information from many sources, more choice in patient treatments, more choice of providers. In such a consumer society, Kickbusch (2009) argues active health citizenship is a critical empowerment strategy that enables people to make sense of and discriminate between such choices.

4.10 The first approach is health education, telling the patient what health risks he faces as a result of his drinking habits. The second approach is health education and promotion – more enabling and patient-oriented and seeking to understand his perspective. The third approach is medically oriented and seeks a result (lower blood pressure), with little active involvement from the patient.

4.11 The underlying principle of health education is to facilitate people to make their own choices about health behaviour. For those who believe the roots of ill health lie in social structures, this emphasis on choice is merely illusory. In Chapter 6 we explore further the limits to freedom of choice and how far an ethical principle such as the promotion of autonomy can govern our practice as health educators.

4.12 A key difference between these two interventions is their aims. In the coronary care unit, the nurse is actively engaged in disease prevention – to prevent a further heart attack. The community youth worker aims to equip young people with the information and skills for a healthy lifestyle. In both cases the health promoter aims for behaviour change, more obviously so in the coronary care unit. Both use similar educational methods of providing information, encouraging clients to reflect on their attitudes and experience, and providing opportunities to practise skills.

4.13 Schools are cautious about giving advice to parents, as they do not want to be seen as interfering. Advice can be given in leaflets and children can be encouraged to prepare food in cook–eat sessions.

Personal social and health education sessions could include discussions of what makes a healthy lunch and why it is important. Nutritional standards for school meals were revised in 2015 in England, 'junk food' has been removed from vending machines and schools allow only water as a drink (see www.childrensfoodtrust.org.uk). The 'healthy choice' thus became a necessary one. The dilemma of whether policy measures such as this are coercive is discussed in Chapter 6.

4.14 Depending on your role, it is likely that it includes elements of advocacy, or working on behalf of clients or the public. This can include helping patients navigate their way through available services. Public health advocacy is planning and using the media to promote public health policies or initiatives.

4.15 The scope for encouraging patient or client participation will depend on your role. Giving information (e.g. about a healthy diet) or encouraging networking (e.g. informing patients about local carers' support groups) is relevant for health professionals with individual caseloads. For staff with a more strategic or managerial role, including patient participation as a professional goal, supporting staff to achieve this goal and using the media to promote this goal may all be part of their remit.

4.16 You might have included:
- listening in an open way to a client's views and using as a starting point his or her knowledge, attitudes and beliefs
- making links between the client's situation and those of others in the community
- providing information about informal support available in the community
- negotiating future action with the client to ensure that it is reasonable, appropriate and realistic.

4.17 The aim is clearly to reduce teenage pregnancies, as in number 1. There are many different strategies that may be relevant and contribute to this goal, each of which may be prioritized for various reasons. Your role (e.g. service provider or researcher; employed by education or health services) will also impact on what initiatives are considered appropriate. For example, providing education and counselling to prevent teenage pregnancies, as in the educational aims numbered 2, 5 and 6, may be a health promotion priority, in which case the interventions numbered 7, 8, 9 and 11 might be appropriate. Providing more effective contraception and early abortion services may be part of the strategy, as in aim 4 and interventions 10 and 16. Assessing patterns and trends to determine the impact of interventions will be important. Strategies will be multidisciplinary, so stakeholders need to work in partnership, as in intervention 15. Providing dedicated services for teenage parents may be considered relevant, as in aim 3 and intervention 13. Initiatives may also be divided between those that belong in the education sector (e.g. interventions 8 and 9) and those that belong in the health sector (e.g. interventions 16 and 17). Finally, building capacity in both the health and education sectors may be a long-term vision and priority, as in interventions 15 and 17.

References

Abel, T., 2007. Cultural capital in health promotion. In: McQueen, D.V., Kickbush, I. (Eds.), Health and Modernity: The Role of Theory in Health Promotion. Springer, New York, pp. 43–73.

Amos, A., 1993. In her own best interests: women and health education, a review of the last 50 years. Health Education Journal 52, 3.

Blythe, M., 1986. A century of health education. Health and Hygiene 7, 105–115.

Cohen Committee, 1964. Health Education. Report of a Joint Committee of the Central and Scottish Health Services Councils. HMSO, London.

Cribb, A., Dines, A., 1993. What is health promotion? In: Dines, A., Cribb, A. (Eds.), Health Promotion: Concepts and Practice. Blackwell Scientific, Oxford.

Department of Health, 1987. Promoting Better Health. HMSO, London.

Department of Health, 1992. The Health of the Nation. HMSO, London.

Department of Health, 1999. Saving Lives: Our Healthier Nation (White Paper). Stationery Office, London. Available online at: https://www.gov.uk/government/publications/saving-lives-our-healthier-nation (accessed 25.02.15).

Department of Health, 2004. Choosing Health: Making Healthier Choice Easier. Stationery Office, London. Available online at: http://webarchive.nationalarchives.gov.uk/+/dh.gov.uk/en/publicationsandstatistics/publications/publicationspolicyandguidance/dh_4094550 (accessed 25.02.15).

Department of Health, 2010. Healthy Lives, Healthy People. Stationery Office, London. Available online at: https://www.gov.uk/government/uploads/system/uploads/attachment_data/file/216096/dh_127424.pdf (accessed 25.02.15).

Department of Health and Social Security, 1976. Prevention and Health: Everybody's Business. HMSO, London.

Duffy, B., Quigley, A., Duxbury, K., 2010. National health? In: Citizens' Views of Health Services around the World. Ipsos Social Research Institute. Available online at: http://www.ipsos-mori.com/DownloadPublication/1395_sri-national-health-citizens-views-of-health-services-december-2010.pdf (accessed 09.08.14).

Gott, M., O'Brien, M., 1990. Attitudes and beliefs in health promotion. Nursing Standard 5, 30–32.

HM Government, 1998. Independent Inquiry into Inequalities in Health (Acheson Report). Stationery Office, London.

Kellehear, A., O'Connor, D., 2008. Health promoting palliative care. Critical Public Health 18, 111–115.

Kickbusch, I., 2001. Health literacy: addressing the health and education divide. Health Promotion International 16, 289–297.

Kickbusch, I., 2006. Health literacy: engaging in a political debate. Editorial. International Journal of Public Health 54, 1–2. Available online at: http://heapro.oxfordjournals.org/content/16/3/289.full.pdf+html (accessed 22.09.15).

Lalonde, M., 1974. A New Perspective on the Health of Canadians. Government of Canada, Ottawa.

Marmot, M., 2010. Fair Society, Healthy Lives. DH, London. Available online at: http://www.instituteofhealthequity.org/projects/fair-society-healthy-lives-the-marmot-review (accessed 10.08.14).

Marteau, T., Ogilvie, D., Roland, M., Suhrcke, M., Kelly, M.P., 2011. Judging nudging: can nudging improve population health? BMJ 342, 263–265.

McKinlay, J.B., 1979. A case for refocussing upstream: the political economy of health. In: Jaco, E.G. (Ed.), Patients, Physicians and Illness. Macmillan, Basingstoke.

Milio, N., 1986. Promoting Health through Public Policy. Canadian Public Health Association, Ottawa.

Naidoo, J., Wills, J., 2010. Public Health and Health Promotion: Developing Practice, second ed. Baillière Tindall, London.

Nutbeam, D., 1998. Health Promotion Glossary. World Health Organization, Geneva. Available online at: http://heapro.oxfordjournals.org/content/13/4/349.full.pdf (accessed 25.02.15).

Nutbeam, D., 2000. Health literacy as a public health goal: a challenge for contemporary health education and communication strategies into the 21st century. Health Promotion International 15, 259–267.

Office for National Statistics, 2012. Conceptions in England and Wales. Stationery Office, London. Available online at: http://www.ons.gov.uk/ons/dcp171778_353922.pdf (accessed 10.02.15).

Raphael, D., 2008. Grasping at straws: a recent history of health promotion in Canada. Critical Public Health 18 (4), 483–495.

Sanders, D., Stern, R., Struthers, P., Thabale, J., Ngulube, Onya, H., 2008. What is needed for health promotion in Africa: band-aid, live aid or real change? Critical Public Health 18 (4), 509–519.

Seedhouse, D., 1997. Health Promotion: Philosophy, Prejudice and Practice. Wiley, Chichester.

Sparks, M., 2011. Building healthy public policy: don't believe the misdirection. Health Promotion International 26 (3), 259–262. Available online at: http://heapro.oxfordjournals.org/content/26/3/259.full.pdf+html (accessed 22.09.15).

Sutherland, I., 1987. Health Education: Half a Policy. National Extension College, Cambridge.

Tannahill, A., 1985. What is health promotion? Health Education Journal 44, 4.

Thaler, R., Sunstein, C., 2009. Nudge: Improving Decisions about Health, Wealth and Happiness. Yale University Press, New Haven, CT.

Tones, B.K., 1986. Health education and the ideology of health promotion: a review of alternative approaches. Health Education Research 1, 3–12.

Tones, K., 1990. Why theorise: ideology in health education. Health Education Journal 49, 1.

Townsend, P., Davidson, N., 1982. Inequalities in Health: The Black Report. Penguin, Harmondsworth.

Townsend, P., Whitehead, M., Davidson, N. (Eds.), 1992. Inequalities in Health: The Black Report and the Health Divide, second ed. Penguin, London.

US Department of Health and Human Services, 2000. Healthy People 2010. Available at: http://www.healthypeople.gov/default.htm (accessed 27.02.15).

Welshman, J., 1997. Bringing beauty and brightness to the back streets: health education and public health in England and Wales 1890–1940. Health Education Journal 56, 199–209.

Williams, G., 1984. Health promotion – caring concern or slick salesmanship. Journal of Medical Ethics 10, 191–195.

Wills, J., Douglas, J., 2008. Health promotion still going strong? Critical Public Health 18 (4), 431–434.

Wilson-Barnett, J., 1993. The meaning of health promotion: a personal view. In: Wilson-Barnett, J., Macleod Clark, K. (Eds.), Research in Health Promotion and Nursing. Macmillan, Basingstoke.

Winslow, C.E.A., 1920. The untilled field of public health. Modern Medicine 2, 183–191.

World Health Organization, 1977. Health for All by the Year 2000. World Health Organization, Geneva.

World Health Organization, September 6-12, 1978. Declaration of Alma Ata, International Conference on Primary Health Care, Alma Ata. World Health Organization, Geneva. Available online at: http://www.who.int/publications/almaata_declaration_en.pdf (accessed 25.02.15).

World Health Organization, 1984. Health Promotion: A Discussion Document on Concepts and Principles. World Health Organization, Geneva. Available online at: http://apps.who.int/iris/bitstream/10665/107835/1/E90607.pdf (accessed 22.09.15).

World Health Organization, 1985. Targets for Health for All. World Health Organization, Geneva.

World Health Organization, 1986. Ottawa Charter for Health Promotion. World Health Organization, Geneva. Available online at: http://www.who.int/healthpromotion/conferences/previous/ottawa/en/ (accessed 25.02.15).

Chapter Five

Models and approaches to health promotion

Learning Outcomes

By the end of this chapter you will be able to:
- analyse different approaches to health promotion
- understand different conceptual and analytical models of health promotion and how they might be applied
- appreciate the importance of theory-based approaches to planning health promotion.

Key Concepts and Definitions

Model A simplified description or graphic representation of reality (processes, organizations, beings). Models are often used to hypothesize the outcomes of specific inputs or processes.

Theory An idea or proposition, often using general principles, used to explain something specific.

Medical model This model uses medical concepts of health and sickness rooted in physical or psychological changes that can be measured and quantified.

Social model This model uses sociological concepts to theorize about health and illness. Health is normal social functioning, whereas illness is any impairment (physical or psychological) of social functioning.

Empowerment The act of acquiring power and the ability to make decisions and take control over one's life.

Importance of the Topic

The diversity in concepts of health, influences on health and ways of measuring health lead, not surprisingly, to a number of different approaches to health promotion. If health is seen as the absence of disease, clinical interventions will be seen as appropriate. If health is viewed as the product of interaction and interdependence between the individual and the environment, then legislative or regulatory interventions will be seen as appropriate. Chapter 4 began to explore the concepts of health education and health promotion. In this chapter, five different approaches will be discussed:
- medical or preventive
- behaviour change
- educational
- empowerment
- social change.

These approaches are examined in terms of their different aims, methods and means of evaluation. The approaches have different objectives:
- to prevent disease
- to encourage people to adopt healthy behaviours

- to ensure that people are well informed and able to make health choices
- to help people to acquire the skills and confidence to take greater control over their health
- to change policies and environments in order to facilitate healthy choices.

All the approaches reflect different ways of working. Identifying the different approaches is primarily a descriptive process. The framework is descriptive – it does not indicate which approach is best, nor why a practitioner might adopt one approach rather than another. There are also a number of theoretical frameworks or models of health promotion which are outlined, discussed and assessed in relation to practice in the latter part of this chapter.

It is common for a practitioner to think that theory has no place in health promotion, and that action is determined by work role and organizational objectives rather than values or ideology. We have argued elsewhere that practitioners should be aware of the values implicit in the approach they adopt: 'Values thus determine the way in which the world is seen and the selection of activities and priorities and how strategies are implemented' (Naidoo and Wills, 2010: p. 13).

Models of health promotion are not guides to action but attempts to delineate a contested field of activity, and to show how different priorities and strategies reflect different underlying values. They are useful in helping practitioners think through:

- aims
- implications of different strategies
- what would count as success
- one's own role as a practitioner.

The medical approach

Aims

This approach focuses on activity which aims to reduce morbidity and premature mortality. Activity is targeted towards whole populations or high-risk groups. This kind of health promotion seeks to increase medical interventions which will prevent ill health and premature death. The approach is frequently portrayed as having three levels of intervention.

1. *Primary prevention* – prevention of the onset of disease through risk education, e.g. immunization, or reducing exposure to risk factors, e.g. the use of statins to reduce blood cholesterol.
2. *Secondary prevention* – preventing the progression of disease through early diagnosis, e.g. screening.
3. *Tertiary prevention* – reducing further disability and suffering in those already ill, preventing recurrence of an illness, e.g. rehabilitation, patient education and palliative care.

The medical approach to health promotion is popular for several reasons.

1. It has high status because it uses scientific methods, such as epidemiology (the study of the pattern of diseases in society).
2. In the short term, prevention and the early detection of disease are much cheaper than treatment of people who have become ill. Of course, in the long term this may not be the case, as people live longer, experience degenerative conditions and draw pensions for a longer period.
3. It is an expert-led, or top-down, type of intervention. This kind of activity reinforces the authority of medical and health professionals, who are recognized as having the expert knowledge needed to achieve the desired results.
4. There have been spectacular successes in public health as a result of using this approach, for example the worldwide eradication of smallpox as a result of the vaccination programme.

As we saw in Chapter 1, the medical approach is conceptualized around the absence of disease. It does not seek to promote positive health, and can be criticized for ignoring the social and environmental dimensions of health. In addition, the medical approach encourages dependency on medical knowledge and removes health decisions from the people concerned. Thus healthcare workers are encouraged to persuade patients to cooperate and comply with treatment.

Public health medicine is the branch of medicine which specializes in prevention, and most day-to-day preventive work is carried out by the community health services, which include specialist community public health nurses and district nurses.

Methods

The principle of preventive services such as immunization and screening is that they are targeted to groups at risk of a particular condition. While immunization requires a certain level of take-up for it to be effective, screening is offered to specific groups. For example, cervical screening every 3 to 5 years is offered to all women aged 25–64.

For screening to be effective for a condition or disease:

- the disease should have a long pre-clinical phase, so a screening test will not miss its signs
- earlier treatment should improve the outcomes
- the test should be sensitive, i.e. it should detect all those with the disease
- the test should be specific, i.e. it should detect *only* those with the disease
- it should be cost-effective, i.e. the number of tests performed should yield a number of positive cases, making it an economically sound intervention.

The UK National Screening Committee oversees screening policies and gives advice based on available evidence. (For more details visit www.screening.nhs.uk.)

Preventive procedures need to be based on a sound rationale derived from epidemiological evidence. The medical approach also relies on having infrastructure capable of delivering screening or an immunization programme. This includes trained personnel, equipment and laboratory facilities, information systems which determine who is eligible for the procedure and record uptake rates, and, in the case of immunization, a vaccine which is effective and safe. It can thus be seen that the medical approach to health promotion can be a complex process, and may depend on the establishment of national programmes or guidelines.

Learning Activity 5.1 The criteria for screening

Would it be appropriate to have a national screening programme for depression?

Having screening or immunization facilities available is effective only if people can be persuaded to use them.

Learning Activity 5.2 Increasing the uptake of screening

What methods can you think of that are used to increase the uptake of preventive screening services?

Recent outbreaks of vaccine-preventable diseases (e.g. polio in the Russian Federation and measles in Wales) reflect the challenges to public health authorities in obtaining optimum levels of vaccination. A key factor is gaining public trust through media campaigns, face-to-face communication and support materials to address the population's perception on the necessity, safety and efficacy of a vaccine.

Evaluation

Evaluation of preventive procedures is based ultimately on a reduction in disease rates and associated mortality. This is a long-term process, and an example of a more popular measure capable of short-term evaluation is an increase in the percentage of the target population being screened or immunized.

Case Study 5.1 Measles outbreak in Swansea

The medical approach is not always successful. A major outbreak of 700 cases of measles occurred in Swansea, Wales, in November 2012, despite a UK child vaccination campaign that had been running since 1994 and had resulted in 17,440 people aged 10–18 being vaccinated for the first time. An inquiry into the outbreak by the National Assembly for Wales concluded that Andrew Wakefield's (1998) study linking the measles, mumps and rubella (MMR) vaccine with autism, which had been exposed as fraudulent (Godlee et al., 2011), had affected parents' willingness to consent to MMR. Local media had run a high-profile negative campaign against vaccination in 1998. Uptake of MMR among 2-year-olds in Wales fell from 91 percent in 1996 to 80 percent in 2003. Thus children who had not been routinely vaccinated at that time were now of secondary-school age and had no protection against these diseases.

Learning Activity 5.3 The medical approach to health promotion

What might be some of the critiques of the medical approach?

Behaviour change

Aims

This approach aims to encourage individuals to adopt healthy behaviours, which are seen as the key to improved health. Chapter 8 shows how making health-related decisions is a complex process and, unless a person is ready to take action, it is unlikely to be effective. As we saw in the previous chapter, seeking to influence or change health behaviour has long been part of health education.

The approach is popular because it views health as a property of individuals. It is then possible to assume that people can make real improvements to their health by choosing to change their lifestyle. It also assumes that if people do not take responsible action to look after themselves, then they are to blame for the consequences.

 Learning Activity 5.4 Barriers to behaviour change

What are the reasons why people may not be able to put a healthy diet into practice?

It is clear that there is a complex relationship between individual behaviour and social and environmental factors. Behaviour may be a response to the conditions in which people live, and the causes of these conditions (e.g. unemployment, poverty) are outside individual control.

Methods

The behaviour change approach has been the bedrock of activity undertaken by the lead agencies for health promotion. Campaigns persuade people to desist from smoking, adopt a healthy diet and undertake regular exercise. This approach is targeted towards individuals, although mass means of communication may be used to reach them. It is most commonly an expert-led, top-down approach, which reinforces the divide between the expert who knows how to improve health and the general public who need education and advice. However, this is not inevitable. Interventions may be directed according to a client's stated needs when these have been identified. For example, social marketing techniques (see Chapter 12) focus on finding out what consumers want and need, and then providing it. The national archive for public information films (http://www.nationalarchives.gov.uk/films/) provides examples of some of the ways the public have been encouraged to change their health behaviour over the years.

Many healthcare workers educate their clients about health through the provision of information and one-to-one counselling. Patient education about a condition or medication may seek to ensure compliance – in other words, a behaviour change – or it may be more client-directed and employ an educational approach (see Chapter 9).

Evaluation

Evaluating a health promotion intervention designed to change behaviour would appear to be a simple exercise. Has the health behaviour changed after the intervention? But there are two main problems: change may only become apparent over a long period, and it may be difficult to isolate any change as attributable to a health promotion intervention.

 Research Example 5.1 The effectiveness of behaviour change approaches in relation to weight management

A systematic review of interventions using behaviour change methods to prevent weight gain found mixed results (Hardeman et al., 2000). Only one randomized controlled trial that included various methods – a correspondence programme, goal setting, self-monitoring and being prepared for contingencies – reported significant positive results. The review concluded that progress in this field would be facilitated by:

- the explicit use of methods of behaviour change that have been successful in other contexts (e.g. individual goal setting, the use of incentives, feedback on behaviour change)
- explicit description of interventions in write-ups
- a longer follow-up of the behaviour being targeted, to assess if any changes made are adhered to in the long term.

Another systematic review examined the evidence for using social media such as blogs to promote healthy diet and exercise (Williams et al., 2014). This review did not show high levels of participation, but concluded that it might be helpful in one-to-one interventions with tailored feedback and in providing personal support.

As shown in the research example above, behaviour change approaches, while popular with politicians and policymakers, are often unsuccessful. Behaviour, as we have seen, is a response to the social context in which people live, and therefore attempts to simply change those health behaviours may be victim blaming. Population-based behaviour change approaches, such as mass-media campaigns, assume a homogeneity which may not exist amongst the receivers of the health promotion messages.

The educational approach

Aims

The purpose of this approach is to provide knowledge and information, and to develop the necessary skills so that people can make an informed choice about their health behaviour. The educational approach should be distinguished from a behaviour change approach in that it does not set out to persuade or motivate change in a particular direction. However, education *is* intended to have an outcome. This will be the client's voluntary choice, and it may not be the one the health promoter would prefer.

The educational approach is based on a set of assumptions about the relationship between knowledge and behaviour: that by increasing knowledge, there will be a change in attitudes which may lead to changed behaviour. The goal of a client being able to make an informed choice may seem unambiguous and agreed upon. This ignores, however, not only the very real constraints that social and economic factors place on voluntary behaviour change, but also the complexities of health-related decision-making (see Chapter 9).

Methods

Psychological theories state that learning involves three aspects:

- cognitive (information and understanding)
- affective (attitudes and feelings)
- behavioural (skills).

An educational approach to health promotion will provide information to help clients to make an informed choice about their health behaviour. This may be through the provision of leaflets and booklets, visual displays or one-to-one advice. It may also provide opportunities for clients to share and explore their attitudes to their own health, perhaps through group discussion or one-to-one counselling. Educational programmes may develop clients' decision-making skills through role plays or activities designed to explore options. Clients may take on roles or practise responses in 'real-life' situations – for example, clients taking part in an alcohol programme may role-play situations where they are offered a drink. Educational programmes are usually led by a teacher or facilitator, although the issues for discussion may be decided by the clients. Educational interventions require the practitioner to understand the principles of adult learning and the factors which help or hinder learning.

Case Study 5.2 Water education in Africa

Projectwet is a water education programme for teachers, funded by USAID, to reduce the spread of waterborne diseases in Africa. Materials are developed to be incorporated into the curriculum, thereby empowering community action such as conservation, water quality and using groundwater to solve water issues (www. projectwet.org).

Evaluation

Increases in knowledge are relatively easy to measure. Health education programmes using mass-media campaigns, one-to-one education and classroom-based work have all shown success in increasing information about health issues, or the awareness of risk factors for a disease. Information alone is, however, insufficient to change behaviour and, as we shall see in Chapter 8, even the desire and ability to change behaviour are no guarantee that the individual will do so.

Empowerment

Aims

The World Health Organization (1986) defined health promotion as enabling people to gain control over their lives. This approach helps people to identify their own concerns and gain the skills and confidence to act upon them. It is unique in being based on a 'bottom-up' strategy, and calls for different skills from the health promoter. The health promoter needs to become a facilitator whose role is to act as a catalyst, getting things going and freeing up resources, and then to withdraw from the situation.

Learning Activity 5.5 Defining empowerment

- What do you understand by the term 'empowerment'?
- Can a practitioner empower a client?
- Are there health promotion actions which can disempower someone?

When we talk of empowerment, we need to distinguish between *self*-empowerment and *community* empowerment. Self-empowerment is used in some cases to describe those approaches to promoting health which are based on counselling and use nondirective, client-centred methods aimed at increasing people's control over their own lives. For people to be empowered they need to:

- recognize and understand their powerlessness
- feel strongly enough about their situation to want to change it
- feel capable of changing the situation by having information, support and life skills.

Empowerment is also used to describe a way of working which increases people's power to change their 'social reality'. Chapter 10 includes a discussion of community development as a way of working which seeks to create active, participating communities which are *empowered* and able to challenge and change the world about them. This may or may not include political consciousness raising, such as that advocated by the radical educationist Paulo Freire (1972).

Methods

Many health, education and social care practitioners use empowerment strategies, which may be referred to as client-centred approaches, advocacy or self-care. Laverack (2005) states that the challenge for practitioners is to use their own power (power over) to help clients to gain power (power from within).

Case Study 5.3 Empowering through reminiscence

Reminiscence is an example of a communication strategy which encourages older people to tell their story and recall past events. This provides opportunities for them to say what kind of care they want. It shifts the balance of the relationship to the client or patient, and helps build trust and understanding. In dementia care, older people can be encouraged to retrieve their past experience and maintain their personhood. Some ethnic groups with strong oral traditions use reminiscence to preserve their cultural identity (Coleman and O'Hanlon, 2004).

Community development is a similar way of working to empower groups of people by identifying their concerns, and working with them to plan a programme of action to address these concerns. Some health promoters have a specific remit to undertake community development work; most do not. Community development work is time-consuming, and most health promoters have clearly defined priorities which take up all their time. Funding for this kind of work is invariably insecure and short term; and the communication, planning and organizational skills necessary for the approach may not be included in professional training. For many health promoters, relinquishing the expert role may be difficult and uncomfortable. Ways of working with communities are discussed more fully in Chapter 10.

There are numerous examples of social movements in health promotion and of health activitists using empowerment approaches. Laverack (2013) gives examples of those seeking to:

- develop healthy public policy (e.g. prostitute collectives)
- tackle the social determinants of health (e.g. members of the community visiting elderly neighbours)
- use the media (e.g. the BUGA UP campaign – Billboard Utilizing Graffitiists Against Unhealthy Promotions)
- use coalitions and networks (e.g. for the homeless).

Evaluation

Evaluation of empowering activity is problematic, partly because the process of empowerment and networking is typically long term. This makes it difficult to be certain that any changes detected are due to the intervention and not some other factor. In addition, positive results of such an approach may appear to be vague and hard to specify, especially when compared to outcomes used by other approaches, such as targets or changes in behaviour which are capable of being quantified. Evaluation includes the extent to which specific aims have been met (outcome evaluation) and the degree to which the group has gelled, or been empowered, as a result of the intervention (process evaluation). Evaluation therefore needs to include qualitative methods that reveal people's perceptions and beliefs as well as quantitative methods that demonstrate outcomes such as behaviour change.

Social change

Aims

This approach, which is sometimes referred to as radical health promotion, acknowledges the importance of the socio-economic environment in determining health. Its focus is at the policy or environmental level, and the aim is to bring about changes in the physical, social and economic environment which will have the effect of promoting health. This may be summed up in the phrase 'to make the healthy choice the easier choice'. A healthy choice exists, but to make it a realistic option for most people requires changes in its cost, availability or accessibility. Chapter 11 discusses the processes involved in creating healthy public policies.

 Learning Activity 5.6 Social change approaches and healthy eating

Several studies have shown that a healthy diet which includes fruit and vegetables costs more than the typical diet of a low-income family (Cade et al., 1999). What should be the focus of health promotion interventions on healthy eating?

Methods

The social change or radical approach is targeted towards groups and populations, and involves a top-down method of working. Change may be in organizations (e.g. nutritional standards for school meals), communities (e.g. age-friendly cities) or policies and laws (e.g. smoke-free legislation). Although there may be widespread consultation, the changes being sought require commitment at the highest levels. Chapter 11 discusses healthy public policy and how legislation has had an enormous impact on the nation's health. The successful implementation of policy and legislation requires the support of the public, which is achieved through education, lobbying and social marketing. Chapter 9 discusses social marketing in greater detail.

For most health promotion workers, the scope for this type of activity will be more limited than for the traditional medical or behaviour change approaches. The necessary skills for working in this way, such as lobbying, policy planning, negotiating and implementation, may not be included in professional training. Working in such a way may be interpreted as being beyond the brief of the job, too political or someone else's remit. There is, however, scope for professional organizations to become involved as stakeholders in social change processes. For example, health practitioners' professional bodies were involved in lobbying for a total smoking ban in public places, alongside pressure groups such as ASH (Action on Smoking and Health).

Evaluation

Evaluation of the social change approach includes outcomes such as legislative, organizational or regulatory changes which promote health, e.g. regulations governing food labelling, a ban on tobacco sponsorship and advertising and a ban on smoking in public places.

The extent of partnership working and the profile of health issues on common agendas may also be used to demonstrate a greater degree of commitment to social change for health. These outcomes are typically long-term, complex processes, making it difficult to prove a link to particular health promotion interventions.

Learning Activity 5.7 Social change approaches in practice

Are there parts of your work which are aimed at social change? Have you sought to influence policies and practices which affect health?

Learning Activity 5.8 Approaches to healthy eating

Table 5.1 uses the example of healthy eating to show how different approaches to health promotion will have different aims and use different methods. Choose one of the current public health priorities (reducing obesity, encouraging sensible drinking or improving mental health and well-being). Consider how health promotion interventions in this area will be affected by working with the five identified approaches to health

promotion: medical, behaviour change, educational, empowerment, social change.
- In each case what would working within this approach entail in terms of:
  - aims or focus?
  - methods?
  - worker–client relationship?
- How would you evaluate your success using each approach?
- With which approach would you feel most comfortable?

Models of health promotion

The schema of different approaches to health promotion in Table 5.1 is primarily descriptive. It is what health promoters do, and it is possible to move into and out of different approaches depending on the situation. A more analytic means of identifying types of health promotion is to develop models of practice. All models, be they building models, diagrammatic maps or theoretical models, seek to represent reality in some way and try to show in a simplified form how different things connect. Implicit in the use of models is a theoretical framework that explains how and why the elements in the model are connected. Themes, conceptual maps and models structure our thinking and action about a problem, and provide a rationale for acting or developing an approach. Models of health promotion may help to:
- conceptualize or map the field
- interrogate and analyse existing practice
- plan and chart the possibilities for interventions (Naidoo and Wills, 2010).

Using a model can be helpful because it encourages you to think theoretically and come up with new strategies and ways of working. It can also help you to prioritize and locate more or less desirable types of interventions.

There has been a proliferation of models in health promotion literature, with large areas of overlap but little consensus on terminology or underlying criteria. Thus we find that Caplan and Holland (1990) use 'theories of knowledge' and 'theories of society' (see Figure 5.1). Beattie (1991) uses criteria of

Table 5.1 Approaches to health promotion: the example of healthy eating

Approach	Aims	Methods	Worker/client relationship
Medical	To identify those at risk from disease	Screening, individual risk assessment, e.g. measurement of body mass index	Expert led; passive, conforming client
Behaviour change	To encourage individuals to take responsibility for their own health and choose healthier lifestyles	Persuasion through one-to-one advice and information; mass-media campaigns, e.g. five-a-day dietary messages	Expert led; dependent client; possible victim-blaming ideology
Educational	To increase knowledge and skills about healthy lifestyles	Information and exploration of attitudes through individual or small-group work; development of skills, e.g. cooking healthy meals	May be expert led; may also involve client in negotiation of issue for discussion
Empowerment	To work with clients or communities to meet their perceived needs	Advocacy; negotiation; networking; facilitation, e.g. community horticulture projects	Health promoter is facilitator; client becomes empowered
Social change	To address inequalities in health based on class, race, gender or geography, adopting a population perspective	Development of organizational policy, e.g. hospital catering policy; public health legislation, e.g. food labelling lobbying; fiscal controls, e.g. subsidy to farmers to produce lean meat	Entails social regulation and is top down

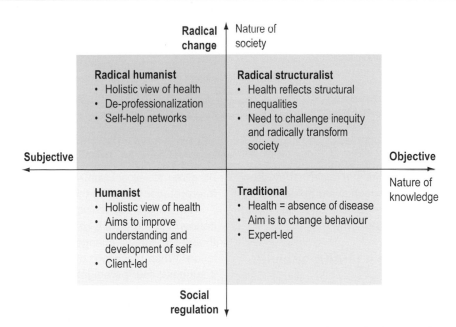

Fig. 5.1 ● Four paradigms or perspectives of health promotion. (Adapted from Caplan, R., Holland, R., 1990. Rethinking health education theory. Health Education Journal 49,10–12.)

'mode of intervention' (authoritative–negotiated) and 'focus of intervention' (individual–collective) to generate four paradigms (see Figure 5.2). The terminology for models also varies. For example, French (1990) calls a social change approach 'politics of health', while Caplan and Holland (1990) distinguish between a radical model and a Marxist model. This can be extremely confusing for the reader.

The following two models derive from sociological and social policy frameworks. They adopt a structural analysis which draws attention to the material and social influences on health and the social structures

Mode of intervention
Authoritative
Mode of thought
Objective knowledge

Health persuasion
- To *persuade* or encourage people to adopt healthier lifestyles
- Practitioner is in the role of expert or 'prescriber'
- Conservative political ideology
- Activities include advice and information

Legislative action
- To *protect* the population by making healthier choices more available
- Practitioner is in the role of 'custodian' knowing what will improve the nation's health
- Reformist political ideology
- Activities include policy work, lobbying

Focus of intervention

Individual   Collective

Personal counselling
- To *empower* individuals to have the skills and confidence to take more control over their health
- Practitioner is in the role of 'counsellor' working with people's self-defined needs
- Liberation or humanist political ideology
- Activities include counselling and education

Community development
- To *enfranchise* or *emancipate* groups and communities so they recognize what they have in common and how social factors influence their lives
- Practitioner is in the role of 'advocate'
- Radical political ideology
- Activities include community development and action

Mode of intervention
Negotiated
Mode of thought
Participatory, subjective knowledge

Fig. 5.2 ● Using Beattie's model to analyse practice. (Based on Beattie, A., 1993. The changing boundaries of health. In: Beattie, A., Gott, M., Jones, L., Sidell, M. (Eds.), Health and Wellbeing: A Reader. Macmillan/Open University, Basingstoke.)

which contribute to inequalities in health. They show how health promotion approaches are influenced by political ideology and different value positions about power, responsibility and autonomy.

Caplan and Holland's (1990) analytic model

This model suggests that there are essentially four paradigms or ways of looking at health promotion. These paradigms can be generated from two dimensions (see Figure 5.1). The first dimension is concerned with the nature of knowledge. Knowledge is seen as based along a continuum which ranges from subjective approaches to understanding through to objective approaches. Objective explanations deriving from science (e.g. health is the absence of disease) are only part of the picture. Emphasis may also

be given to lay accounts and people's own unique interpretations of what their health means to them.

The second dimension relates to assumptions concerning the nature of society. These range from theories of radical change to theories of social regulation. When these two dimensions are put together it suggests four paradigms or perspectives of health promotion, as illustrated in Figure 5.1.

Each quadrant represents a major approach to the understanding of health and the practice of health promotion. They are not necessarily exclusive, but there will be situations when to hold one position or approach precludes the adoption of other approaches. Each quadrant incorporates different theoretical and philosophical assumptions about society, concepts of health and the principal sources of health problems.

1. **The traditional perspective** relates to the medical and behaviour change approaches described

earlier. Knowledge lies with the experts, and the emphasis is on giving information to bring about behavioural change.

2. **The humanist perspective** relates to the educational approach. Individuals are enabled to use their personal resources and skills to maximize their chances of developing what they consider to be a healthy lifestyle.

3. **The radical humanist perspective** relates to the empowerment approach. Health promotion is designed to raise consciousness, and part of the emphasis is on the exploration of personal responses to health issues. Alongside this, individuals are encouraged to form social, organizational and economic networks.

4. **The radical structuralist perspective** holds that structural inequalities are the cause of many health problems, and the role of health promotion is to address the relationship between health and social inequalities.

The model is useful in showing that practice is the outcome of deeper social conflicts and values.

Beattie's (1991) analytic model

Beattie offers a structural analysis of the health promotion repertoire of approaches. He suggests that there are four paradigms for health promotion (see Figure 5.2). These are generated from the dimensions of mode of intervention, which ranges from authoritative (top down and expert led) to negotiated (bottom up and valuing individual autonomy). Much health promotion work involving advice and information is determined and led by practitioners. Equally, policy work may also be expert led, with the priorities determined by epidemiological data. Here, there are objective explanations for health as opposed to approaches which privilege subjective accounts of what health means. The other dimension relates to the focus of the intervention, which ranges from a focus on individuals who are responsible for their own health to a focus on the collective and the roots of ill health.

Beattie's typology generates four strategies for health promotion.

1. **Health persuasion.** These are interventions directed at individuals and led by professionals. An example is a primary healthcare worker encouraging a pregnant woman to stop smoking. This approach is based on the premise that the expert knows best. Health persuasion may range from straightforward signposting to brief interventions that seek to motivate a person to change.

2. **Legislative actions.** These are interventions led by professionals but intended to protect communities. Examples are lobbying for tighter controls on food labelling, and controlling the number of licenced premises that serve alcohol in a neighbourhood.

3. **Personal counselling.** These interventions are client led and focus on personal development. The health promoter is a facilitator rather than an expert. An example is a youth worker helping young people to identify their health needs and then working with them individually or in groups to increase their confidence and skills. Another example is motivational interviewing (see Chapter 9), which is widely used in primary care settings.

4. **Community development.** These interventions, in a similar way to personal counselling, seek to empower or enhance the skills of a group or local community. An example is a community worker working with a local tenants' group to increase opportunities for further education and active leisure pursuits. The community development process is based on principles of social justice, and can therefore be viewed as a radical approach to health promotion.

Figure 5.2 shows how Beattie's model can point up the following aspects:

- goals and activities
- client–practitioner relationship
- political ideologies.

Each of the four strategies corresponds to a different political perspective. Thus conservative reformist perspectives see health promotion as attempting to correct or repair what is seen as a deficit in the conservative perspective (e.g. lack of information) or an aspect of deprivation in the reformist perspective (e.g. difficulties of access). These perspectives give rise to authoritative and prescriptive approaches. Libertarian and radical perspectives both see health promotion as seeking to empower or enfranchise individuals. The radical perspective, in addition, seeks to mobilize and emancipate communities. Each of these perspectives also casts the practitioner in a different role in relation to clients.

Beattie's model is useful for health promoters because it identifies a clear framework for deciding a strategy, and yet reminds them that the choice of these interventions is influenced by social and political perspectives.

 Learning Activity 5.9 Applying Beattie's model of health promotion

Take one of the following programme objectives, and use Beattie's model to plot the different strategies which might be employed to reduce:
- smoking among pregnant women
- drinking among young people
- accidents among older people.

Tannahill's (Downie et al., 1996) descriptive model

This model of health promotion is widely accepted by healthcare workers. Tannahill talks of three overlapping spheres of activity: health education, health protection and prevention.

Health education – communication to enhance well-being and prevent ill health through influencing knowledge and attitudes.

Prevention – reducing or avoiding the risk of diseases and ill health primarily through medical interventions.

Health protection – safeguarding population health through legislative, fiscal or social measures. This is not how the term 'health protection' is currently used, which is to control infections.

Tannahill's diagrammatic representation (Figure 5.3) shows how these different approaches relate to each other in an all-inclusive process termed 'health promotion'.

The model is primarily descriptive of what goes on in practice. It is useful for the health promoter to see the potential in other areas of activity, and the scope of health promotion. It does not, however, give any insight into why a practitioner may choose one

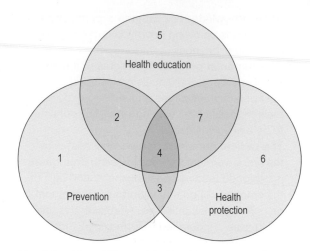

Fig. 5.3 ● Tannahill's model of health promotion. (From Downie, R.S., Tannahill, C., Tannahill, A. 1996. Health Promotion: Models and Values, second ed. Oxford Medical Publications, Oxford.)
1. Preventive services, e.g. immunization, cervical screening, hypertension case finding, developmental surveillance, use of nicotine chewing gum to aid smoking cessation.
2. Preventive health education, e.g. smoking cessation advice and information.
3. Preventive health protection, e.g. fluoridation of water.
4. Health education for preventive health protection, e.g. lobbying for seat-belt legislation.
5. Positive health education, e.g. life-skills work with young people.
6. Positive health protection, e.g. workplace smoking policy.
7. Health education aimed at positive health protection, e.g. lobbying for a ban on tobacco advertising. Downie et al. (1996).

approach over another. It suggests that all approaches are interrelated, but, as we have seen, they reflect distinctive ways of looking at health issues.

Tones's (Tones and Tilford, 2001) empowerment model

This model claims to be an empowerment model which has as its cardinal principle the goal of enabling people to gain control over their own health. It prioritizes empowerment, which is seen as both the core value and the core strategy underpinning and defining the practice of health promotion.

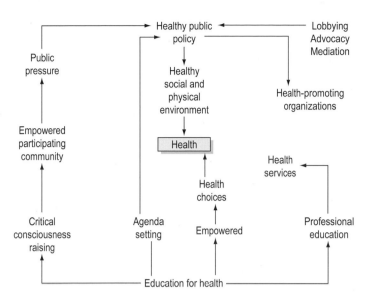

Fig. 5.4 ● The contribution of education to health promotion. (Adapted from Tones, K., Tilford, S., 2001. Health education: Effectiveness, Efficiency, Equity, third ed. Nelson Thornes, Cheltenham.)

Tones makes a simple equation that health promotion is an overall process of healthy public policy × health education (see Figure 5.4). These twin approaches underpin health promotion practice.

Tones considers education to be the key to empowering both lay and professional people by raising consciousness of health issues. People are then more able to make choices and create pressure for healthy public policies. An example of this is the media attention on school dinners generated by Jamie Oliver. This created public pressure, which in turn led to the introduction of school meal standards and universal free school meals for infants in England. We have seen how there is a distinction between self-empowerment and community empowerment. Tones argues that there is a reciprocal relationship between the two. Changes in the social environment achieved through healthy public policies will facilitate the development of self-empowered individuals. People who have the skills to participate effectively in decision-making are better able to access resources and shape policy to meet their needs. The support of individuals is also necessary for implementing change. Empowerment, as opposed to prevention or a radical political approach, is the main aim of health promotion in Tones's model. Working for empowerment enhances individual autonomy and enables individuals, groups and communities to take more control over their lives.

Theories in health promotion

So far in this chapter we have looked at models of health promotion, which are visual representations seeking to explain this emerging area of thinking and practice. The terms theory and model are often used interchangeably. Theories are organized sets of knowledge applicable in a variety of circumstances. In most disciplines the building of theory and progress towards understanding a phenomenon are an accepted part of research. Theories seek to analyse, explain or predict a particular phenomenon or why something happens, and the ways in which change takes place in individuals, communities, organizations or societies. Theories are then the backbone of the processes used to plan, implement and evaluate health promotion interventions, as they remind us what we are trying to do, how

Table 5.2 Health promotion action areas and associated theories

Level of activity	Key areas for change	Theories or models	Chapter in this book
Individual	How can we motivate individuals to change?	Health belief model	9
		Stages of change/model	
	How do individuals learn?	Social learning theory	
	What is the influence of social norms?	Theory of planned behaviour	
	Why do individuals relapse or not comply?	Theory of reasoned action	
Community	Why do some people adopt new ideas readily while others are more conservative?	Diffusion of innovation theory	10
		Community mobilization	
Organizational change	Why do some organizations resist change?	Theories of organizational change	13–17
	What factors in settings create health?	Settings' theories: socio-ecological, salutogenesis	
Population	How do we market or design effective communication to the general public?	Social marketing theory	12

activities are supposed to work and what needs to be in place for them to work. Health promotion draws on a number of disciplines for its theory (Naidoo and Wills, 2015).

- Teaching and learning theory, e.g. social learning theory assists in the development of health education campaigns.
- Communication theory, e.g. social marketing theory is used in some areas of health promotion.
- Sociological theory, which assists in understanding issues related to gender, ethnicity, social divisions and social change.
- Psychological theory, which assists in understanding individual constructs like self-esteem, self-efficacy, locus of control and the different stages of the life cycle. These ideas are valuable in understanding the attitudes and needs of clients.
- Theories of organizational change, which assist in explaining the development and implementation of public policy.

As health promotion is essentially about enabling change at different levels, a theory-driven approach provides a direction and justification for activities. Table 5.2, adapted from Nutbeam et al. (2010), matches the focus of interventions to theories or models that seek to explain change processes at the appropriate level. This facilitates action

informed by theory (rather than by tradition or knee-jerk response).

Chapter 1 in our associated textbook *Public Health and Health Promotion: Developing Practice* (Naidoo and Wills, 2010) discusses the role of theory in more detail.

 Case Study 5.4 Using theory in health promotion planning

Consider the example of partner notification as a priority in sexual health promotion. It is known that there is a reluctance to notify partners if a person has an STI (sexually transmitted infection) for fear of introducing conflict into a relationship, although people are more likely to inform 'steady' partners than casual ones. Studies show anxiety about raising the issue and how to persuade a partner to go for testing and possible treatment. It is also known from case audits that partner notification is frequently not discussed (National AIDS Trust, 2012).

A psychosocial/behavioural theory may predict that:
- a greater intention to notify would be associated with higher levels of self-efficacy and a greater likelihood of notifying all partners.

Organizational theory may predict that:
- the lack of case notes on partner notification may reflect organizational structures and processes rather than actual activities.

Conclusion

A number of quite different activities are subsumed under the label 'health promotion'. For example, there can be many approaches to tackling an issue such as teenage pregnancy:

- medical approach: providing contraception
- behavioural approach: contraceptive advice
- educational approach: sex education
- empowerment approach: life skills, including negotiation, assertiveness and communication
- social change approach: review of services and benefits (education and training, financial, housing) available to young women.

Attempts to organize these activities into different categories have generated a plethora of models and typologies. The most obvious starting point is to describe the variety of current practices, and this is the approach taken at the beginning of this chapter.

However, there are limitations to this method, and it may be criticized as being insufficiently analytical. Theorists who have taken this one step further have identified key criteria which serve to locate different forms of practice, both existing and potential. Adopting a more analytical approach enables judgements to be made about more and less desirable forms of practice, and opens up these judgements for debate. If health promotion is to progress as a discipline and an activity in its own right, a strong theoretical framework is necessary.

The search to clarify models and typologies of practice may appear to be academic and unrelated to the 'here and now' of your activities to promote health. However, we would argue that for practice to grow beyond a reactive response to demands made by others, practitioners need to have an idea of all available options and reflect on which approaches are most congruent with their own beliefs and values. It is only when we can contemplate different ways of promoting health that we can make judgements as to what is possible and what is preferable. Recognizing that the two are not always synonymous may be frustrating in the short term, but must in the long term contribute towards the effectiveness and efficiency of health promotion.

Learning Activity 5.10 Using health promotion models to plan strategy

The smoking rate among women on low incomes increases with:

- greater disadvantage
- more children to care for
- children in poorer health
- caring alone
- carrying extra responsibility for family members.

Using one of the models discussed earlier, map those health promotion interventions which you would regard as:

- most appropriate for women smokers on a low income
- most likely to be adopted
- ones you would use.

If the answers to these three criteria are different, what might account for this?

Summary

This chapter has examined five different approaches to health promotion: the medical or preventive approach; the behaviour change or lifestyle approach; the educational approach; the empowerment and community development approach; and the social change or radical approach. In practice, the edges between them may be blurred. However, they do differ in significant ways. They encompass different assumptions concerning the nature of health, society and change. The preferred methods of intervention, necessary skills and means of evaluation all differ. Many health promoters will find that the approach they adopt is dictated, in part at least, by their job role and functions. This chapter stresses the importance of examining your approach to health promotion and identifying any changes you may wish to make.

Questions for further discussion

- Which approaches to health promotion do you favour?
- Which approaches do you adopt in your work? What are the most important reasons for adopting these approaches?

Further reading and resources

Cragg, L., Davies, M., Macdowall, W., 2013. Health Promotion Theory. McGraw Hill, London. *A useful synthesis of theory and its application.*

Laverack, G., 2005. Public Health: Power, Empowerment and Professional Practice. Palgrave Macmillan, Hampshire. *This book explores the concept of power and discusses the potential and dilemmas for professional practitioners seeking to empower their clients, in both individual and community settings.*

Naidoo, J., Wills, J., 2010. Public Health and Health Promotion: Developing Practice, third ed. Baillière Tindall, London. *Chapter 1*
examines the body of health promotion theory, the key principles which inform practice and why their application may be difficult.*

Tones, K., Tilford, S., 2001. Health Education: Effectiveness, Efficiency and Equity, third ed. Nelson Thornes, Cheltenham. *Chapter 1 explores the values underpinning three different models of health promotion: radical–political, self-empowerment and preventive.*

Wills, J., 2012. Understanding and using theory and models. In: Jones, L., Douglas, J. (Eds.), Public Health: Building Innovative Practice. Open University, Buckingham. *A brief summary of health promotion models and theories.*

 ## Feedback to learning activity

5.1 Depression would not be recommended as suitable for a national screening programme as there is no validated test or assessment for it. NICE (National Institute for Health and Clinical Excellence) guidelines (2009) do not recommend anti-depressants as the primary intervention for mild to moderate depression, so there is no specific treatment to give for cases of early identified depression.

5.2 Community-based interventions can enable the public to understand the meaning and relevance of screening. Other methods include communication through call-recall systems that send personal invitations. Barriers to uptake, such as poor access, have been addressed through mobile clinics. See www.commvac.com for a taxonomy of interventions to improve communication about childhood vaccination.

5.3 A medical approach to an issue:
- does not seek to understand or address the underlying cause, which is probably related to social determinants of health
- does not seek to promote positive health
- encourages a dependence on medical solutions, including technology and medication
- probably removes decision-making from lay people.

5.4 The reasons why people may not be able to achieve a healthy diet include:
- cost, e.g. of fruit and vegetables, lean meat and fish
- negative perceptions, e.g. healthy food is not tasty
- beliefs, e.g. that their current diet is already healthy
- lack of knowledge, e.g. about portion sizes or the different food groups in their diet
- lack of cooking skills

- lack of availability of healthy foods
- family or peer pressure, e.g. to eat the same (unhealthy) diet as friends and family.

5.5 Empowerment is a complex, albeit popular, concept. Empowerment is the giving of power or control, and may occur at individual, organizational or community levels. Empowerment is both a process and an outcome. Practitioners can empower clients by providing information and skills. Health promotion actions, even if they will lead to better health, can be disempowering if decisions are taken with no consultation. See Woodall et al. (2010) for a review of the evidence on empowerment and well-being.

5.6 You may have included some of the following:
- changes in pricing structures, such as reducing the price of wholemeal bread compared to white bread
- working with food manufacturers and distributors to promote food labelling, making it easier for customers to identify low-fat, low-sugar foods
- farming subsidies which encourage the production of lean meat
- the provision of healthy food in workplaces and hospitals
- ensuring that the existing nutritional standards for school meals, which promote healthy food including fruit and vegetables, are maintained.

5.7 Organizational development, environmental health measures, economic or legislative activities and public policies on housing, education or the provision of services may all be examples of health promotion aimed at social change.

Partnership working with other agencies enables the socio-economic and environmental determinants of health to be targeted, e.g. health, education and environment practitioners may work together to lobby for the provision of safe outdoor recreation areas.

Practitioners may seek to address the root causes of ill health by developing health profiles, conducting health equity audits, working in partnerships with other agencies, social commentary and research.

5.8 Assuming you are a health worker with individuals on your caseload, and you chose behaviour change to reduce obesity, this would involve working with individuals or small groups with the goal of reducing weight. Methods might include education (about the calories in different foods) and behaviour change (avoiding calorific snacks, exercising more). You would want your patient/s to acknowledge your expertise and knowledge, but would also want them to feel empowered by their knowledge. You would evaluate your success by recording weight loss among your caseload.

5.9 What you may find is that there is a preponderance of strategies in one quadrant. The approach which used to be most popular was health persuasion, but increasingly there are more examples of state-led legislative interventions.

5.10 It is likely that there may be a discrepancy between the model you as a health professional would adopt, and the model that might be most effective or acceptable to the woman living on a low income. As a health professional you might feel most comfortable with the health education or prevention models, providing information or Nicorette to the young mother. Such an approach vindicates your authority and expertise. However, the young mother might feel more comfortable with a health protection model, which introduces restrictions on smoking in public places but does not target her behaviour at home. Health professionals are constrained by their workload and budget, and their primary role is to provide care for individual patients rather than to lobby for societal changes regarding health behaviours (such as smoking bans in public places).

References

Beattie, A., 1991. Knowledge and control in health promotion: a test case for social policy and social theory. In: Gabe, J., Calnan, M., Bury, M. (Eds.), The Sociology of the Health Service. Routledge, London.

Beattie, A., 1993. The changing boundaries of health. In: Beattie, A., Gott, M., Jones, L., Sidell, M. (Eds.), Health and Wellbeing: A Reader. Macmillan/Open University, Basingstoke.

Cade, J., Upmeier, H., Calvert, C., Greenwood, D., 1999. Costs of a healthy diet: analysis from the UK women's cohort study. Public Health Nutrition 2, 505–512.

Caplan, R., Holland, R., 1990. Rethinking health education theory. Health Education Journal 49, 10–12.

Coleman, P.G., O'Hanlon, A., 2004. Ageing and Development. Arnold, London.

Cragg, L., Davies, M., Macdowall, W., 2013. Health Promotion Theory. McGraw Hill, London,.

Downie, R.S., Tannahill, C., Tannahill, A., 1996. Health Promotion: Models and Values, second ed. Oxford Medical Publications, Oxford.

Freire, P., 1972. Pedagogy of the Oppressed. Penguin, Harmondsworth.

French, J., 1990. Boundaries and horizons, the role of health education within health promotion. Health Education Journal 49(1), 7–10.

Godlee F., Smith, J., Marcovitch, H., 2011. Wakefield's article linking MMR vaccine and autism was fraudulent. British Medical Journal 342, c7452. doi: 10.1136/bmj.c7452.

Hardeman, W., Griffin, S., Johnston, M., Kinmonth, A.L., Wareham, N.J., 2000. Interventions to prevent weight gain: a systematic review of psychological models and behaviour change methods. International Journal of Obesity 24 (2), 131–143.

Laverack, G., 2005. Public Health: Power, Empowerment and Professional Practice. Palgrave Macmillan, Hampshire.

Laverack, G., 2013. Health Activism: Foundations and Strategies. Sage, London.

Naidoo, J., Wills, J., 2010. Public Health and Health Promotion: Developing Practice, third ed. Baillière Tindall, London.

Naidoo, J., Wills, J., 2015. In: Health Studies: An Introduction. Palgrave Macmillan, Basingstoke.

National AIDS Trust, 2012. HIV Partner Notification: A Missed Opportunity? NAT, London. Available online at: http://www.nat.org.uk/media/Files/Policy/2012/May-2012-HIV-Partner-Notification.pdf (accessed 24.10.13).

Nutbeam, D., Harris, E., Wise, M., 2010. Theory in a Nutshell. McGraw Hill, Sydney.

Tones, K., Tilford, S., 1994. Health Promotion; Theory Models and Approaches, 2nd Edition. Nelson Thornes, Cheltenham.

Wakefield, A.J., Murch, S.H., Anthony, A., Linnell, Casson, D.M., Malik, M., et al., 1998. Ileal lymphoid nodular hyperplasia,non-specific colitis, and pervasive developmental disorder in children [retracted]. Lancet 351,637–641.

Williams, G., Hamm, M., Shulhan, J., Vandermeer, B., Hartling, L., 2014. Social media interventions for diet and exercise behaviours: a systematic review and meta-analysis of randomised controlled trials. British Medical Journal Open 4 (2).

Woodall, J., Raine, G., South, J., Warwick-Booth, L., 2010. Empowerment and Health and Wellbeing: Evidence Review. Available online at: www.apho.org.uk/resource/view. aspx?RID=96495 (accessed 24.02.15).

World Health Organization, 1986. Ottawa Charter for Health Promotion. WHO, Geneva. Available online at: http://www. who.int/healthpromotion/conferences/previous/ottawa/en/ (accessed 28.02.15).

Chapter **Six**

6

Ethical issues in health promotion

Learning Outcomes

By the end of this chapter you will be able to:
- analyse critically the ethical values and principles underpinning health promotion
- discuss some ethical issues in promoting health
- defend health promotion as an ethically sound activity.

Key Concepts and Definitions

Ethics A branch of philosophy that focuses on defining moral principles and what concepts and behaviours are morally right or wrong.

Morality Principles and beliefs about what is right and wrong or good and bad behaviour.

Autonomy A person's ability to be independent and free, and make his or her own decisions.

Social justice Justice or fairness regarding the opportunities, privileges and distribution of wealth within a society.

Beneficence (doing good) Actions taken to benefit and help other people.

Non-maleficence (doing no harm) Actions that are not intended to harm other people.

Importance of the Topic

Health promotion involves working to improve people's health. This requires a series of value judgements about what better health means for the individual and society, and about whether, when and how to make a health promotion intervention. This book uses the perspectives of social science to help you explore your role and aims in health promotion. In this chapter we consider some of the prevailing problems for a health promoter from a philosophical perspective.

- The extent to which individuals can be held responsible for their own health.
- Whether it is justified to institute health promotion interventions which have not been sufficiently evaluated.
- The extent to which health promotion should influence the public to choose what is deemed to be the healthy (and, by implication, correct and good) choice.
- The legitimacy of the state to influence the environment to encourage healthy behaviour.

In particular, the chapter focuses on the limits to individual freedoms and how these are balanced against the health of the community. The chapter outlines the key ethical principles of beneficence (doing good), non-maleficence (doing no harm), justice, telling the truth and respect for people and their autonomy.

The need for a philosophy of health promotion

Debate in health promotion has centred on discussion of practice and some attempts to develop a theoretical base. However, there has been relatively little discussion concerning the philosophy of health and yet it is an essential part of the way in which we understand the world.

Health promotion involves decisions and choices that affect other people and require judgements to be made about whether particular courses of action are right or wrong. There are no definite ways to behave. Health promotion is, according to Seedhouse (2009), 'a moral endeavour'. Philosophical debate helps to clarify what it is that one believes in most and how one wants to run one's life. It can and does help practitioners to reflect on the principles of practice, and thus to make practical judgements about whether to intervene and which strategies to adopt.

Philosophy has three main branches.
1. Logic – the development of reasoned argument.
2. Epistemology – enquiry into the nature and grounds of knowledge and meanings.
3. Ethics – enquiry into how we ought to act and conduct ourselves.

Morals refer to those beliefs about how people 'ought' to behave. These debates about right and wrong, good and bad, and duty are part of everyday discourse. Is it wrong to tell a lie? Is it justified to kill another? Is it our duty to look after ageing parents? Judgement about the morality of these actions may derive from our personal values and moral beliefs, which in turn derive from religion, culture, ideology, professional codes of practice or social etiquette, the law and our life experience. The function of ethical theory is not to provide answers, but to inform these judgements and help people work out whether certain courses of action are right or wrong, and whether one ought to take a certain action.

Western philosophy has been shaped by two theories of ethics – deontology and consequentialism.

Deontology comes from the Greek word *deonto*, meaning duty. Deontologists hold that we have a *duty* to act in accordance with certain universal moral rules. Consequential ethics are based on the premise that whether an action is right or wrong depends on its end result.

Duty and codes of practice

Deontologists hold that there are universal moral rules that it is our duty to follow. Many of the philosophical discussions about the nature of duty are based on the theories of Immanuel Kant. The essence of Kant's thinking is encapsulated in the categorical imperative which can help us to discover, through reason, if a rule or moral principle exists (Kant, 1909).

The major features of Kant's theory are as follows.
1. Act as if your action in each circumstance is to become law for everyone, yourself included, in the future. In other words, if everyone always behaved this way, would the overall effect be good? If it would, then this is the rule to apply in all similar situations. The biblical 'Do unto others as you would they do unto you' becomes a universal moral imperative.
2. Always treat human beings as 'ends in themselves' and never merely as 'means'. A moral rule, then, is one that respects all people.

Deontological theories make decision-making apparently easy, because as long as we obey the rules then we must be doing the right thing, regardless of the consequences.

 Learning Activity 6.1 The ethics of antenatal screening

How ethical is antenatal screening?

Many healthcare workers have codes of practice which set out guidelines for the fulfilment of duties. For example, doctors take the Hippocratic oath, which requires them as a first principle to avoid doing harm. The Nursing and Midwifery Council (www.nmc-uk.org) states the duty to respect life, the duty to care and the duty to do no harm. Kant (1909) would have added 'the duty to be truthful in all declarations is a sacred, unconditional command of reason, and not to be limited by any expediency'.

Sindall (2002) argues that health promotion has not engaged in the kind of debate necessary to establish the principles, duties and obligations to which health promoters would need to agree to work in the field. Codes of conduct are simply devices offering a framework in which to practice; they do not help practitioners involved in the messy and complex everyday world of healthcare (Duncan, 2015). For example, Article 3 of the nursing code declares that the registered nurse, midwife or specialist community public health nurse must obtain consent before any treatment or care, but the concept of informed consent is complex.

 Learning Activity 6.2 Defining informed consent

What do you understand by the concept of informed consent? What difficulties might there be in complying with this aspect of the code of practice?

Consequentialism and utilitarianism: The individual and the common good

The other classical school of ethics is consequentialism, and utilitarianism is its best-known branch. Consequentialism differs from deontological theories because it is concerned with ends and not only means. The utilitarian principle is that a person should always act in such a way that will produce more good or benefits than disadvantages. Utilitarians such as John Stuart Mill and Jeremy Bentham aimed for the greatest good or pleasure for the greatest number of people. Utilitarians can thus respond to all moral dilemmas by reviewing the facts and weighing up the consequences of alternative courses of action. This can, of course, prove difficult. What exactly is a good end? How does one

predict whether an outcome will be favourable? One of the main problems with utilitarianism is that if the aim of all actions is to achieve the greatest good, does this justify harm or injustice to a few if society benefits? Smoking restrictions offer an example, where the health of society takes precedence over the right of the individual to smoke.

Health promotion raises many questions over its ends and means.

- Good health is a relative concept, so whose definition should take precedence? Is it ethical for a practitioner to persuade someone to adopt his or her perception of a healthier lifestyle?
- What means are justifiable to promote good health in the population? Should the interests of the majority always prevail?
- Since most ill health is avoidable, should those who knowingly adopt unhealthy behaviours be refused treatment?

In Chapter 11 the concern over 'social engineering' in health promotion is discussed in relation to public policy used to promote health, and whether government intervention has risked becoming government intrusion. Many interventions are justified as being in the interests of a 'healthy society', yet they may not have been requested or desired.

 Learning Activity 6.3 The ethics of healthy public policy

Consider these examples of healthy public policies and whether, in your view, they are ethical.
- Fluoridation of tap water.
- Subsidy of lead-free petrol.
- Ban on smoking in green areas run by local government, e.g. parks, sports grounds, beaches.
- Complete ban on drinking and driving (requiring a 0mg blood alcohol level for drivers).
- Compulsory testing of all visitors to the UK for human immunodeficiency virus (HIV) infection.
- Ban on the use of hands-free mobile phones in cars.
- Government subsidy of child-minding places.
- Nutritional standards for all school meals.
- Compulsory immunization for all children entering education.

Ethical principles

Ethical principles can help to clarify the decisions that have to be taken at work. Sometimes decisions may be guided by trying to do the best for the greatest number of people; at other times they may be guided by an overriding concern for people's right to determine their own lives; and sometimes decisions may be guided by other ethical principles or a professional code of conduct.

There are four widely accepted ethical principles (Beauchamp and Childress, 2013).

1. Respect for autonomy (a respect for the rights of individuals and their right to determine their lives).
2. Beneficence (the commitment to do actions that are of benefit).
3. Non-maleficence (the obligation not to harm other people; if there is doubt, precaution should prevail).
4. Justice (the obligation to act fairly when dealing with competing claims for resources or rights).

These principles provide a framework for consistent moral decision-making. However, situations rarely involve a single option, but can encapsulate increasingly complex and sometimes conflicting choices between these principles. Seedhouse (2009) has developed the principles into an ethical grid which provides health promoters with an easy-to-follow guide on which to ground their work on moral principles (Figure 6.1).

The ethical grid

The grid provides a tool for practitioners, helping them to question basic principles and values, and be clear about what they mean and intend to do. It suggests ways in which practitioners can work through proposed actions. In any situation we should be asking ourselves certain questions.

1. Central conditions in working for health
   a. Am I creating autonomy in my clients, enabling them to direct their own lives?
   b. Am I respecting the autonomy of my clients, whether or not I approve of their chosen direction?

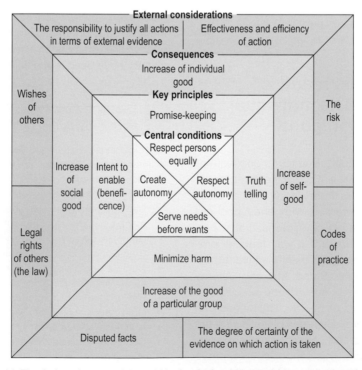

Fig. 6.1 ● The ethical grid. The limit to the use of the grid is that it should be used honestly to seek to enable enhancement of people's potentials. (From Seedhouse, D., 1988. Ethics: The Heart of Health Care. Wiley, Chichester.)

c. Am I respecting all people as equal?

d. Do I work with people on the basis of needs first?

2. Key principles in working for health

a. Am I doing good and avoiding harm?

b. Am I telling the truth and keeping promises?

3. Consequences of ways of working for health

a. Will my action increase the individual good?

b. Will it increase the good of a particular group?

c. Will it increase the good of society?

d. Will I be acting for the good of myself?

4. External considerations in working for health

a. Are there any legal implications?

b. Is there a risk attached to the intervention?

c. Is the intervention the most effective and efficient action to take?

d. How certain is the evidence on which this intervention is based?

e. What are the views and wishes of those involved?

f. Can I justify my actions in terms of all this evidence?

Health promotion involves working to improve people's health. This requires a series of value judgements about what health means for the individual and society, and about whether, when and how to intervene.

Learning Activity 6.4 The ethics of incentivizing change

In the USA a charity has offered young women addicted to heroin or crack cocaine and who have frequent pregnancies resulting in abortions, stillbirths or addicted babies a sum of money to be sterilized. Use Seedhouse's ethical grid illustrated in Figure 6.1 to consider whether or not such action is morally justified.

Learning Activity 6.5 Ethical dilemmas

In the following scenarios, decide what ethical issues are involved, and what action you would take and why.

1. You are nursing a 50-year-old who has chronic obstructive pulmonary disease. The patient has smoked 40 cigarettes a day since he was 17. He has become very distressed by advice to stop smoking.

2. A child has recently died from glue-sniffing at a local secondary school. The community police officer is keen to visit all local schools to show a video depicting a group of children who sniff glue and get into all kinds of trouble.

3. As part of a local mental health strategy, a general practice has introduced questionnaires to detect early indicators of mental health problems at all its clinics. A middle-aged, single, unemployed man regularly attends the diabetic clinic. His questionnaire indicates that he has sleep disturbance and high levels of anxiety.

Autonomy

Autonomy derives from the Greek word *autonomous*, meaning self-rule. It refers to people's capacity to choose freely for themselves and be able to direct their own lives. Since people do not exist in isolation from each other, there will be restrictions on individual autonomy and autonomous people have a sense of responsibility: they cannot do entirely as they like. Thus people do not have complete freedom of choice. The limits to an individual's autonomy are when that individual's action affects others in a negative way. Beyond this, traditional notions of liberal individualism see autonomy as essential to all human beings. It is only constrained by:

- reason and the ability to make rational choices
- the ability to understand one's environment
- the ability to act on one's environment.

In addition, a person needs to be free from pressures such as fear and want, and have the personal and social circumstances to make any chosen action possible.

Autonomy must, therefore, be thought of not as an absolute but as attainable, to a greater or lesser extent. Not everyone has autonomy. When people's capacity for rationality is affected in some way, decisions are often taken on their behalf on the basis that 'they do not know what's best for them'. Thus people with a learning disability or mental illness, young children and older people with mental confusion are often assumed to be unable to make a rational choice. It was not until the twentieth century that women were deemed able to make a rational choice in a democratic election. The Children Act of 1989 first recognized the rights and capacity of children to have a say in their care.

 Learning Activity 6.6 Ethical dilemma: the sexual rights of people with learning disabilities

The rights of young people with profound learning disabilities to determine their sexual health is a contested area.

- Should young people with a severe learning disability have sexual relationships?
- Should they decide whether or not to use contraception?
- Should they decide if they wish to have children?

What do we mean by autonomy? In part, we must mean respecting our clients as persons and helping them to cope with the consequences of their choices. Seedhouse (2009) makes a distinction between creating autonomy and respecting autonomy, which he regards as the central conditions when working for health.

Creating autonomy is making an effort to improve the quality of a person's autonomy by trying to enhance what that person is able to do. In health promotion work, this is often called empowerment. It may involve giving information to enable clients to make choices or developing the clients' skills in analysing situations and making decisions by increasing self-awareness and assertiveness. As stated elsewhere in this book, it is of prime importance in health promotion practice to recognize the limits to individual autonomy, and that social and economic circumstances can constrain individual health choices. Health promoters may claim they are creating autonomy by explaining the health hazards of smoking and thereby enabling individuals to make an informed choice to quit. Yet the autonomy of smokers may be compromised by addiction, social circumstances in which cigarettes may serve as a 'drug of solace', advertising, peer pressure and so on.

Respecting autonomy is respecting a person's chosen direction, whether or not it is approved – for example, respecting a pregnant woman's autonomy to smoke. Creating and respecting autonomy are closely related. People cannot express a free wish if they are not aware of the possibilities open to them, and thus it may, in some circumstances, be ethically justifiable not to respond to a client's expressed wishes but to attempt to open up other options.

 Learning Activity 6.7 Self-determination and health promotion

Is self-determination compatible with the health promoter's goal of seeking health improvement?

 Learning Activity 6.8 Creating autonomy

Think of some examples from your work when you have attempted to *create* autonomy in your clients so they are able to express their wishes and wants.
At what point did you decide that the client is autonomous and to *respect* his or her wishes?

Chapter 10 explores a community development way of working which aims to empower people with regard to their own health agenda. It explores this dilemma of control and autonomy, and to what extent community development workers impose, collaborate with or genuinely facilitate local or community health needs. Chapter 9 looks at ways practitioners support individuals to change, and whether such approaches are intent on empowering individuals or merely getting them to change.

Perhaps the starkest example of the ethical problems associated with respecting autonomy is that which confronts the health worker when a patient or client chooses not to follow advice or treatment which is known to be beneficial. It would seem straightforward that this is the client's right, and the health worker should respect the client's autonomy in choosing such action if the client is properly informed and understands any risks involved. However, the health worker is committed to 'doing good' and may feel it is his or her duty to persuade the client. This is particularly so if the client's decision has implications for other people. Certainly this is paternalistic, and putting the health worker's need to do good above the client's wish for autonomy. Yet by not seeking to persuade or motivate the client, the practitioner may, by omission, be doing harm.

Respecting autonomy involves respecting another person's rights and dignity such that the person reaches a maximum level of fulfilment as a human being. In the context of health promotion and healthcare this means that the relationship with patients or clients is based on a respect for them as people with individual rights. It follows that we must then see them as 'whole people' – with physical, social, emotional and spiritual needs – as fundamentally equal and also as unique individuals.

 Learning Activity 6.9 Ethical dilemma: refusing treatment

A patient who has undergone heart bypass surgery continues to smoke after the operation.
- Is it justifiable to refuse further treatment?
- What factors do you take into account in making your judgement?

Rights in relation to healthcare are usually taken to include:
- the right to information
- the right to privacy and confidentiality
- the right to appropriate care and treatment.

Health workers are often placed in the position of deciding whether to inform patients or relatives of an adverse prognosis. Although the patient's right to information is usually considered paramount, there are occasions when the health worker's duty of beneficence – to do good and avoid harm – may outweigh this right.

Beneficence and non-maleficence

Beneficence means doing or promoting good as well as preventing, removing and avoiding evil or harm. The common good is often put before individual good. Wearing a seat-belt may halve the risk of death to the driver, but the odds that a particular individual will ever benefit are not great, as few people will be killed on the roads. Rose (1981) termed this the 'prevention paradox', according to which a measure that brings large benefits to the community offers little to each participating individual. The alternative to a mass approach

is to focus on risk groups, but this may stigmatize certain groups (Naidoo and Wills, 2010).

 Learning Activity 6.10 Ethical dilemma: vaccination

- Is getting vaccinated an individual choice?
- Is it right to require individuals to participate in an immunization programme for the sake of the communal benefit of herd immunity?
- Should people be able to refuse a vaccination if they believe it to be dangerous?
- Should the state be able to make immunization compulsory?

In such circumstances the duty to care has to be extended to include the concept of informed consent. The individual must be informed, and understand the information and implications of any action which is taken to be beneficial. In this way the health worker can be said to be avoiding harm.

In the field of drug education, harm reduction has been adopted as a way of working. This is perhaps more realistic than the encompassing principle of doing no harm. The healthcare worker recognizes that clients may not wish to change their behaviour, and therefore seeks to encourage a safer way of life and reduce harm. Drug workers may give clients clean needles and condoms, and provide information about emergency first aid to reduce the risks of HIV infection and accidents.

 Case Study 6.1 Tobacco and harm reduction

NICE (National Institute for Health and Clinical Excellence) public health guidance (PH45 2013) recommends a harm-reduction approach for people who are highly dependent on nicotine and who may not be able to stop smoking in one step. Nicotine is highly addictive, but it is the toxins and carcinogens in tobacco smoke that are most harmful. A harm-reduction approach would include:
- using a licensed nicotine product
- cutting down
- temporary abstinence.

Learning Activity 6.11 Ethical dilemma: condoms in prisons

Should condoms be provided in prisons?

The example of screening illustrates the complexities of ethical decision-making, and how attempting to follow the key ethical principles of doing good and avoiding harm is not a simple process. Most preventive services are offered with an explicit promise that they will do some good and an implicit understanding that they will do no harm. Yet what is the nature of that good? Screening, for example, only tells people that they are healthy at the present time. A negative result does not mean that illness will not develop the following year. Screening cannot promise a good outcome. Early detection can mean more effective or less radical treatment in some cases, but there may be no medical benefit and no treatment available. This used to be the case with HIV infection. However, anti-retroviral drug therapies may prevent or delay illness in some people with HIV.

Learning Activity 6.12 Ethical dilemma: screening

Consider a screening process with which you are familiar. In what ways is screening beneficial? Is screening harmful in any way?

Ethically, screening represents the tension between beneficence and non-maleficence. Poorly conducted screening can cause psychological harm by, for example, giving false-positive results. Unfortunately, the pressure to ensure adequate take-up and to demonstrate success of a service means screening is often 'sold' to the public and consent is often presumed, making refusal seem impossible.

Justice

Philosophers suggest three versions of justice.
1. The fair distribution of scarce resources.
2. Respect for individual and group rights.
3. Following morally acceptable laws.

Thus justice requires that people are treated equally. But what is meant by equal? Does it mean according to equal need? Or according to merit? Or according to equal contribution? Or ensuring non-discriminatory practices?

For example, the equal distribution of resources can mean different things. It could mean that resources should be distributed equally in mathematical terms. Or should they be distributed according to how much was contributed – thus those who have and can put in most get out most? Or should we apply the Marxist adage of 'From each according to his ability, to each according to his needs'? Chapter 7 discusses the politics of health promotion.

The National Health Service was established on the basis of free medical care to all those who need it. In an era of scarce resources, demand far exceeds supply. Need is an obvious criterion for distributing care, but it is not sufficient. Tudor Hart (1971), whose inverse-care law was described in Chapter 2, observed that those who needed healthcare most received least. As we shall see in Chapter 18, although we may use some objective measurement for the assessment of individual health needs, such as the ability to self-care or to perform certain tasks, this does not overcome the subjective value judgement that is involved in making these decisions. In recent years health economists have tried to establish some other sort of objective and measurable criteria to compare competing claims – possibly the relative financial costs of treatment, or an assessment made on quality-adjusted life years, which are described in Chapter 3.

Issues of social justice are glaringly evident in health promotion. We noted earlier the evidence of wide differences in health status between different groups in society. While health promoters may be unable to alter society's inequities, they may nevertheless be able to work on programmes which acknowledge that people's abilities to achieve health differ, avoid victim blaming and tackle discriminatory practices.

Being fair to everyone might seem to suggest adopting public health measures which iron out differences in resources, healthcare or environmental quality. Yet any kind of state intervention means addressing the issue of individual rights versus the common good. For instance, would it be just for top wage earners to pay 50 percent income tax to finance public spending on health and welfare? Chapter 7 examines different political perspectives on health promotion, and the fundamental differences between right and left of the political spectrum towards health and welfare.

Telling the truth

The process of health education and giving information in health promotion also involves complex ethical decisions. Seedhouse (2009) identifies telling the truth and keeping promises as principles which the health promoter should hold on to when deliberating a course of action. As we saw earlier, the individual's right to information and the health promoter's duty to tell the truth may conflict with the duty of beneficence.

Practitioners want people to make healthy choices. When convinced of the 'good' of an action, practitioners may seek to persuade, perhaps through raising clients' anxiety or selecting the information or evidence. Yet ethical health promotion also includes a commitment to enhancing autonomy. As we saw in Chapter 4, the essential nature of health promotion is that it is based on a principle of voluntarism. It should not seek to coerce or persuade, but rather to facilitate an informed choice.

 Learning Activity 6.13 Ethical dilemma: opportunistic health promotion

Is it ethical to carry out opportunistic health education in primary healthcare? For example, a patient goes to her GP with back pain. The doctor uses the opportunity for some health education, and takes the patient's blood pressure and family history.

All education may involve some persuasion, and it is too simplistic to suggest that a desire to empower and create autonomy rules out persuasion. This means, however, that the health promoter must ensure that clients *seek* advice and help, and

are not persuaded against their will. Yet many health promoters would argue that the only way to balance this need to empower people *and* facilitate healthier choices is to make this easier through policy decisions and frameworks (see Chapter 11). This takes us back to the argument that developing healthy public policy prioritizes the public good over individual freedom of choice, and may not even be mandated by public opinion.

There may also be debate about the point at which enough information has been collected to justify legislative or coercive means of health promotion. The UK government's ban on unpasteurized green-top milk and France's ban on tomato ketchup are examples where government action has been criticized for removing choice and leading to negative effects on employment and economic activity. Yet government inaction in the field of regulation and labelling of food has also been criticized for removing people's right to make decisions based on information. In Chapter 7 we explore how information about what is deemed 'healthy' is often influenced by political decisions and vested interests.

 Learning Activity 6.14 Ethical dilemma: sponsorship and health promotion

There is an increasing trend towards sponsorship for health promotion activities. This ranges from health research sponsored by a tobacco company trust to the sponsorship of health information by drug companies, sanitary-wear manufacturers, condom manufacturers or a local healthfood shop.
Is sponsorship compatible with health promotion?

Because the knowledge base of health promotion is changing, there are few areas where recommendations can be made on a factual basis. It is possible to think of numerous examples in recent years where information on the risks or benefits of certain behaviours has changed.

- The advice to exercise for 30 minutes each day, and that these minutes may be built up over the course of the day, is likely to be disputed by new US physical activity guidelines.

- The importance of reducing saturated fat for those with normal cholesterol levels is disputed.
- Potatoes are no longer thought to be fattening, but rather are a good bulk food and source of fibre.
- Moderate amounts of alcohol are now thought to have a beneficial effect on the heart.

Learning Activity 6.15 Ethics and evidence

Should the public be made aware of debates over the evidence for health promotion advice?
Should interventions be employed when the evidence for their effectiveness is in doubt?

Conclusion

Do practitioners whose work involves decisions affecting the lives of others engage in a moral deliberation about the best course of action? In general, most combine features of utility and deontology. They respect autonomy, try to be honest and fair and avoid victim blaming. At the same time they try to achieve the best overall solution to any given situation. Yet situations can involve complex layers of decision-making generating many ethical dilemmas. Screening, for example, a frequently unchallenged linchpin of preventive health promotion, raises key issues about its benefits for an individual versus the increase of the social good, as well as questions about the extent to which screening is honestly presented. Before we can make any sort of ethical judgement, we need to be clear about the values and principles which underpin our actions. If we return to the questions asked earlier in this chapter, what do we mean by doing good and avoiding harm? At what point should we switch from creating autonomy to respecting autonomy? What do justice and equity mean in health promotion practice?

Tools to enable clear thinking around ethical issues, such as codes of practice or the Seedhouse (2009) ethical grid, provide a way to clarify decision-making and make the process more transparent. But dilemmas remain, and following different principles (each of which is sound and desirable) may lead to contradictory courses of action. While there may

never be absolute answers in ethical decision-making, a way forward is to be clear about which principles and duties you value most, and to encourage an open debate about ethical principles and how these translate into health promotion practice.

Summary

Health promoters need to be clear that what they do involves certain values and principles about what is 'good' health and health promotion. Beneficence, justice and respect for persons and their autonomy are fundamental ethical principles in health promotion. Their application in practice, however, is often problematic. Every situation or potential intervention involves a judgement not only of its possible effectiveness but also of its morality – whether it is 'right' or 'wrong'. In this chapter we have defined these key ethical principles and considered how they are manifested in common dilemmas for the health promotion practitioner.

Questions for further discussion

- Is it ethical to attempt to persuade or 'sell' health? Is this part of your practice with patients or members of the public?
- How would you balance ethics (voluntarism and autonomy) against evidence in, for example, the case for compulsory vaccination?

Further reading and resources

Cribb, A., Duncan, P., 2002. Health Promotion and Professional Ethics. Blackwell, Oxford. *An exploration of ethical issues and their impact on practice. Case studies explore value conflicts and issues such as codes of practice.*

Duncan, P., 2015. Ethics and law. In: Naidoo, J., Wills, J. (Eds.), Health Studies: An Introduction, third ed. Palgrave Macmillan, Basingstoke, pp. 401–431. *An introduction to the key principles of ethics and law as applied to health. The chapter includes a detailed analysis of the ethics of banning junk-food advertising.*

Holland, S., 2007. Public Health Ethics. Polity, Cambridge. *An interesting and useful introduction to the ethical dilemmas involved in protecting and promoting public health. The book introduces aspects of moral and political philosophies, and debates key issues such as screening and immunization.*

Feedback to learning activities

6.1 This screening programme is in place to reduce the birth prevalence of a chromosomal disorder. The assumption underlying screening for conditions such as Down's syndrome is that parents with a positive result will decide to terminate the pregnancy. Some positive-testing parents who do not choose termination may indirectly benefit from the test because they will be better able to adjust to the condition of their baby.

The Kantian objection is that the screened population becomes a mere means to achieve the public health goal of reducing chromosomal disorders in the population.

As Holland (2007, p.182) points out, there is a contradiction in offering termination for a fetal abnormality while maintaining a positive societal attitude towards disability.

6.2 Patients have different capacities to understand the nature of treatment or intervention. Patients may feel they will be judged or other interventions withheld if they refuse. Consent is so obviously presumed in many cases, e.g. in the 'invitation' to screen or test, that refusal can seem impossible. Practitioners may also not communicate risk clearly, so patients are not fully informed when they consent.

6.3 Some of these actions are intended to protect the population from possible harm. For example, fluoridation of water is a public health strategy. The loss of individual choice is overridden by the proven benefits for all of such an action. Others are promoting evidence-based health interventions, although their universal application can restrict the actions of some people. Smoking bans restrict individual choice but benefit the whole population.

6.4 You probably concluded that offering money as an inducement for sterilization is a coercive measure that does not respect the autonomy of the individual. Although it may give women greater control over their reproduction, having more money may result in increased drug use. Sterilization is an irreversible procedure about which women need to be fully and freely informed. This action is not, then, one which increases morality. It is a quick-fix solution which fails to deal with the root causes of drug addiction.

6.5
1. Although your patient is distressed by advice to quit smoking, your duty to tell the truth and do good would suggest that such advice needs to be given. Addressing the reasons why he is so distressed, and providing support, are ethically sound actions.
2. You need to balance the possible negative effect of showing the video with its possible positive outcomes. The negative impact might be to dramatize drug-taking (and make it more appealing) and to blame the student who died for his/her actions. The positive impact may be to deter children from drug-taking. It might be more effective and ethically sound to integrate education about drug-taking into the normal curriculum, rather than have an external person deliver the messages.
3. Your duty to do good would suggest you need to intervene and try to help this patient with his anxiety and sleep disturbance. As long as this is done in a respectful way that acknowledges his autonomy, such an intervention will be ethically sound.

6.6 In recent years the courts have ruled that a young woman with a learning disability should be sterilized to avoid the possible trauma of pregnancy and childbirth or abortion, for which it was considered she would not be prepared. This decision was also deemed to be in the best interests of a possible child, who would not be able to be brought up by the young woman. The rights of people with learning disabilities to determine whether, how and with whom to have sex and intimate relationships is a long-running campaign. According to section 1 of the Mental Capacity Act, a person must be assumed to have capacity until it is established that he/she does not, and a person is not to be treated as unable to make a decision.

6.7 Respecting clients' autonomy can be difficult for health promoters. There is often a tendency to give advice, to exert pressure on them to make the 'right' decision or to persuade clients to change their behaviour. The challenge for health promoters is to accept a role of partner and enabler rather than expert and controller. This means the following.
1. Not imposing their own solutions to the clients' problems.

Continued

2. Not instructing clients on what to do because they take too long to work it out for themselves.

3. Not dismissing clients' ideas without providing an adequate explanation or the opportunity to try them out.

6.8 Children and young people may be encouraged to express their wishes as part of growing up. People with mental health problems may also be encouraged to express their wishes. Autonomy is usually deemed appropriate for fully functioning adults – those aged 18 and over who have capacity.

6.9 A healthcare professional following a code of conduct ought to treat the patient if that is what the patient wants and if some treatment is available which will provide net benefit to the patient. The healthcare professional may also fulfil her/his duty by advising that the most effective way of regaining and maintaining health is to alter one's lifestyle. But coercion will generally be contraindicated by the requirement to respect people's autonomy, and withdrawal of care from those who reject one's advice will generally be contraindicated by a doctor's personally and professionally undertaken duty of care, or obligation of beneficence.

6.10 Although it could be argued that people have a duty not to infect others and not simply to reap benefits of herd immunity, the risks of vaccination are contested. Coercion therefore seems unjustified (Holland 2007).

6.11 In England and Wales condoms can be prescribed by the prison medical officer where there is risk of HIV transmission. Condoms are not available in the prisons of Northern Ireland.

The argument in favour of condoms being made available in prisons is based on reducing risk: prisoners are disproportionately affected by HIV and other blood-borne viruses such as hepatitis C. Condoms are tools for prevention and risk reduction. Needle exchanges and the provision of clean needles are available in some European prisons but not in UK prisons.

6.12 Screening is usually deemed to be of benefit, as it identifies people with an illness at an early stage when treatment is likely to be more effective, e.g. cancer screening. However, there are some negative aspects to screening.

- Screening is never wholly routine and inclusive. It is targeted at identified risk groups and therefore excludes certain categories of people, usually on the grounds of age.
- Screening is spaced because of economic considerations, and therefore people may develop the disease in the intervening period.

Screening can lead to some harm.

- The screening process may foster anxieties and be uncomfortable or painful.
- The call and recall procedures may be poorly handled, and the informing of results may take some time.
- Laboratory protocols may not be rigorous enough, leading to the need for repeat tests.
- Screening uses high-sensitivity methods which can result in a high number of false-positive results. These people will be subjected to unnecessary worry and distress, and in some cases treatment.
- Screening uses methods which are less than 100 percent specific, therefore some people will go away falsely reassured.

6.13 The patient had not sought a health check, and nor was she made aware beforehand of the implications if her blood pressure was found to be raised. The patient had not freely chosen to have her blood pressure checked in this way. Although she gave her consent, it might not be regarded as fully informed.

6.14 Sponsorship may be acceptable when it comes from enterprises compatible with health promotion principles and practices, and when the acceptance of income does not divert practitioners from meeting more demonstrable health needs.

6.15 There is no definitive answer to this question. Evidence does change – in 2015, for example, considerable press was devoted to challenging public health advice to reduce saturated fat based on a research study suggesting that this advice was premature (http://openheart.bmj.com/content/2/1/e000196.full). The evidence supporting some public health measures, e.g. mandatory vaccination of healthcare workers, is not strong, and if an argument is made for a compulsory policy or key message that hinges on controversial evidence, public health's reputation becomes damaged. The media have a role to play in providing responsible and knowledgeable reporting of risk that enables the public to make informed decisions.

References

Beauchamp, T.L., Childress, J.F., 2013. Principles of Biomedical Ethics, seventh ed. Oxford University Press, Oxford.

Duncan, P., 2015. Ethics and law. In: Naidoo, J., Wills, J. (Eds.), Health Studies: An Introduction, third ed. Palgrave Macmillan, Basingstoke, pp. 401–431.

Holland, S., 2007. Public Health Ethics. Polity, Cambridge.

Kant, I., 1909. On the Supposed Right to Tell Lies from Benevolent Motives. Cited in: Rumbold G 1991 Ethics in nursing and midwifery practice. Distance Learning Centre, South Bank University, London.

Naidoo, J., Wills, J., 2010. Public Health and Health Promotion: Developing Practice. Baillière Tindall, London.

Rose, G., 1981. Strategy of prevention: lessons from cardiovascular disease. British Medical Journal 282, 1847–1851.

Seedhouse, D., 2009. Ethics: The Heart of Health Care, third ed. Wiley, Chichester.

Sindall, C., 2002. Does health promotion need a code of ethics? Health Promotion International 17 (3), 201–203. Available online at: http://heapro.oxfordjournals.org/content/17/3/201.full.pdf+html (accessed 23.09.15).

Tudor Hart, J., 1971. The inverse care law. Lancet 1, 405.

Chapter Seven

7

The politics of health promotion

Learning Outcomes

By the end of this chapter you will be able to:
- analyse critically issues of power and politics in health promotion policy and practice
- understand different ideological positions in relation to health promotion.

Key Concepts and Definitions

Politics is the achieving and exercising control over human communities, e.g. states.

Government The group of people with the authority to govern a state or country.

Ideology A set of ideas or beliefs which underlies and justifies the actions of governments, corporations or religious groups, or attempts to undermine these entities.

Power The ability or right to control people or things.

Neoliberal An economic or political approach that favours the free market and deregulation.

Social policy Planned government activities to regulate society.

Importance of the Topic

Politics and health promotion are often thought of as separate activities. However, different approaches to health promotion reflect different political positions. This chapter outlines the diversity of social and political philosophies, which helps us to understand how health promotion has developed in the social and political context of the late twentieth and twenty-first centuries. Understanding our own values helps us to see the logical consequences for health promotion. The political dimensions of health promotion in relation to its organization, its methods and the content of its activities are then explored.

What is politics?

Heywood (2007) identifies a fourfold classification of politics.

1. Politics as government – party politics and state activities.
2. Politics as public life – the management of community affairs.
3. Politics as conflict resolution – negotiation, compromise and conciliation strategies.
4. Politics as power – the production, distribution and use of scarce resources.

Although these are separate concepts, they are arguably united by the fourth definition – politics as power – that is the main focus of this chapter. In democratic countries, people use their vote to give power to the political party of their choice. The elected party then governs public life and thus wields power on behalf of the populace. Power includes not only material or physical resources but also psychological and cultural aspects, which may be equally effective in limiting or channelling people.

Power is distributed unequally worldwide, and globalization has contributed to increasing the divide between high-income regions, e.g. Europe, the USA and Canada, and low-income regions such as sub-Saharan Africa. For example, 6.3 million children under the age of five die each year, almost all in poor countries or poor areas of middle-income countries (World Health Organization, 2014) and over half of these deaths are caused by malnutrition and lack of access to safe water and sanitation (Labonte and Schrecker, 2007).

 Learning Activity 7.1 A question posed by Aristotle

If A made the flute,
B plays it best and
C will die if s/he can't have it,
who should have the flute?

Political ideologies

One of the arenas in which power relationships are manifest is social policy, which may be defined as planned government activities designed to maintain, integrate and regulate society. This includes both welfare and economic policies, and ranges from national legislation to local policy developments within local authorities. (See Chapter 11 for a discussion of developing healthy public policy.)

Government policies are determined according to its beliefs and ideas – its ideological position. Different political positions give rise to certain types of policy interventions. Analysts have identified many different frameworks and pointed to the shift in ideologies since the 1960s (Bambra et al., 2015). The old mid-twentieth-century spectrum of political belief from the hard-line left (Marxism) via socialism and liberalism to the right wing (conservatism) no longer describes accurately the political beliefs and ideologies of nations and parties. Globalization, the demise of Soviet rule over Eastern Europe and the permeation of national boundaries through international trade have instigated new political beliefs, in particular the rise of neoliberalism and neoconservatism. The relationship between ideology and welfare provision is summarized in Table 7.1.

Views on health and health promotion reflect a complex mix of values and beliefs, which in turn reflect different political ideologies. The central proposition of this chapter is that health, and therefore health promotion, is political. Health promotion takes place in the policy area and embodies ideological values. Bambra et al. (2005) describe ideology as a system of interrelated ideas and concepts that reflect and promote the political, economic and cultural values and interests of a particular societal group. Thus in the 1970s and 1980s feminist, Black and development perspectives were prominent ways of thinking. In the 1990s environmental, faith and disability perspectives became prominent. The ideological viewpoints of different political parties vary widely. Key beliefs in relation to promoting health on which people differ concern:

- the extent of personal responsibility
- the role of government legislation and intervention
- the role of the economy, and whether or not it should be regulated by governments

Table 7.1 A typology of health and welfare ideologies

Political ideology	Socialism	Social democracy	Nationalist; neoliberalism	Neoconservatism
Political party	Marxist/socialist	Social democrats	New Right	Conservatives
Role of state	Collectivist, state control	Collectivist	Anti-collectivist	Anti-collectivist
View of economy	Regulated	Mixed	Market deregulation and state decentralization	Free market
View of society	Equality of opportunity and economic and political freedom are safeguarded by the state; the state should enable individual self-fulfilment and social justice through redistribution	The state should provide a safety net, although people should be encouraged to fend for themselves	The individual is central; state intervention in economic affairs should be reduced and market economics prevail	Society is made up of self-interested individuals; inequalities in wealth are inevitable and desirable because they stimulate innovation and success; market forces ensure people's needs are met in a satisfactory manner; state intervention should be minimal
View of healthcare	Universal and free state provision to promote social cohesion and redistribution, plus individual provision if desired	State provision to safeguard the vulnerable alongside individual choice and private provision	Paternalistic state should provide a safety net of healthcare provision, alongside individual responsibility	Individual responsibility and freedom of choice; needs are best met through free-market consumerism
Core values	Equality; collective responsibility; humanitarianism; social harmony	Individualism; social justice; collectivism	Individualism; social justice; freedom; responsibility; authority; nationalism	Tradition; individualism; freedom; self-discipline; choice; competition

- legitimate means to encourage choices and decisions
- the nature of society and the extent to which people are connected to each other
- the extent to which inequalities should be reduced.

On the right of the political spectrum there is a belief in individual self-determination and an antipathy to government intervention, which not only restricts freedom but also inhibits enterprise. Conservatism sees inequality as inevitable and beneficial, in that differences stimulate people to succeed, resulting in innovation and productivity. Neoconservatism stresses the need to restore traditional values and a shared culture.

Neoliberalism has evolved since the 1960s as an attempt to combine the twin goals of social justice and economic growth. Neoliberalism is committed to reducing state intervention in the economy, and advocates market deregulation as the means to economic growth and social welfare. Such views are associated with the rugged individualism of Margaret Thatcher, who famously asserted, 'there is no such thing as society, only individuals and their families'.

Socialism is based on a belief in equality, fellowship and community, or a sense of responsibility for others. The government has a key role to play in ensuring everyone's basic needs are met, redistributing material resources and promoting a sense of social stability and cohesion. Social democracy, while embodying the same core beliefs, also embraces the notion of individual choice within a free market.

Case Study 7.1 Sustainable development and health promotion

Since the 1980s 'green' parties with the aim of moving environmental concerns up the political agenda have emerged in most industrialized countries. Most political parties claim to be concerned with the environment but their actions suggest otherwise, and there is little support for radical change to protect the environment. There is also a lack of integrated policymaking that addresses social, economic and environmental needs. Economic growth has not been accompanied by the equitable distribution of wealth or addressing environmental priorities, and there has been variable progress in health (Haines et al., 2012).

Health promotion and sustainable development are linked through the interactions of the physical environment, e.g. pollution, and the social environment, together with a reduction in poverty and associated diseases (Haines et al., 2012). Health contributes to development and is a prerequisite for people to reach their full potential. The world's ecosystem provides the foundation for population health.

Globalization

Globalization, defined primarily as the economic processes of free trade supporting a global marketplace, is another reason for the shifting positions of political parties. No political party can ignore the immense power of global capitalism, which reaches across the world, ignoring national or regional boundaries. McDonald's, Microsoft and Philip Morris are known worldwide for promoting junk food, internet communication and tobacco respectively. Proponents of globalization argue it is more efficient and allows poorer countries to benefit from the technological advances of more developed countries. Critics argue that globalization destabilizes national economies, reduces everything to a market value and increases inequalities of wealth and health. It has been argued that the socio-economic determinants of health have become globalized, leading to increased inequalities between rich and poor countries as well as within countries (Labonte and Schrecker, 2007). Whatever the stance adopted, health promotion needs to develop and function within an increasingly global economy and world.

Learning Activity 7.2 The politics of free trade

Globalization is based on free trade. Is free trade good for health?

Globalization in politics is mirrored by globalization in health. Health risks are now increasingly global in their scope and spread, fuelled by the displacement of people (through war and natural disasters), global trade and movement of people and products. For example, the spread of human immunodeficiency virus/acquired immunodeficiency syndrome (HIV/AIDS), severe acute respiratory syndrome (SARS) and the Ebola virus requires continued vigilance and concerted action by nations and international agencies. Chapter 11 discusses some of the challenges of developing a global public health policy on issues such as environmental degradation and the fragmentation of labour markets that contribute to lower standards of occupational health and safety, and also to a loss of workers in poorer countries. The political challenge for health promotion is to foreground health as a valued goal and a key component of the global public good.

This century has seen a considerable investment in global public health, e.g. the eight Millennium Development Goals promulgated by the United Nations (which include halving extreme poverty rates and halting the spread of HIV/AIDS by 2015) and the World Health Organization (WHO) Commission on the Social Determinants of Health (CSDH). The CSDH, launched in 2005 and headed by Michael Marmot, was a group of policymakers, researchers and civil society organizations whose aim was to give support in tackling the social causes of poor health and avoidable health inequalities (health inequities). But the dominant theme in global health initiatives is the reduction of risk factors rather than development. Health is often reduced to the prevention of a threat to the population, as in the Ebola outbreak of 2014, when the main concern in Western countries was to prevent immigrants bringing Ebola into their territories, followed by a focus on finding an effective treatment for the disease. The promotion of positive health and the prevention of poverty and disease do not rank highly in political terms. However, there are exceptions to the rule, and the Framework Convention on Tobacco Control, first ratified in 2005, is an example of positive global public health (see Chapter 11).

Health as political

In the WHO Alma Ata declaration (World Health Organization 1978) health was seen as both a human right and a global social issue. The Universal Declaration of Human Rights adopted by the United Nations in 1948 proclaimed that 'everyone has the right to a standard of living adequate for the health and well-being of oneself and one's family, including food, clothing, housing, and medical care'. The right to healthcare, including reproductive choices, is asserted in the constitution of South Africa, which includes a human rights charter. Economic globalization has threatened these views of health as a human right. The People's Health Movement (www.phmovement.org) is a group of political activists and advocates opposed to globalization. This group argues that it is health, not the economy, that should be prioritized.

Within nation-states, the political context affects all areas of government policy that have an impact on health, both directly and indirectly. Bambra et al. (2015) argue that health is political because power is exercised over health and its correlates (such as citizenship and organization). The American national health promotion and disease prevention programme, Healthy People 2020 (www.healthypeople.gov), identifies the following as some of the social determinants of health:

- availability of resources to meet daily needs
- access to healthcare
- education and job training
- transport options
- public safety
- incidence of crime, violence and disorder
- socio-economic conditions
- language/literacy
- access to emerging technologies.

Evidence suggests that these social determinants are the best predictors of individual and population health, that they structure lifestyle choices and that they interact to produce health. This, in turn, leads to the notion of health as political and the outcome of national and international policy decisions. A strong welfare state that provides people with access to the social determinants of health is arguably the best means to promote health.

Learning Activity 7.3 Politics and health

Can you take politics out of health? Why might people say this?

The politics of health promotion structures and organization

Internationally and nationally, health promotion has enjoyed varying levels of support throughout the twentieth and twenty-first centuries. The first International Conference on Health Promotion in 1986 led to the adoption of the Ottawa Charter for Health Promotion (World Health Organization, 1986), whose five action areas – building a healthy public policy, creating supportive environments, developing personal skills, strengthening communities and reorienting health services – are still used widely. This was followed by conferences in Adelaide (1988), Sundsvall (1991), Jakarta (1997), Mexico (2000), Bangkok (2005), Nairobi (2009) and Helsinki (2013) which identified additional areas for action. The Bangkok Charter (World Health Organization, 2005) outlines four key commitments.

1. Strong intergovernmental agreements to improve health.
2. Health determinants need to be addressed by governments.

3. Empowered communities and civil societies.
4. Good corporate practice to promote health in the workplace, communities and worldwide.

A brief history of political ideologies and their impact on health promotion developments in England is provided in Case Study 7.2.

 ### Case Study 7.2 A brief history of health promotion in England

1800–1900: Public health movement
- The movement arose out of a conservative tradition of reluctant collectivism: that the state had to intervene to ensure national efficiency, economic advantage and social stability.

1900–1940: Health education
- A liberal, *laissez-faire* agenda which allowed voluntary organizations to provide preventive health education.

1940–1970s: Rise of prevention
- A broadly conservative ideology: the emphasis was on individual responsibility for health with information and advice being provided by health professionals; this was coupled with state intervention to provide a safety net for the most vulnerable.

1980s: The rise of the individual
- Despite calls for a coherent national programme to tackle widespread inequalities in health and the WHO Ottawa Charter, New Right ideology dominates the health service and individual freedom is emphasized.

1990s: The rise of the market
- Emphasis is on public accountability to the consumer in services, and the need to consult lay views.

- Collaboration is advocated as a means of efficiency and to reduce demands on the health service.
- Despite an environmental consciousness, this is not seen as an agenda for government action.

1997–2011: Community, responsibility and equality
- Acknowledgement of the role of socio-economic factors in health.
- Emphasis on public participation in care and services.
- Promotion of community cohesion.
- Emphasis on the free market, individual choice and the commodification of health as a means to satisfy needs.

2011 onwards: Citizens, responsibility and choices
- The public health function shifts to local government, acknowledging wider influences on health.
- Localism leads to areas deciding their own priorities.
- 'Ambitions' rather than performance targets are set for key priorities such as tobacco control, obesity and alcohol.
- 'Nudging' rather than state intervention is used to encourage healthy practices.
- Focus on well-being.

Several commentators have argued that health promotion in the UK has been subsumed by public health (Orme et al., 2007; Scott-Samuel and Springett, 2007). Health promotion has always struggled to have a visible presence, and its position within the National Health Service has led to it being viewed as a 'Cinderella' service subordinated to healthcare provision and the medical model. Since 1997 and the election of the New Labour government, health promotion has been sinking from view, with the disappearance of both its specialist workforce and its lead organization in England (Scott-Samuel and Wills, 2007). Health promotion is now termed 'health

improvement' and is just part of the remit of a range of other agencies and staff, including public health practitioners, the National Institute for Health and Clinical Excellence (NICE), health trainers and community development agencies. In many other countries the ascendance of neoliberalism combined with traditional biomedical approaches inhibits the wholesale adoption of the Ottawa Charter principles for health promotion (Raphael, 2008; Wills et al., 2008). For example, in Canada an epidemiological focus on population health has displaced health promotion. The term 'health promotion' is, however, still used worldwide.

Learning Activity 7.4 Wicked problems

The notion of 'wicked problems' in health is widely referred to. What does this mean to you?

Health promotion activities are structured by the prevailing policy framework, which has the effect of legitimizing certain approaches and excluding others. Until 1997 in the UK a combination of free-market economics with authoritarianism favoured medical preventive approaches and those which focus on individual lifestyles. Health promotion was seen as a means to prevent morbidity and mortality from specified diseases. Education and advice were the key strategies. Primary care practitioners would identify individuals at risk from a database of the practice population, and carry out lifestyle interventions.

Neoliberal ideology sees a more interventionist role for government, although the free-market economy is also emphasized as the means to meet needs. There is an emphasis on partnership working and consumer choice, attempting to transfer free-market economic relationships into the service sector. However, there is also recognition that state support and intervention are required to mitigate the inequalities in health driven by socio-economic inequalities (Bambra and Scott-Samuel, 2005). This runs parallel to a pervasive life-course discourse that locates health in the hands of the individual. (See Chapter 2 for more discussion of socio-economic inequalities in health.)

The politics of health promotion methods

The methods used in health promotion are often viewed as a technical choice. Health promotion specialists are seen as possessing the expertise to decide what methods will prove most effective given the circumstances. However, we shall argue that methods imply political perspectives, and that the choice of which methods to use is not a politically neutral decision.

 Learning Activity 7.5 Political philosophies

The following statements reflect particular political philosophies. Can you identify these political philosophies? Which statements do you agree with?

1. There should be a safety net of economic and social support for the needy.
2. Energy and enterprise should be rewarded, not stifled by high taxation.
3. All people in a society have a commitment and a responsibility to others.
4. Inequality is inevitable, and necessary for development and growth.
5. High levels of benefits make people dependent on support.
6. Certain public services are essential and should be run by the state.
7. Macropolitics is of less significance than issues, particularly those affecting local communities.
8. People cannot be equal, but everyone should have the same chances.
9. Shared values and a common culture are vital to the maintenance of social cohesion.
10. A person's lot in life is determined by luck and accident of birth.

Health promotion has at its disposal a large repertoire of methods, which are discussed in greater detail in Part Two of this book. Figure 7.1 illustrates how different political philosophies privilege different methods and approaches.

The individual paternalist approach (Conservative)

This approach is expert-led by professionals, and is focused on the individual. It has a long history, remaining perennially popular. The virtue of professional training is that it gives patients and clients confidence and a clearly demarcated role. Methods focused on the individual send a clear message about personal responsibility for health. Such methods rely on the belief that individuals can make significant changes in their lifestyle or environment. The focus on the individual also implies that everyone has equal resources and means of complying with health

113

Mode of intervention
Paternalist

Individual paternalist (Conservative)
People need help and support to take care of their health but health problems are essentially an individual responsibility
• Advice
• Information giving
• Education

Collective paternalist (Marxist, socialist)
The government needs to take responsibility for protecting public health and reducing inequalities
• Advocacy and legislation to redistribute power and resources in favour of the disadvantaged
• Activism to increase wages and improve working conditions

Focus of intervention
Individual

Focus of intervention
Collective

Individual participatory (New Right)
Everyone should have the opportunity to determine their own lives and health
• Counselling
• Education
• Group work

Collective and individual participatory (New Left)
Key factors are community, equality, responsibility and empowerment
• Group work
• Community development
• Lobbying skills, sharing and training

Mode of intervention
Participatory

Fig 7.1 ● Political philosophies and health promotion methods. (Adapted from Beattie, A., 1993. The changing boundaries of health. In: Beattie, A., Gott, M., Jones, L., Sidell, M. (Eds.) Health and Wellbeing: A Reader. Macmillan/Open University, Basingstoke.)

promotion messages. This may be viewed as ineffective or incorrect, and there has been much criticism of these methods as 'victim blaming' and misconceived (Naidoo, 1986). However, such a viewpoint is also politically inspired, which may go some way to explaining its endurance.

By ignoring structural factors which affect the life chances and perceptions of different groups of people, the fact that people's personal identities are bound up with their membership of such groups is obscured. Such an approach also ignores the structured inequalities in health status that are linked to socio-economic status. This approach reinforces professional power by stating that individuals need to comply with expert advice.

The notion of individual free choice is a central tenet of the free-market economy. In economic terms, individualism becomes translated into consumerism,

or the right to purchase goods. This approach is linked to the commodification of health, which becomes advertised as a tangible asset that can be bought. For example, sales of organic food and health-club memberships have risen sharply in the UK, due in large part to their promotion as routes to health and well-being. This process in turn further exacerbates inequalities in health, as only the richest people can afford these healthier lifestyle choices.

 Learning Activity 7.6 Is there a healthy choice?

Do you think there is such a thing as a 'healthy choice'? Is it your role to inform patients and clients about healthy choices?

The individual participatory approach (New Right/Neoliberal)

Neoliberalism emphasizes the role of individuals in determining their own choices. The individual participatory approach differs from the paternalistic individual approach by being premised on a different, and more equal, relationship between the health promoter and the client. This approach includes negotiated methods such as counselling, education and group work which take into account people's beliefs, attitudes and knowledge. The client is an active partner in the process, and the end goal is enhanced client autonomy. Many professional groups have shifted their practice in recent years and tried to become more client-centred. Many health promoters feel more comfortable using these methods. Patient or public engagement has as its overarching principle 'no decisions about me without me'. This needs to be seen within the context of a political shift in the relationship between the state and the citizen, whereby the citizen is not just a consumer but is also a co-producer.

 Learning Activity 7.7 Critique of the neoliberal approach to health promotion

What criticisms can be offered of the individual participatory (neoliberal) approach in terms of promoting the nation's health?

The collective and individual participatory approach (New Left)

Methods which focus on the collectivity are more likely to be allied to social democratic or socialist political ideologies. The emphasis here is on understanding the processes which shape health outcomes, and assisting people to develop the skills to shape and challenge these processes. The New Left political ideology retains a belief in the supremacy of the free market, leading to a focus on individuals and consumerism. The unifying factor is a stress on participation and active involvement, whether of communities or individual consumers. Being well integrated into a community (sometimes called communitarianism) is increasingly recognized as an independent source of health as well as self-esteem.

Governments have sought to encourage social inclusion and collective participation through neighbourhood and community initiatives, for example neighbourhood regeneration and renewal interventions. There has been some attempt by Conservatives to develop a one-nation type of social solidarity, exemplified in England by the term 'big society', which would take power away from politicians and devolve power to the people.

The collective paternalist approach (Marxist, socialist)

The collective paternalist methods of working are associated with Marxist and socialist political beliefs. These beliefs include the primacy of socio-economic status in predicting social status, culture and life chances. Socialism sees individual identity as shaped by social interaction and membership of social groups. The owners of the means of production (the middle class) and those who only have their labour power to sell (the working class) have conflicting economic goals (to maximize profits or maximize wages, accordingly). Class conflict is seen as inevitable according to this perspective.

Karl Marx's (1875) famous phrase, 'from each according to his ability, to each according to his need', sums up the socialist goal of equality and social solidarity. Appropriate action uses methods such as the active redistribution of power in favour of the disadvantaged. Such action can be top down (e.g. advocacy on behalf of lower socio-economic groups or equity audits to expose inequalities) or bottom up (e.g. trade union activism to increase wages and improve working conditions). Other methods may include promoting social cohesion through community development (see Chapter 10). Wilkinson and Pickett (2009) present a strong case for arguing that more egalitarian societies have healthier populations, even if they are poorer than wealthy capitalist societies.

The methods adopted by practitioners in response to particular issues reflect political values about:

- humanity – the rights of people
- responsibility – whether health is in the hands of the individual or a result of particular social patterns which are reproduced and maintained by social policies
- the role of the practitioner – whether practitioners should hold power in the form of professional expertise, or whether knowledge should be defined and shared by people themselves
- the role of the citizen – whether citizens have the autonomy and resources to exercise free choices, or they are constrained by social and national norms and the exercise of professional power
- the role of government – whether the state should take an active role in protecting its citizens' health, or responsibility for health should lie with the individual
- the role of the economy – whether there is a free market and competition, or a regulated economy overseen by government.

 Learning Activity 7.8 The political values underpinning an HIV prevention programme

Consider the following methods which might be adopted in an HIV and sexually transmitted infection (STI) prevention programme with vulnerable young people.
1. Enhancing self-esteem.
2. Peer education.
3. Educational media campaigns.
4. Young people's sexual health clinic run by nurses.
5. Funding for a telephone helpline run by a voluntary self-help group.
6. Easier and more open access to condoms.
7. More opportunities for young people to gain work experience and skills.
8. Creation of hostels and sheltered housing for homeless young people.

What political values are being reflected in each approach?

This discussion has presented the view that the methods chosen to promote health are not politically neutral. Certain methods fit into, maintain and reproduce the ideological assumptions of certain political perspectives. However, it is important not to overstate this view. Methods and ideology are not deterministically linked in a cause-and-effect manner. A variety of methods across all four ideological perspectives may be used by health workers who espouse a particular political viewpoint. There may be convincing reasons for adopting an eclectic methodology to promote health. But it is a fallacy to assume that methods are a technically neutral aspect of a health promoter's activity.

The politics of health promotion content

The previous sections have examined the view that the structure, organization and methods used in health promotion have a political dimension. It is sometimes argued that although the process of promoting health is a political activity, the content of health promotion is neutral. Our position is that health promotion content is inevitably political. The framing of suitable agendas and the construction of what information is relevant are not value-neutral activities; on the contrary, they imply certain political values.

 Learning Activity 7.9 Health promotion for the twenty-first century

What are health promotion priorities for the twenty-first century?

Perhaps the clearest example of the political nature of health promotion is the debate surrounding the social determinants of health. As outlined in Chapter 2, a wealth of research evidence from the 1980s linked poverty and disadvantage with ill health, but different governments reacted differently. For almost two decades (1979–1997) the Conservative UK government refused to recognize the evidence on social inequalities and health, referring instead to 'variations in health status between different socio-economic groups within the population' (Department of Health, 1992, p. 121). By denying the evidence, a non-interventionist policy could be adopted which argued that the free market is the best means of meeting health needs. By contrast, the Labour government elected in 1997 acknowledged the link between social inequalities and disadvantage and health, and adopted targets to reduce health inequalities (Department of Health, 2003). The Marmot Review, *Fair Society, Healthy Lives* (Marmot, 2010), clearly signals its political stance: 'reducing health inequalities is a matter of fairness and justice' and 'economic growth is not the most important measure of our country's success' (see www.instituteofhealthequity.org).

Several research studies have confirmed that social democratic countries with strong welfare states, egalitarian ideologies and redistributive policies produce healthier populations, as indicated by lower infant mortality and low-birth-weight rates and increased life expectancy (Navarro and Shi, 2001; Chung and Muntaner, 2006, 2007; Navarro et al., 2006).

Case Study 7.3 The political discourse of obesity

The discourse of obesity frames concerns as a societal panic and obesity as a consequence of immoral behaviour. The necessity for urgent action is highlighted (Campos et al., 2006). If obesity is framed as a lifestyle choice (as is most common in public health discourse), then it becomes a matter of individual responsibility. This may fuel stigmatization against minorities and people living in poverty, who are more likely to be obese. Foucault describes how governments govern people to act in certain ways through the construction of knowledge (Coveney, 1998). Thus obesity is referred to as a threat or a risk, and citizens are expected to be responsible and active consumers.

Practitioners are called upon to base their work on evidence. The rise of evidence-based practice can be linked to New Right ideas about the accountability of practitioners and services to the 'consumer'. It could also be linked to socialist paternal collectivist ideas, identifying what works best and then requiring practitioners to follow set protocols. Evidence-based practice usually refers to a scientific notion of evidence that prioritizes randomized controlled trials as providing the best evidence (see Chapter 3).

However, this stance may be criticized for ignoring service users and their values, desires and wants. It may also neglect political and social issues that are too complex to factor into this model of decision-making. Evidence needs to engage with people's views and beliefs rather than pursue abstract notions of health or ill health.

Monaghan et al. (2003, p. 37) claimed that 'political ideology still informs the values that guide government such as, in this case, a concern with the health and wellbeing of the people. We are now, however, in an era where an evidence-based rather than ideological approach seems the most appropriate method of policy formulation.' More than a decade later, the same tension remains between ideology and objective science, and their contribution to health promotion.

Social scientists (Bauchspies et al., 2005; David, 2005) point out that science is a social activity like any other, subject to similar constraints. Health-related research does not take place in ivory towers. Researchers have to bid for funds, and provide findings which are acceptable to funders and the academic community. The process of research is not immune to political considerations: what evidence filters through to the general public as the scientific consensus on health topics is also the result of political processes. The very idea of scientific consensus in social science is debatable, as there is no issue where there is 100 percent agreement of the 'scientific facts'. For example, there is an ongoing debate about whether it is social capital or income that is responsible for the better health status of the more advantaged groups.

Being political

We have seen how health promotion arises from and reinforces political values and beliefs, and takes place in a political context. Health promoters hold values and beliefs which are underpinned by established sets of ideas or ideologies. Many health promoters are engaged in practice which accords (more or less) with their personal values. The medical model of health provides a clear role for practitioners because it recognizes their expertise. It also gives a clear role for individuals to act to protect their own health. Some health promoters may find that their professional role at times comes into conflict with their political beliefs and values. A belief in collective health goals and the need to empower people to be involved and take control over factors influencing their health may be at odds with a health promotion role bound by corporate contracts and the need to meet targets.

 Learning Activity 7.10 Radical health promotion

The following are suggestions for developing radical health promotion practice. How many do you think are feasible for you? Be clear and honest about your own political standpoint.

- Develop an equal relationship with clients, where beliefs and values are respected and information shared.
- Try to ensure real community involvement in policies and decision-making.
- Try to address health as a collective issue, making explicit the facts about health inequalities and supporting collective action around health issues.
- Vet the health education materials you use to ensure they do not reproduce stereotypes or assumptions about gender, class, race, disability, age or sexuality.
- Engage in action research in which researchers and researched are partners.
- Develop a support network with like-minded health workers, where perspectives can be shared and issues discussed.
- Be honest to yourself and others about the limitations of your work role.

Adapted from Adams and Slavin (1985); O'Neill (1989).

Conclusion

Politics, or the process and study of the distribution of power in society, underpins all human activities, including health promotion. The political scene is in a state of constant flux, with the twenty-first century witnessing the rise of neoliberalist ideology and globalization. These processes and values are embedded in the context in which health promoters practice. An understanding of and engagement with politics in its widest sense are necessary in order to practice reflectively and in accordance with one's personal values and beliefs.

There is often resistance to the idea that health promotion is a political activity. Accepting the premise that politics is involved in health promotion may be seen as muddying the waters, for it transforms a situation of relative certainty to one of uncertainty. It is no longer sufficient to rely on professional training to ensure effective health promotion. A whole range of different considerations needs to be taken into account, some of which threaten and call into question the whole notion of professional expertise.

However uncomfortable the process may be, an awareness of the political nature of health promotion is vital to its effectiveness (O'Neill, 1989). Accepting the status quo is not an apolitical position but a deeply political one. What exists is not inevitable, but the result of complex forces and historical processes. Things might be otherwise. Health promotion is centrally concerned with a vision of better health for all. This vision may be informed by scientific knowledge and technical know-how, but its overall shape is determined by personal values and beliefs. Part of the task of health promoters is to uncover and hold up to scrutiny their values and beliefs. It is hoped that this chapter and Chapter 6 will help health promoters in this task.

Summary

This chapter has examined the political implications of health promotion structures, organization, methods and content. The central proposition is that health promotion is a political activity, and to attempt to deny this lessens one's understanding and the possibility of effective action. It has been demonstrated that mainstream health promotion activity is predicated on certain political values. The late twentieth and twenty-first centuries have witnessed a shift in the political values underpinning health promotion practice in England and many other countries, triggered by the growth of neoliberalist ideologies and the process of globalization. A non-interventionist role focused on individual advice and giving information sits alongside a commitment to tackle the social origins of health.

The role of the practitioner is still crucial, although it could be argued that the practitioner's function needs to expand to include client advocacy and empowerment, with more emphasis on national and international networking and collaborative working across sectors and professions. Whether this shift in practice can occur, given increasing demands on healthcare services, is problematic. Many practitioners may feel that the broad political framework is now more supportive of health promotion. However, the task of practicing in accordance with one's political beliefs remains a challenge.

Questions for further discussion

- To what extent do you regard your practice in health promotion as political activity?
- How have your political values and beliefs informed your practice?

Further reading and resources

Bambra, C., Smith, K., Kennedy, L., 2015. Politics. In: Naidoo, J., Wills, J. (Eds.), Health Studies, third ed. Palgrave, Basingstoke, pp. 265-293. *Chapter 7 provides a clear overview of politics as a discipline, and applies its methodology and concepts to health issues.*

Baggott, R., 2010. Public Health Policy and Politics, second ed. Wiley Blackwell, Oxford. *This book explores the UK political environment and addresses health promotion and public health issues.*

Feedback on learning activities

7.1 Aristotle thought that justice was giving each person his/her due or what he/she deserved. The purpose of the flute is to be played, and played well. Therefore, according to Aristotle, B should have the flute. However, other views produce different answers. If people's well-being is the priority, C should have the flute. If material ownership of goods is the priority (as in a capitalist state), then A should have the flute.

7.2 Free trade or trade liberalization, such as the proposed Transatlantic Trade and Investment Partnership (TTIP) between the European Union and the USA, may result in lower standards on food safety. Trade policy also affects the food chain, and the TTIP would result in increased imports and a reduction in locally sourced food. This would impact on the environment as well as on the quality of food. Critics of TTIP argue that it would increase corporate power and reduce the ability of governments to promote health through the regulation of markets or environmental protection.

7.3 Health is inextricably bound up with politics. For example, access to health services depends on political decisions such as funding and access criteria. In 1948 the NHS was created in post-war England, the first national healthcare system available on the basis of need rather than wealth or fees. A Labour government was in power at this time. This political decision had the effect of freeing healthcare from politics, although socio-economic health inequalities persist in the UK. In contrast, in many other countries access to healthcare services varies according to wealth. In some countries, such as South Africa, the level of healthcare is largely dependent on ethnic status. People may want to take politics out of health because they want health services provided on the basis of need.

7.4 'Wicked problems' are highly resistant to resolution, perhaps because they are difficult to define, are multicausal, have no clear solution or may be the responsibility of more than one government department (World Health Organization, 2008). In 1997 UK Prime Minister Tony Blair referred to the need for joined-up government. Health in All Policies is a global strategy which aims to integrate health considerations into policymaking across all the sectors that influence health, such as transport and housing (see Chapter 8).

7.5
1. Most social democrats support a system of welfare.
2. Conservatives believe in reducing taxation.
3. The New Left has tried to encourage communitarianism.
4. Neoliberalism, in its support for the free market, regards inequality as inevitable.

Continued

5. Neoliberals and conservatives wish to roll back the state, partly to reduce dependency.
6. A principle of socialism is that essential services, e.g. railways and electricity, should be run by the state.
7. Liberals, in particular, support ideas of localism.
8. Equal opportunity is a key principle of liberalism.
9. Conservatives are concerned that high levels of immigration threaten a country's stability, and want to support a nation-state.
10. Conservatives believe that everyone has a chance to succeed.

You can identify your political compass and where you stand at www.politicalcompass.org/test.

7.6 Healthy choices, such as organic fruit and vegetables and daily physical activity, tend to be expensive and time-consuming. It can be argued that not everyone is able to make these choices. It may be a practitioner's role to advocate healthy choices, but unless your clients can afford these, this may be unethical. It might be more productive to find out what your clients believe to be healthy choices, and then discuss with them whether these are indeed healthy choices and, if so, how they may be put into practice.

7.7 It may be argued that individually negotiated methods are most used and valued by the relatively privileged, healthy and articulate sections of society. Those with the greatest need are least likely to be able to access this kind of health promotion intervention. The focus on the individual maintains the free-market consumerist ethos criticized in this chapter.

7.8 These initiatives reflect different views about the factors that contribute to sexual ill health or teenage pregnancy, and whether these relate to the individual or the social context in which young people live. They also reflect views about the extent to which individuals are responsible for their own health. Initiatives that rely on the individual or an accredited professional to achieve their goal (e.g. 4) or the provision of information to enable individual choice (e.g. 3) reflect conservative political values. Initiatives that rely on an enabling environment to achieve their goal (e.g. 5 to 8) are more in tune with left-wing political values. Initiatives that seek to empower people (e.g. 1 and 2) are more consonant with liberal political values.

7.9 The Jakarta Conference (World Health Organization, 1997) identified the following priorities for worldwide health:
- urbanization
- demography (ageing population and population growth)
- chronic disease
- sedentary lifestyle
- resistance to antibiotics
- substance misuse
- violence (domestic, civil and international warfare)
- communicable disease
- environmental degradation
- globalization.

The Priority Public Health Conditions Knowledge Network of the Commission on the Social Determinants of Health (http://whqlibdoc.who.int/publications/2010/9789241563970_eng.pdf) analysed the impact of social determinants on specific health conditions and explored possible interventions to improve health equity by addressing social determinants of health. The health conditions identified were alcohol-related disorders, cardiovascular diseases, child health, diabetes, food safety, HIV/AIDS, maternal health, malaria, mental health, neglected tropical diseases, nutrition, oral health, sexual and reproductive health, tobacco and health, tuberculosis and violence and injuries.

7.10 These suggestions for radical health promotion practice are now thirty years old. But they reflect the core principles of health promotion: to strive for social justice, to work in partnership and to engage in co-production with patients, clients or the community. Depending on your role, you may be able to incorporate all or some of the suggestions for radical health promotion practice. Some of the suggestions (e.g. developing an equal relationship with clients) refer to everyday practice, whereas others (e.g. engage in action research) refer to activities over and above everyday practice. To ensure good practice, health promotion practitioners need to be aware that it is a political activity and that they work in a macro-political context.

References

Adams, L., Slavin, H., 1985. Checklist for personal action. Radical Health Promotion 2, 47.

Bambra, C., Scott-Samuel, A., 2005. The Twin Giants: Addressing Patriarchy and Capitalism. Politics of Health Group, UK. Available online at: http://www.pohg.org.uk/.

Bambra, C., Fox, D., Scott Samuel, A., 2005. Towards a new politics of health. Health Promotion International 20 (2). Available online at: http://heapro.oxfordjournals.org/content/20/2/187.full.pdf+html (accessed 25.02.15).

Bambra, C., Smith, K., Kennedy, L., 2015. Politics. In: Naidoo, J., Wills, J. (Eds.), Health Studies, third ed. Palgrave, Basingstoke, pp. 265–293.

Bauchspies, W., Croissant, J., Restivo, S., 2005. Science, Technology and Society: A Sociological Approach. Wiley-Blackwell, Oxford.

Beattie, A., 1991. Knowledge and control in health promotion: a test case for social policy and social theory. In: Gabe, J., Calnan, M., Bury, M. (Eds.), The Sociology of the Health Service. Routledge, London, pp. 162–201.

Beattie, A., 1993. The changing boundaries of health. In: Beattie, A., Gott, M., Jones, L., et al. (Eds.), Health and Wellbeing: A Reader. Macmillan/Open University, Basingstoke.

Campos, P., Saguy, A., Ernsberger, P., Oliver, E., Gaesser, G., 2006. The epidemiology of overweight and obesity: public health crisis or moral panic? International Journal of Epidemiology 35 (1), 55–60. Available online at: http://ije.oxfordjournals.org/content/35/1/55.full.pdf+html (accessed 23.09.15).

Chung, H., Muntaner, C., 2006. Political and welfare determinants of infant and child health indicators: an analysis of wealthy countries. Social Science and Medicine 63, 829–842.

Chung, H., Muntaner, C., 2007. Welfare state matters: a typological multilevel analysis of wealthy countries. Health Policy 80, 328–339.

Coveney, J., 1998. The government and ethics of health promotion: the importance of Foucault. Health Education Research 13 (3), 459–468.

David, M., 2005. Science in Society. Palgrave Macmillan, Houndsmill.

Department of Health, 1992. The Health of the Nation. HMSO, London.

Department of Health, 2003. Tackling Health Inequalities: A Programme for Action. Stationery Office, London. Available online at: http://webarchive.nationalarchives.gov.uk/20130107105354/http://www.dh.gov.uk/en/Publicationsandstatistics/Publications/PublicationsPolicyAndGuidance/DH_4008268 (accessed 28.02.15).

Haines, A., Alleyne, G., Kickbusch, I., Dora, C., 2012. From the earth summit to Rio +20: integration of health and sustainable development. Lancet 379 (9832), 2189–2197.

Heywood, A., 2007. Key Concepts in Politics, third ed. Palgrave, Hampshire.

Labonte, R., Schrecker, T., 2007. Globalization and social determinants of health: introduction and methodological background (part One of Three). Globalization and Health 3, 5.

Marmot, M., 2010. Fair Society, Healthy Lives. Institute of Health Equity, London. Available online at: http://www.instituteofhealthequity.org/projects/fair-society-healthy-lives-the-marmot-review (accessed 27.02.15).

Marx, K., 1875. Critique of Gotha. International Publishers, NYC, US.

Monaghan, S., Huws, D., Navano, M., 2003. The Case for a New UK Health of the People Act. Nuffield Trust, London. Available online at: http://orca.cf.ac.uk/67412/1/the-case-for-a-new-uk-health-of-the-people-act-apr03.pdf (accessed 28.02.15).

Naidoo, J., 1986. Limits to individualism. In: Rodmell, S., Watt, A. (Eds.), The Politics of Health Education. Routledge and Kegan Paul, London, pp. 17–37.

Navarro, V., Shi, L., 2001. The political context of social inequalities and health. Social Science and Medicine 52, 481–491. Available online at: http://www.jhsph.edu/research/centers-and-institutes/johns-hopkins-primary-care-policy-center/Publications_PDFs/2001%20SSM%202.pdf (accessed 23.09.15).

Navarro, V., Muntaner, C., Borrell, C., et al., 2006. Politics and health outcomes. Lancet 368, 1033–1037.

O'Neill, M., 1989. The political dimension of health promotion work. In: Martin, C.J., McQueen, D.V. (Eds.), Readings for a New Public Health. Edinburgh University Press, Edinburgh, pp. 222–234.

Orme, J., de Viggiani, N., Naidoo, J., et al., 2007. Missed opportunities? Locating health promotion within multi-disciplinary public health. Public Health 121, 414–419.

Raphael, D., 2008. Grasping at straws: a recent history of health promotion in Canada. Critical Public Health 18 (4), 483–495.

Scott-Samuel, A., Springett, J., 2007. Hegemony or health promotion: prospects for reviving England's lost discipline. Journal of the Royal Society of Health 127, 210–213.

Scott-Samuel, A., Wills, J., 2007. Health promotion in England: sleeping beauty or corpse? Health Education Journal 66, 115–119. Available online at: http://hej.sagepub.com/content/66/2/115.full.pdf+html (accessed 23.09.15).

Universal Declaration of Human Rights, 1948. UN Department of Public Information, Geneva. Available online at: http://www.un.org/en/documents/udhr/ (accessed 28.02.15).

Wilkinson, R.G., Pickett, K., 2009. The Spirit Level: Why More Equal Societies Almost Always Do Better. Penguin, London.

Wills, J., Evans, D., Scott-Samuel, A., 2008. Hungry for change: politics and prospects for health promotion in England. Critical Public Health 18 (4), 521–531.

World Health Organization, 1978. In: Declaration of Alma-Ata. International Conference on Primary Health Care, Alma-Ata, USSR. WHO, Geneva. Available online at: http://www.who.int/publications/almaata_declaration_en.pdf (accessed 25.02.15).

World Health Organization, 1986. Ottawa Charter for Health Promotion. WHO, Geneva. Available online at: http://www.who.int/healthpromotion/conferences/previous/ottawa/en/ (accessed 25.02.15).

World Health Organization, 1997. New players for a new era: leading health promotion into the 21st century. In: 4th International Conference on Health Promotion, Jakarta, Indonesia 21–25 July 1997. Conference report. World Health Organization, Geneva/Ministry of Health, Indonesia Available online at: http://www.who.int/healthpromotion/conferences/previous/jakarta/declaration/en/ (accessed 28.02.15).

World Health Organization, 2005. The Bangkok Charter for Health Promotion in a Globalized World. WHO, Geneva. Available online at: http://www.who.int/healthpromotion/conferences/6gchp/bangkok_charter/en/ (accessed 28.02.15).

World Health Organization, 2008. Closing the Gap in a Generation: Health Equity through Action on the Social Determinants of Health. Final report of the Commission on Social Determinants of Health. WHO, Geneva. Available online at: http://whqlibdoc.who.int/publications/2008/9789241563703_eng.pdf (accessed 29.02.15).

World Health Organization, 2014. Children: Reducing Mortality. Fact sheet No. 178. Available online at: http://www.who.int/mediacentre/factsheets/fs178/en/ (accessed 28.02.15).

Part Two

Strategies and methods

The Ottawa Charter for Health Promotion (World Health Organization, 1986) remains one of the most influential policy documents in the history of health promotion. It established the fundamental guiding principles and values of health promotion and described five key action areas.

1. Building healthy public policy.
2. Creating supportive environments.
3. Strengthening communities.
4. Developing personal skills.
5. Reorienting health services.

Each of these areas is the focus of a chapter in Part Two. Together, these five areas encompass the goals of health promotion: to go 'upstream' and have an impact on the socio-economic and environmental determinants of health; to focus on population health; to emphasize prevention rather than treatment; and to build capacity in communities and individuals. But while social and physical determinants of health were highlighted in the Ottawa Charter, little attention was given to global, environmental and economic issues; this reflects the reality of the 1980s, when such issues were not on the agenda (Hills and McQueen, 2007). However, many of these issues can be addressed using the strategies outlined in the Ottawa Charter.

Improving the health of the population depends on many factors. Among the most important are:

- tackling socio-economic inequalities in health
- making health everybody's business
- making the healthy choice the easy choice.

These principles, and the values they encompass, underpin the Ottawa Charter's strategies. Tackling socio-economic inequalities in health promotes equity and moves upstream, from a focus on blaming individuals to tackling the policies that shape environments.

The Ottawa Charter called for support for personal and social development through providing information, educating about health and enhancing life skills. By so doing, health promotion increases the options available to people to exercise more control over their own health and their environments, and to make choices conducive to health. Individual skills therefore include not just knowledge about health issues, but also practical life skills such as negotiation, setting realistic and achievable targets and building self-esteem, all of which have an impact on the ability to make lasting behavioural changes.

Although not specifically flagged up in the Ottawa Charter, using the media is a core health promotion strategy and one that may be put to many different uses.

Media coverage may be sought to promote individual life-style campaigns, to lobby for policy change or to highlight the importance of socio-economic determinants of health. Using the media therefore contributes to all the other strategies, and is the subject of Chapter 12.

Community development is one of the most fundamental strategies that informed the development of the concept and principles of health promotion, and featured as a strategy in the Ottawa Charter. It was conceived as a process that draws on existing human and material resources in the community to enhance self-help and social support, and to develop flexible systems for strengthening public participation in, and direction of, health matters. A focus on communities provides a route to tackle the social determinants of health through, for example, improving access to education, employment and housing. Strengthening communities is therefore a key strategy in moving upstream. The theoretical and policy base for community action has been informed more recently by research into community capacity building and concepts such as social capital.

Building healthy public policy and ensuring health is in all policies is an increasingly important strategy for health promotion, and one that is currently being used in relation to an expanding number of issues, e.g. tobacco control, active travel systems and food labelling. It combines diverse but complementary approaches, including legislation, fiscal measures, taxation and organizational change. It requires an interventionist role by government, advocacy by practitioners and coordinated and joint action by different sectors. Globalization presents new challenges for international action.

Reorienting the health services, from treatment towards prevention, is the subject of Chapter 8. In some respects this strategy has proved most taxing and impervious to change. There is always a demand that exceeds supply for health services, so trying to shift services away from immediate treatment to long-term prevention is extremely difficult. Treatment is high profile, media friendly and politically popular. Prevention is low profile, and its long timescale for effects to be evident makes it politically unpopular.

Creating supportive environments is the subject of Part Three, where different environments are discussed in separate chapters.

The Ottawa Charter stated that all of these actions would be required to promote health, and illustrated this in a spiral image (Figure 1). At the heart are the skills of enablement, mediation and advocacy. Increasingly, health promotion activities are conducted in combination in a comprehensive approach using a mix of such strategies and at multiple (national, regional, community) levels of action.

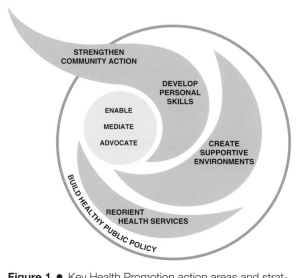

Figure 1 ● Key Health Promotion action areas and strategies. (WHO: 1986 Ottawa Charter for Health Promotion. Permission request to: http://www.who.int/about/licensing/copyright_form/en/. Referred to as 'Health Promotion logo (Ottawa)': http://www.who.int/healthpromotion/conferences/previous/ottawa/en/index4.html.)

References

Hills M., McQueen D.V,. 2007. At issue: two decades of the Ottawa Charter Promotion and Education (Suppl. 2): 5.
World Health Organization, 1986. Ottawa Charter for Health Promotion. WHO, Geneva.

Chapter Eight

Reorienting health services

Learning Outcomes

By the end of this chapter you will be able to:
- understand why reorienting health services is a key action area
- discuss the challenges associated with reorienting health services
- debate what should be the balance of investment between care, cure, prevention and health promotion.

Key Concepts and Definitions

Health system All public and private organizations, institutions and resources needed to improve, maintain and restore health.

Prevention The action of stopping something from happening. Disease prevention means actions taken at primary, secondary or tertiary levels to prevent disease occurring or worsening.

Primary care The day-to-day care provided by health workers in the community. Primary care workers are usually the first point of contact for patients, and provide continuing care as well as coordinating other specialist care as required.

Integrated care Joined-up care across health and social care boundaries.

Importance of the Topic

Many agencies, services and practitioners contribute to the promotion of health, and this chapter outlines the role of these stakeholders and different occupational groups. A reorientation of health services towards prevention was one of the key action areas of the Ottawa Charter (World Health Organization, 1986), yet it is the least successfully applied. Health promotion poses several ambitious challenges for the healthcare sector: to extend the core business of health services from clinical outcomes to quality of life; to extend the focus from patients and relatives to staff and the wider community; and to integrate prevention into care and cure practices. To do so can only be achieved through organizational and funding changes. This chapter discusses these challenges, the practitioners and agencies involved in promoting health, and how their contribution to health promotion can be mainstreamed and validated. The provision of healthcare and social care services differs widely from country to country, and this chapter focuses on the UK experience.

Introduction

Historically, the cure and treatment of illness have taken precedence over the prevention of ill health or the promotion of positive health in an organization. Most people thinking of health services think of hospitals and family doctors, a focus on treatment, developments in surgery, and new techniques and more effective medicines. There is widespread acceptance that prevention is better than cure, and it is the only rational way forward for public health. Yet a review of the sustainability of the National Health Service (NHS) in 2007 claimed that £1.5 million is spent on prevention and health promotion in the UK each year, which is the sum spent on the NHS in one-and-a-half days (Wanless et al., 2007). Part of the reluctance to invest in prevention is because the benefits accrue over time, thus with limited resources and pressure to demonstrate results, the focus of health services becomes skewed towards care.

While the contribution of health services to longevity is clear, as we saw in Chapter 2 many factors unconnected with health services have a profound impact on health. For many health promotion practitioners, the contribution of healthcare services in addressing the determinants of health is marginal (Wise and Nutbeam, 2007). However, health services do have a unique and significant contribution to make towards population health. This chapter argues that health services, defined as 'all the activities whose primary purpose is to promote, restore, or maintain health' (World Health Organization, 2000), are critically important in progressing health and human development.

Learning Activity 8.1 Health systems and equity

The Commission on the Social Determinants of Health (World Health Organization, 2007, p. viii) considered the contribution of health systems to equity. Do you agree with the following statement?

'[Health systems] fail to apply their expertise to address the social determinants of health; fail to contribute to social empowerment in the interests of health equity; institutionalize health care arrangements that create financial and geographic barriers to access for disadvantaged groups; alienate disadvantaged groups through culturally insensitive and sometimes antagonistic health worker and institutional practices; and impoverish the poor whilst allowing the rich to capture greater levels of public health care spending.'

Chapter 4 outlined the case made for health promotion by the Ottawa Charter of 1986, which stated that healthcare should encompass traditional education, disease prevention and rehabilitation services but also 'health enhancement by empowering patients, relatives and employees... enabling people to increase control over, and to improve, their health'. Not only would this involve 'open[ing] channels between the health sector and broader social, political, economic and physical environmental components', but it would also demand a 'change of attitude and organization of health services which refocuses on the total needs of the individual as a whole person'.

Learning Activity 8.2 Reorienting health services

Reorienting health services is the least successfully applied of the Ottawa Charter's key action areas (Wise and Nutbeam, 2007). What might be the reasons behind this?

There is some evidence of change, and of a recognition of the need to move towards a national *health* service and away from being a sickness service. The focus has shifted from treatment for acute conditions to the management of chronic conditions and the maintenance of optimum health. In recent years concepts such as 'self-management', 'collaborative' care, 'shared decision-making' and 'the expert patient' have become integrated into the management of chronic lifestyle conditions like diabetes. Our companion volume *Public Health and Health Promotion: Developing Practice* (Naidoo and Wills, 2010) discusses these moves towards involvement and participation by patients and the public in health service planning and delivery in Chapter 6.

A major incentive for the reorientation of health services is economics. Increased longevity and expectations, coupled with the rising costs of health services, have led to a concern about the cost-effectiveness of services. There is growing evidence of the economic case for shifting focus from treatment to health promotion. A major UK review to examine healthcare funding needs (Wanless, 2002) concluded that the 'fully engaged scenario', in which people self-manage their health and the NHS embraces prevention, is the most cost-effective. However, the review found that in many countries less than 4 percent of the health budget is allocated to public and primary health.

The goals of reorienting health systems are:

- to achieve a better balance between prevention and treatment
- to focus on population health outcomes alongside the focus on individual health
- to achieve a better health status for the population as a whole
- to achieve more cost-effective services
- to integrate services maximizing the contribution of the entire workforce.

Promoting health in and through the health sector

In addition to its obvious role of providing healthcare services, the NHS plays a major role in promoting health.

- The NHS is a major employer – 1.3 million people in the UK (NHS Confederation at www.nhsconfed.org/resources/key-statistics-on-the-nhs).
- It purchases a wide range of goods and is a potential support to local economies. Its purchasing power is estimated as £17 billion per year on, among other things, food, furniture, medical supplies, cleaning and office equipment, road vehicles and building materials (Coote, 2002).
- It is a major user of energy and producer of waste and carbon emissions. About 2.4 million tonnes of resources, excluding water and oxygen, are consumed in the NHS, with about 15 percent being discarded as waste and 1 percent remaining

as stock. The NHS carbon footprint is annually 25 million tonnes of carbon dioxide equivalents in procurement, building, energy and travel.

- It is a direct provider of health promotion services.
- It is a means of communicating with large numbers of people, whether as patients, family members, carers, employees, policymakers, suppliers or health professionals
- It is a highly valued social institution providing social cohesion in all countries.

The NHS is a social setting, just like a school or workplace (see Part Three). It has its own organizational procedures, values and ethos and cultural norms. For it to embrace health (rather than the treatment of disease) as its goal requires a change in all these elements.

 Learning Activity 8.3 The potential for health promotion

Considering the potential for health promotion, in what ways does the health service provide:

- opportunity?
- access?
- credibility?
- competence?

The health service is an important setting for health promotion because it offers a range of health professionals the opportunity to integrate promotion into their practice, and thus to fulfil the early promise of a comprehensive and health promoting health service.

There are several unique characteristics of the health service setting that make it ideal for promoting health. Use of health services is universal – everyone at some point in their lives comes into contact with health service providers. For many more vulnerable groups, such as people with long-standing limiting illness, contact is long term and frequent. In the UK 97 percent of the population are registered with a general practitioner (GP) and 70 percent consult their GP at least once a year. Health practitioners enjoy high levels of trust and credibility among the general population, and thus have the ability to affect people's knowledge, attitudes and beliefs. The NHS is the country's largest single employer, and therefore workplace initiatives may affect a significant percentage of the UK workforce and their families. All these factors provide good reasons for prioritizing the health services as a setting for health promotion. Chapter 16 discusses the hospital as a health promoting setting.

Primary healthcare and health promotion

The 1978 Alma Ata declaration (World Health Organization, 1978) defined primary care:

> *Primary health care seeks to extend the first level of the health system from sick care to the development of health. It seeks to protect and prevent the problems at an early stage. Primary health care services involve continuity of care, health promotion and education, integration of prevention with sick care, a concern for population as well as individual health, community involvement and the use of appropriate technology.*

Primary care is often used interchangeably with primary medical care, as its focus is on clinical services provided predominantly by GPs, as well as by practice nurses, primary/community healthcare nurses, early childhood nurses and community pharmacists.

Primary healthcare (PHC) incorporates primary care, but has a broader focus through providing a comprehensive range of generalist services by multidisciplinary teams that include not only GPs and nurses but also allied health professionals and other health workers. PHC services also operate at the level of communities. The Royal College of General Practitioners (www.rcgp.org.uk) identifies the functions of the PHC team as:

- diagnosis and management of acute and chronic conditions and treatment in emergencies, when necessary in the patient's home
- antenatal and postnatal care, and providing access to contraceptive advice and provision
- prevention of disease and disability

- follow-up and continuing care of chronic and recurring disease
- rehabilitation after illness
- care during terminal illness
- the coordination of services for those at risk, including children, the mentally ill, the bereaved, the elderly, the handicapped and those who care for them.
- helping patients and their relatives to make appropriate use of other agencies for care and support, including hospital-based specialists.

 Learning Activity 8.4 Primary care provision

There are 60,000 primary care physicians in France, about 1.7 per 1,000 people, which is double the number in the UK. There are just over two primary care nurses, including health visitors, per doctor in France, which is about half the ratio of the UK.

What effect might this have on the promotion of health?

Primary healthcare principles

The PHC approach is characterized by the following principles.

- A holistic understanding of health as well-being, rather than the absence of disease.
- Recognition that the presence of good health is dependent upon multiple determinants – health services are important, but so too are housing, education, agriculture and other services.
- Health services reflect local needs and involve communities and individuals at all levels of planning and provision of services.
- Services and technology are affordable, accessible and acceptable to communities.
- Health services strive to address inequity and prioritize services to the most needy.

Primary healthcare: strategies

PHC strategies need to be consistent with the underlying philosophy of health promotion. In Chapter 5 we discussed various approaches to promoting health, of which education is one. Through education, communities and individuals gain an understanding of the factors influencing their health and can work to gain control over health problems. The term 'empowerment' is often used to describe patient education or any communication with a patient that is client-centred in its orientation. Yet empowering approaches necessitate organizational and environmental change. Figure 8.1 shows how empowerment and health gain can be built into nurse–client contacts.

Much of the health promotion practised in PHC settings is carried out by nurses, and much of this is opportunistic. A client has a consultation or is referred to a member of the PHC team and is identified as 'at risk'. The practitioner takes the opportunity to offer advice, information or a further referral on a health-related issue. In some cases the practitioner may start a series of brief interventions using motivational interviewing to identify the client's readiness to change (see Chapter 9).

Learning Activity 8.5 Opportunistic health promotion

What are the advantages and disadvantages of opportunistic health promotion?

The emphasis of recent policy has been on developing more planned and proactive health promotion activities. The need for a risk assessment becomes a key skill enabling PHC practitioners to target health promotion better. For example, only a minority of those at risk of a sexually transmitted infection (STI) attend genitourinary medicine clinics, whereas the great majority of adults will access primary care in any one year. Matthews and Fletcher (2001) therefore suggest that GPs are likely to encounter patients from across the risk spectrum for STIs, and should develop planned ways of raising the issue of sexual health risks with all patients.

Case Study 8.1 NHS Health Checks

Public health policy identifies a small number of risk factors: poor diet, smoking, high blood pressure, obesity, physical inactivity, alcohol use and high levels of cholesterol. These are addressed through therapeutic, behavioural and structural interventions. Finding and managing those with high risk factors is the first stage. The NHS Health Check is a population-wide approach which was introduced in 2009 and became part of the public health function of local authorities in 2014. The Health Check is a face-to-face risk assessment for cardiovascular disease, stroke and type 2 diabetes. The aim of the Health Check is to be an easily available means of screening to identify those at risk, but implementation has been patchy. In the third year of implementation (2011–2012) only half of the Health Checks offered had been taken up, and the evidence base for general health checks as a public health strategy is not clear (Krogsboll et al., 2012; MacAuley, 2012).

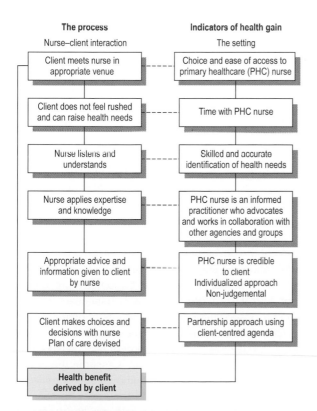

Fig. 8.1 ● Health promoting nurse–client contacts. (Adapted from HEA, 1998.)

The process	Indicators of health gain
Nurse–client interaction	The setting
Client meets nurse in appropriate venue	Choice and ease of access to primary healthcare (PHC) nurse
Client does not feel rushed and can raise health needs	Time with PHC nurse
Nurse listens and understands	Skilled and accurate identification of health needs
Nurse applies expertise and knowledge	PHC nurse is an informed practitioner who advocates and works in collaboration with other agencies and groups
Appropriate advice and information given to client by nurse	PHC nurse is credible to client Individualized approach Non-judgemental
Client makes choices and decisions with nurse Plan of care devised	Partnership approach using client-centred agenda
Health benefit derived by client	

Primary healthcare: service provision

PHC is the first level of healthcare, and is directly accessible to individuals and communities. This means that effective PHC must be locally based, in proximity to the places where people live and work, easy to access and free at the point of delivery. As the first level of healthcare services, PHC services need to be well integrated with the secondary and tertiary healthcare sectors, in order to provide prompt assessment, response, referral and continuity of care for people throughout all levels of the healthcare system. There is an increasing percentage of people, including frail older people, with chronic and complex health conditions that will demand care in the community.

The following examples of PHC services describe the Peckham experiment of the 1930s and the 2007 proposals to reorganize London's healthcare around polyclinics, since halted.

 Learning Activity 8.6 Types of primary healthcare

Do you see any similarities in the following description of two forms of PHC?

The Peckham experiment
The Pioneer Health Centre was started in the 1930s by two doctors concerned about the health of poor people living in south London. The health centre tried to address health in a holistic way, and incorporated a fitness club, theatre, gym, swimming pool, billiards table, children's nursery, a cafeteria serving healthy, cheap food, a library and medical consulting rooms. For one shilling (5 p) a week per family, all of the centre's facilities could be used. In 1938, 600 families belonged. It closed during the Second World War, reopening in 1946 when it added a nursery school, youth club, marriage advisory service, Citizens' Advice Bureau and child guidance. It closed in 1950 because it did not fit into the structure of the emerging NHS. The centre has been revived as Pulse Health and Leisure – a partnership between Southwark Council and Lambeth, Lewisham and Southwark

health authorities funded by £3.2 million of lottery money. Its aim is 'to provide a unique leisure, health and fitness resource that encourages local people to invest in their own health and well-being'. The new partnership thus puts the responsibility for health squarely on the individual.

Polyclinics
Polyclinics, proposed by the Darzi review of healthcare services in London in 2007, would offer not just GP services but also 'antenatal and postnatal care, healthy living information and services, community mental health services, community care, social care and specialist advice all in one place. They will provide the infrastructure (such as diagnostics and consulting rooms for outpatients) to allow a shift of services out of hospital settings. They would be where the majority of urgent care centres will be located. And they will provide the integrated, one-stop-shop care that we want for people with long-term conditions' (Darzi, 2007, p. 11, para. 22). The staff in each centre will include GPs, consultant specialists, nurses, dentists, opticians, therapists, emergency care practitioners, mental health workers, midwives, health visitors and social workers (Darzi, 2007, p. 92, main table). The shift of much healthcare out of hospital settings means that in the future 'the bulk of healthcare activity will take place in polyclinics' (Darzi, 2007, p. 107, para. 71).

One common argument is that adequate provision of PHC services will mean that more specialized hospital-based services are unnecessary. For example, proper management and monitoring of chronic conditions such as diabetes and asthma should help prevent the development of crises which require hospitalization. As stays in hospital become shorter, the role of the primary health team becomes more important. Lord Darzi's (2007) review of healthcare in London proposed shifting huge amounts of hospital care to GPs. However, this proposal was superseded by a plan to devolve commissioning of services to GPs.

Traditional models of PHC that assume the family doctor will build up a detailed knowledge of patients over time and visit patients in their own homes are changing, and may not be relevant for transient and culturally diverse populations. Consultations in general practice in the UK tend to be short (8 to 9 minutes) compared to other countries, and are unable to address adequately the wide range of psychosocial problems experienced by disadvantaged population groups. GPs' awareness of possible referral options in the locality is also limited (Popay et al., 2007), although innovative 'social prescribing' projects exist, such as one in Stockport, in which a GP may refer patients to arts, gardening schemes, learning or a self-help library.

Participation, collaboration, empowerment and equity are core health promotion principles, but incorporating them into health services is a challenge.

Participation

It is now accepted that the public have the right to be consulted and to have a say in the policymaking process (the drivers towards patient and public involvement are discussed in Chapter 6 of our companion volume, Naidoo and Wills, 2010). However, the means of public consultation range from formal to informal, one-off events to ongoing contact, and reactive to proactive. Any of the following activities undertaken to increase public participation and involvement could be said to be public health work.

- Supporting patient participation groups in general practice and including lay people's views in community health profiles.
- Seeking feedback from the community on service provision, and using this to change practice.
- Supporting self-help groups in the community.
- Working with community groups on health issues.

Equity

As we saw in Chapter 2, there is a strong argument for advocating greater social and economic equity as a means of promoting health. This refers to equity of both material resources and power (the ability to achieve desired goals). Equity, or being fair and just, is not the same as equality, which is the state of being equal. While equality may be impossible to achieve,

equity, or providing equal services for people with equal needs and working to reduce known inequalities in health, is a realistic goal.

 Learning Activity 8.7 Promoting equity

What can you do in your health promotion role to promote equity?

Collaboration

Collaboration or partnership working is the third health promotion principle. Collaboration means working together with others on shared projects. Collaboration is necessary because of the many different factors affecting public health, which means that any one agency or organization can have only a limited impact on health. By working together, more fundamental changes can be put into place, with a greater potential to promote health. There is a long history of partnership working to deliver health improvements in England, e.g. through health action zones, local strategic partnerships and community budgets.

Our companion volume *Public Health and Health Promotion: Developing Practice* (Naidoo and Wills 2010) discusses some of the challenges associated with partnership working across organizational boundaries, such as differences in priorities, organizational ethos, funding arrangements, competition for contracts and geographical boundaries. Enabling factors identified include committed individuals, joint funding and pooling of resources, shared education and training opportunities and existing projects which span different agencies.

 Learning Activity 8.8 Health promotion in practice

Think of an intervention in your health promotion practice concerning the health of a service user.
- Reflect on why you did what you did.
- Could you have done something different?

Continued

- Would other health promoters have done the same as you?
- If you adopted a public health approach to your work, what aspects of this intervention would change?
  How could you:
- increase participation?
- promote equity?
- increase collaboration and partnership working?

NHS Health Scotland has developed a framework to support the development of a health promoting service, as shown in Figure 8.2.

The roots of the tree suggest the necessity of understanding the underlying conditions that determine health and ill health:

- biological inheritance
- physical environment
- cultural, social, political and economic circumstances.

This understanding of who is affected, and when and where, enables possible interventions to be identified. The trunk of the tree illustrates the importance of organizational commitment to improving health. The branches describe key areas for health promotion activity and those elements of the setting that contribute to health, e.g. organizational policy and public involvement.

Learning Activity 8.9 Prevention and financial incentives in primary care

To reduce the financial burden on health services there are a number of possible initiatives which aim to prevent ill health. What are the advantages and disadvantages of each?

- Develop campaigns which focus on top public health priorities, seeking to educate the population to behave differently.
- Include health education as part of the core remit of community nurses, to be documented and monitored.
- Pay primary care doctors an incentive fee to call in 'at-risk' patients such as 25–40-year-old men.

- Pay primary care doctors to screen all 'high-risk' patients for specific diseases such as diabetes, kidney disease and stroke.
- Create financial incentives for individuals if they can show they are leading healthy lives by subsidizing insurance schemes.

Most attempts to introduce health promotion into health systems reflect the view that there needs to be incentivization through financing mechanisms or performance management to encourage healthcare organizations to adopt health promotion strategies.

The England Public Health Outcomes framework (2012) sets out objectives in four domains with over 60 indicators for measuring progress (www.phoutcomes.info). Obesity, for example, is a public health priority. Although primary care may offer potential for health promotion, there are numerous barriers to effective health promotion in this setting. Maryon-Davis (2005, p. 97) describes obesity as a frequently intransigent problem for primary care. He cites:

- pressure of time in the consultation
- a lack of appropriately trained primary care staff
- a shortage of community dietitians or nutritionists
- the potentially enormous caseload
- language or cultural barriers
- the intractability of patients' eating habits, exercise behaviour and clinical condition.

Who promotes health?

Learning Activity 8.10 Who promotes health?

'Health is a state of complete physical, social and mental well-being, not merely the absence of disease or infirmity' (World Health Organization 1946). Using this well-known definition of health, make a list of who is involved in promoting and protecting the nation's health.

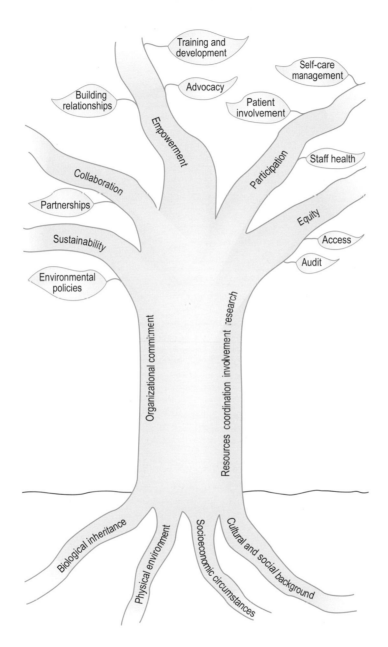

Fig. 8.2 ● The tree of health promotion.

Figure 8.3 illustrates the sectors and range of agencies that can be involved in promoting health. These span international and global interests and national, regional and local levels. Many of these agencies would not regard health as their core business, but their activities can make a significant contribution to the promotion of good health in society. Reorienting the work of such agencies and organizations would mean making explicit their health goals and impact.

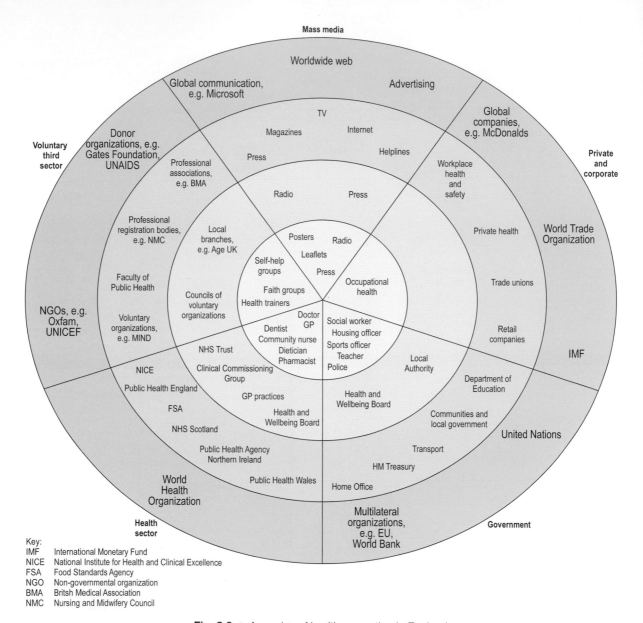

Fig. 8.3 ● Agencies of health promotion in England.

International

Numerous international organizations, such as the World Health Organization, have health promotion as a core function. Other organizations, such as the World Trade Organization, responsible for free trade and investment agreements between nations, can have an impact on resource consumption, environmental stress and wage rates, and thereby on the efforts of countries to reduce inequities. The World Bank provides financial assistance to low-income countries and is a major funder of health projects, including mass-immunization campaigns and anti-malaria projects.

Case Study 8.2 War and public health

Increasing global interdependence has meant that wars are more likely to affect countries geographically far removed from the conflict, through economic repercussions, emigration patterns and even direct forms of action such as terrorism. Almost all wars since the Second World War have been fought in developing countries, which has allowed the West to consider war as an exceptional event rather than a mainstream concern for public health. This is despite the fact that in 1990 war was the sixteenth cause of the global burden of disease (Murray and Lopez, 1997) and predictions were that by 2020 it would take eighth place, putting it ahead of human immunodeficiency virus/acquired immunodeficiency syndrome (HIV/AIDS). Wars have also dramatically shaped the spending of low-income countries, which buy approximately 85 percent of world arms and weaponry. Many of these countries spend more on arms and weapons than on education or health (Levy and Sidel, 2002). The five major developed powers (China, France, Russia, the USA and the UK) produce 90 percent of the world's arms, and the arms trade has a role in the perpetuation of conflict (Bunton and Wills, 2005).

National

Many government departments have an influence on health, and the UK government is committed to 'joined-up' policy. The appointment of a Minister for Public Health in England in 1997 was intended to ensure coordination of health policy across government. Health impact assessments are intended to ensure that the health consequences of a range of policies will be considered during their development stage (see Chapter 11).

A range of agencies within government have a remit for aspects of health, for example:

- the Food Standards Agency – regulation of food labelling, food safety
- the National Institute for Health and Clinical Excellence – gathering of evidence on effective interventions
- the Health Protection Agency (part of Public Health England) – management of health threats, including infectious disease; radiation, chemical and environmental hazards; and emergency response.

In England the lead agency for health promotion is Public Health England. Health Scotland, the NHS Public Health Agency for Northern Ireland and Public Health Wales take on this role in the other UK countries. In other countries there are national centres which may coordinate research and knowledge, contribute to policy advocacy and provide a voice for public health and health promotion practitioners, e.g. the Public Health Agency for Canada.

Increasingly the corporate sector is recognizing the potential of health as a commodity. In recent years there has been a huge expansion in gym membership, exercise equipment, organic foods and farmers' markets. Supermarkets promote foodstuffs on the basis of their health-giving potential. The impact of the corporate sector on health through labour market policies and environmental degradation is increasingly recognized (see Chapter 11 on how public policy is being oriented to health and the encouragement of HiAP – Health in All Policies).

Local

The NHS is locally organized within a centralized policy framework. Figure 8.4 shows the structure of the NHS following its radical reorganization under the Health and Social Care Act 2012.

Currently the NHS in England comprises 211 clinical commissioning groups which commission community-based and hospital services from 261 provider organizations – 161 acute trusts, 56 mental health trusts, 34 community providers, 10 ambulance trusts and 8,000 GP practices.

Key functions that have an impact on health, such as housing, transport and sport and leisure, are all local government responsibilities. Prior to the 1970s the public health function was located in local government, but this was transferred to the NHS in 1974. It reverted back to local government in 2013. Local government is now responsible for improving the health of the local population and for public health services, including sexual health services and drug and alcohol services.

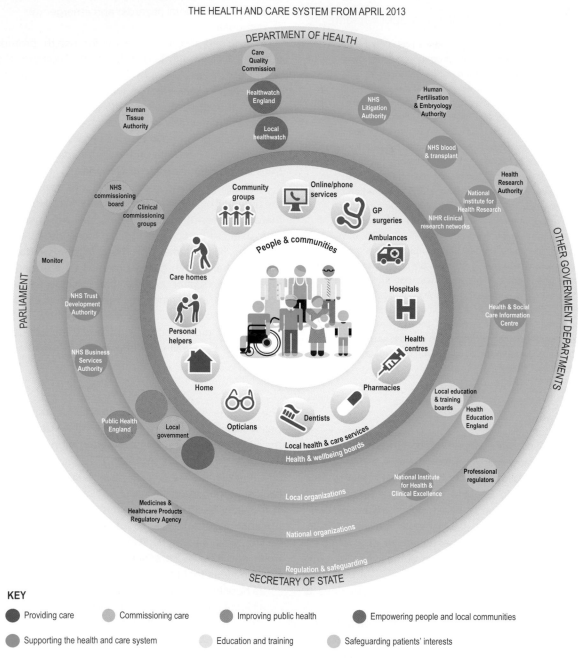

Fig. 8.4 ● The structure of the NHS. (http://www.myhealth.london.nhs.uk/sites/default/files/u4078/nhs-structure.jpg. Open gov't licence/Crown copyright.)

Health and well-being boards are local authority committees that link health and care systems to reduce inequalities and improve health. In 2015 local government took responsibility for 0- to 5-year-olds, and the school nursing and health-visiting services became public health responsibilities.

Public health and health promotion workforce

Public health services require a balance between health promotion, preventive care and illness treatment. This is best achieved through the use of a team drawn from a variety of disciplines, including not only medical and nursing health professionals but also community workers, public health information workers and educators.

The Report of the Chief Medical Officer's Project to Strengthen the Public Health Function (Department of Health, 2001) provided a framework for assessing the contribution of the broader public health workforce to the public health function. In particular the document referred to three main categories of employees.

1. Wider contributors.
2. Practitioners.
3. Specialists.

Reorienting the workforce means identifying health promotion opportunities and also encouraging a way of working which is empowering and enables people to take control over health issues.

Wider contributors

Wider contributors are professionals who have an impact on public health as part of their work, but who may not recognize this, e.g. teachers and social services employees. This part of the workforce is important because they can reach people who are not in contact with health services and refer them on to sources of advice and support. To maximize their contribution, the public health aspects of their work need to be recognized and foregrounded. Teachers provide an example of this failure to recognize the importance of public health and health promotion: although schools are seen as key settings for health promotion in many countries, with national standards and key roles to strengthen the social and emotional well-being of both pupils and staff, health promotion is not part of initial teacher education in many countries (Chapter 13).

There is also a huge informal workforce that contributes to health. Voluntary groups and non-governmental organizations act as service providers, self-help groups, pressure groups and sources of education and information. They are involved in planning and consultation exercises, such as community plans. Voluntary organizations are important in providing specialized information, and being close to the community and isolated and vulnerable groups. They can reflect people's experience of a service and give an indication of other needs, acting as a catalyst for change. The precarious funding of many voluntary organizations means they have to expend a great deal of time and effort securing grants and funding, which can make long-term planning difficult and lead to low morale.

Case Study 8.3 Health trainers and health champions

Health trainers, who may also be called health ambassadors, were introduced as a new kind of workforce in the document *Choosing Health* (Department of Health 2004). Their role is to support people to make healthier choices and change their health-related behaviour. Health trainers are drawn from local communities so they understand the health concerns and experiences of those they support, and have a stake in improving health in the areas where they live. Health trainers may be paid or volunteers.

Health champions are people who, with training and support, voluntarily bring their ability to relate to people and their own life experience to transform health and well-being in their communities. Health champions share learning with patients, resulting in better self-management of health, increased engagement and less reliance on services. The Altogether Better project (www.altogetherbetter.org.uk/health-champions) claims they 'transfer knowledge into the system and increase the intelligence held by services of community issues and assets, identifying opportunities for redesign that services are receptive to because they know and trust our Champions'.

Practitioners

Practitioners are a smaller group of professionals who spend most, or all, of their time in public health practice. Changing contracts and more specific definitions of roles and competencies mean that job remits in primary and social care are in a state of constant flux. Any account of working practice is in danger of being both context-specific and out-of-date in the near future. Increasingly roles are becoming generic, such as those within 'the children's workforce' where the skills, competencies and knowledge required are similar regardless of professional background or role and apply to a very wide range of workers, including personal advisers, health visitors, midwives, youth workers, family workers, substance misuse workers, nursery nurses, educational welfare officers, community children's nurses, school nurses and support staff such as learning mentors working in schools.

A brief description of some key roles follows. It illustrates the importance of health promotion in many job remits, but also the challenges faced and why, for many individual practitioners, health promotion often slips to the bottom of a busy workload.

Specialist community public health nurses

Health promotion is a priority in the role of specialist community public health nurses such as health visitors and school nurses:

> Specialist community public health nursing aims to reduce health inequalities by working with individuals, families, and communities promoting health, preventing ill health and in the protection of health. The emphasis is on partnership working that cuts across disciplinary, professional and organizational boundaries that impact on organized social and political policy to influence the determinants of health and promote the health of whole populations (www.nmc-uk.org).

Increasingly, community nurses are expected to use a population focus, adopting community development methods (see Chapter 10), identifying local needs and supporting community and voluntary groups. Health visitors, family nurses and school nurses are now part of the public health workforce and work closely with other community nurses, GPs and social workers. However, health promotion may not always be coordinated or prioritized because health and social care workers tend to concentrate on their own caseload.

Because community nurses visit people in their own homes, they are able to build a strong relationship with their clients over a period of time. This enables them to carry out much one-to-one education, counselling and opportunistic health education. District nurses, for example, visit people with chronic sickness or disability at home. Much of their work is with older people (one in four people over 75 are on a district nurse caseload), and they carry out opportunistic health education as well as liaising between people living in the community and other relevant health and welfare workers. The individualized basis of patient care offers opportunities for health promotion, but is also a constraint in both limiting time and separating district nursing from a population perspective. One study reports a district nurse commenting: 'Public health... it's like anything isn't it... we just don't realize we are doing it... I think maybe we need to be more aware of just what skills we've got' (Arnold et al., 2004).

 Learning Activity 8.11 Professional roles

What is the health promotion role of a district nurse?

Mental health nurses

Promoting mental health requires a collaborative approach from a diverse and wide-ranging group of stakeholders. Mental health promotion is often associated with the health and social care services involved in delivering care and treatment to people experiencing mental ill health. While treating mental illness is an important component, mental health promotion is concerned with the mental health and well-being of the whole population throughout the life course. Mental health promotion is delivered in a variety of settings, including schools, the workplace, the community at large and within specific communities such as care homes and prisons (see the All Wales Mental Health Promotion Network at www.public-mentalhealth.org).

School nurses

School nurses are part of the community nursing service, but their role varies enormously. Originally it was to focus on the detection and treatment of poor hygiene, infestations and malnutrition, but it has since evolved to become routine health surveillance and screening. In common with health-visiting practice, the current role for school nurses is to move away from routine surveillance towards identifying needs and targeting support, e.g. support for children with chronic diseases or the provision of education and counselling on specialized topics such as sexual health. School nurses may also implement the national Child Measurement Programme on obesity. Some areas adopt a life-course approach, with the school nurse acting as a navigator for children throughout their school journey. The school is recognized as a setting for health promotion and school nurses are a school-based service. Yet there are challenges and barriers for school nurses to extend their role, particularly within schools, where they may not feel part of the organization.

Midwives

Hospital midwives are involved in antenatal education and the delivery of babies. Community midwives visit all new mothers in their area, and provide support and education as well as monitoring the health of mothers and babies.

> *Midwives are in an ideal position to extend support to expectant and new families and to provide a service which helps parents to access information and use it effectively to nurture the health of their family. They also have*

> *an important role in bringing public attention to those issues which are beyond the scope of individuals to change, such as social and environmental obstacles.*
>
> Bowden (2006),p. 14.

A review of public health interventions by midwives (McNeil et al., 2012) identified several effective actions which are already recommended as routine practice, for example education about folic acid supplementation and pelvic floor muscle training to prevent or reduce the risk of urinary incontinence, yet guidelines have not been routinely applied. Other effective interventions were identified which could easily be implemented by a midwife and could potentially impact on public health, such as education programmes for parents of pre-term infants and implementation of specific strategies to reduce caesarean section rates.

General practitioners

General practice has traditionally been a private and personal consultation between doctor and patient. Health promotion consisted of opportunistic advice or information, often limited by time or a concern not to be 'intrusive'. The contracting of GP services provides additional payments to GPs to carry out preventive work such as immunizations, health checks to identify risk and giving advice. Opportunities for planned interventions have increased, and there are numerous examples of exercise referral schemes and lifestyle management programmes.

Practice nurses

Practice nurses are directly employed by GPs. Practice nursing is a relatively new profession, although there are now over 25,000 practice nurses in the UK. Their health promotion role has been largely confined to immunization, taking bloods, cytology, lifestyle advice, travel health and health checks, but increasingly they are staffing minor-illness centres.

Dentists

There is an increasing emphasis on prevention in dentistry, particularly with children. Dentists receive a capitation fee per child, and so have an interest in keeping that child's teeth healthy. Many practices employ a hygienist who gives advice on dental health. Health authorities also have a community dental service which may offer dental health promotion to schools and residential homes.

Pharmacists

The potential of community pharmacies to promote health has been recognized in a national strategy (Department of Health, 2008). Pharmacy staff advise the public on the safe use of medicines, minor ailments and healthy lifestyles. They may also provide specific public health interventions as part of a broader NHS service, for example weight-loss clinics, specialist smoking cessation advice or drug misuse services (see Chapter 16). To maximize their potential, all pharmacies should have areas set aside where members of the public can consult in private with the pharmacist.

Environmental health workers

The role of environmental health is particularly wide-ranging, encompassing statutory powers relating to food hygiene and pollution (of noise and air), specialist work on safety in the workplace and places of entertainment, and work on sustainability and recycling. Because environmental health officers have wide-ranging statutory powers, their work in health promotion is mainly advice on legislation and enabling people to conform to regulations. Their work may thus involve offering training courses or one-to-one advice.

Allied health workers

Many other professions allied to medicine, such as speech and language therapists, chiropodists,

physiotherapists, radiographers and dietitians (known as allied health professionals – AHPs), have a part to play in health promotion, especially patient education.

 Research Example 8.1 Allied health professions and health promotion

Many health professionals have been encouraged to work flexibly and extend their roles to include promoting health and well-being, educating patients and viewing every patient contact as an opportunity for health promotion. Health promotion is a routine component of AHP practice, but is not necessarily well delivered or thought through. The evidence points to a variation between professions, with physiotherapists and dietitians engaging in more highly developed health promotion practice (Needle et al., 2011).

Care workers

Population projections indicate a more rapid ageing of the population. People aged 85 and over will comprise 3.8 percent of the UK population by 2031, and the majority of these will need residential care. Care workers have a key health promotion role to improve fitness and nutrition and thereby minimize illness and dependence. Care workers also have a role in positive mental health promotion and empowering older people to have a degree of control over their lives. Preventing ill health in the frail aged is important, e.g. the prevention of falls and pressure sores. Residential care workers liaise with GPs, social workers, physiotherapists, chiropodists and catering staff.

Specialists

Specialist advisers in public health are usually public health consultants and specialists working at a strategic or senior-management level. They play a role in developing public health programmes and often have specific scientific expertise and accreditation. In many countries they are physicians. Multiprofessional health workers first appeared in Finland, Ireland, the

United States and the United Kingdom. Alongside specialists in public health are public health practitioners, who work in a variety of settings and have varying remits, from health improvement to health protection and health intelligence. These practitioners are mainly employed in public health departments, which are now part of local government and are usually accountable to the Director of Public Health (DPH). They vary widely in size, from a handful to 50 staff. They have the lead role in initiating, coordinating and supporting health education and health promotion activity (termed health improvement – see Chapter 4) within their areas. Activities include:

- assessing local health needs
- contributing to the operational and strategic plans of the local authority
- reviewing service agreements to ensure that they seek to *promote* health
- coordinating the plans and services of different agencies.
  Provider activities include:
- managing health promotion programmes on specific issues such as HIV/AIDS, smoking cessation or coronary heart disease
- providing advice and consultancy to the public and policymakers
- providing training, support and advice to all health promoters and agencies that provide health promotion.

Conclusion

Reorienting health services is a challenging task, and to date little progress has been made. There are many reasons for the intransigence of the health services to change. Both primary and acute care are social systems with their own structures and cultures which determine the ways in which they tackle health and ill health. Partnerships tend to be client-rather than population-focused, and though primary care is based *in* communities, there may be little engagement *with* communities. Health services are driven by a medical model of health rather than a social model, and evaluation is still often seen in terms of reduced morbidity and mortality rather than in terms of health-gain processes and outcomes. The priority is treatment, which means that often patient compliance is valued above patient autonomy and participation. Although progress has been made in prioritizing health promotion, it is still 'bolted on' to core tasks instead of being integral to everyone's work and service delivery. Key health promotion activities, such as addressing health inequalities, are replaced by the need to respond to client demands, which may paradoxically have the effect of reinforcing inequalities by providing more services for more educated and articulate patients. Perhaps the biggest barrier is the growing burden of non-communicable diseases, which leads to health promotion focusing on lifestyle changes.

Chapter 16 discusses what is meant by a health promoting health service and draws attention to some of the challenges highlighted here in enabling patients to engage with the design, implementation and evaluation of health information and services. Reorienting health services and promoting health mean addressing the diverse needs of populations and the ways in which their health is shaped by social determinants.

On the plus side, there is a large pool of potential health promoters, including many practitioners in primary, secondary and tertiary care services. The effective delivery of health promotion would, in the long run, ease the workload of most practitioners, as well as enabling people to enjoy better health and increased longevity. Health promotion underpins many of the activities already being undertaken by practitioners, e.g. collaboration and partnership working. The economic argument for reorienting health services is robust, and provides a compelling case for action. Pulling all these positive factors together is a long-term and daunting task, but many small steps have already been taken. The challenge is to keep the reorienting health services agenda foregrounded and identify ongoing strategies to progress this goal. As Ziglio et al. (2011, p. 218) remark, 'a well functioning health system is one that not only ensures equitable and universal access to a good range of primary and preventive services but also advocates for better social and environmental conditions'.

Questions for further discussion

- What can be done to reorient the healthcare sector to take greater responsibility for health promotion? What in your work experience are the prospects and problems of collaboration with others to promote health?
- How can public health and health promotion professionals engage with the wider workforce to build their capacity and promote health?

Summary

This chapter has discussed the potential of the health-care sector to promote health, and the challenges posed by the medical paradigm. It has outlined the contribution of different agencies and practitioners to health promotion.

Further reading and resources

Scriven, A., Orme, J. (Eds.), 2001. Health Promotion: Professional Perspectives, second ed. Palgrave Macmillan/Open University, Basingstoke. *A useful insight into what health promotion means in different settings. Interesting accounts of practice will help to increase understanding in collaborative partnerships.*

Scriven, A. (Ed.), 2005. Health Promoting Practice: The Contribution of Nurses and Allied Health Professionals. Palgrave Macmillan, Basingstoke. *Discussion of how different roles conceptualize health promotion, and examples of practice.*

Naidoo, J., et al., 2007. Who promotes health? In: Earle, S., Lloyd, C.E., Sidell, M. (Eds.), Theory and Research in Promoting Public Health. Sage/Open University, London, pp. 101–129. *A thorough overview of a range of agencies that promote health.*

The King's Fund is a source of commentary about the health services. It has made a short animated film about the current structure of the NHS: www.kingsfund.org.uk/projects/nhs-65/alternative-guide-new-nhs-england.

The UK's Faculty of Public Health describes the public health function: www.fph.org.uk/what_is_public_health.

 Feedback to learning activities

8.1 Health systems can help to level the health gradient, but they can also inadvertently contribute to inequality. Access to and utilization of services should not depend on socio-economic status, yet people in equal need do not receive equal treatment. Those on higher incomes are more likely to receive specialist, preventive and dental services. The EU Survey on Income and Living Conditions found that financial factors are the most important reason why people miss out on healthcare when they need it (www.cso.ie/en/media/csoie/releasespublications/documents/silc/2012/silc_2012.Pdf). There are geographic barriers for older people and those with limited ability. Limited health literacy can also be a barrier.

8.2 Resistance to reorienting health services is primarily due to the organizational tradition and culture, particularly within the state-funded NHS, of providing treatment and care. This acute-care paradigm means that all too frequently health practitioners view their role as patching people up and sending them home. Prevention is seen as 'helping people to get better by doing what is good for them', with patient compliance as an important objective. Patients who do not take advice may be seen as demanding and, in some cases, refused treatment if they do not follow recommended behaviour change. In countries funded by social contributions, practitioners who are paid a fee for service have little incentive for prevention and activities such as managing chronic disease or health education, which are time-consuming and bring no financial reward.

8.3 The NHS provides excellent access and opportunities for health promotion. Every day over 835,000 people visit a GP; 50,000 visit accident and emergency; 49,000 have an outpatient consultation; 94,000 are admitted to hospital as emergencies; and 36,000 people are in hospital for planned treatment (HSCIS, 2013). In terms of credibility and competence, the 2013 Care Quality Commission satisfaction survey found that 64.2 percent of people definitely had confidence and trust in the last GP they had seen (www.england.nhs.uk/statistics/statistical-work-areas/gp-patient-survey/).

8.4 In many countries, such as France, there has been a move away from PHC in favour of a centralized hospital system. Community care is delivered by medical practitioners with much less involvement in providing a broad PHC with health promotion at its core.

8.5 You may have included some of the following disadvantages of opportunistic health promotion.

- Opportunistic health promotion relies on the decisions of individual practitioners. This leads to patchy and uneven implementation, on a basis of chance rather than proven need.
- Health promotion remains a marginalized luxury, to be tacked on at the end of a consultation if there is time. Lack of time is an important factor limiting the amount of health promotion undertaken by both GPs and nurses.
- Doubts as to the ethics of opportunistic health promotion have been expressed, e.g. raising the subject of smoking with patients consulting for unrelated problems.

You may have included some of the following advantages of opportunistic health promotion.

- Immediate relevance of information.
- Highly motivated patients.
- The ability to adapt and modify the input to suit individual needs.

8.6 Behind both forms of provision is the notion that healthcare needs to be closer to home and include the wide range of services that promote health. While the Peckham experiment had a holistic view of individual and community health needs, the polyclinic is firmly rooted in a medical model of care. Whereas the Peckham centre was rooted within its community, inevitably a polyclinic provides centralized services further away and more difficult to access by the disadvantaged communities who use and need PHC the most.

8.7 Most practitioners see the promotion of equity as a political task beyond their role or competence. However, even small steps contribute to greater equity. For example, ensuring that clients know their benefit entitlement and claim it, helping clients to fill out the necessary forms and supporting the case for a welfare benefits advisory service to receive health authority funding are all aspects of working for equity to improve material circumstances. Identifying inequities in local services, such as

people not registered with general practices, and supporting such groups to gain access to services is also working for equity. Targeting areas of deprivation for more intensive interventions is another example which is frequently found. The arguments and evidence in favour of targeting small areas or population groups are discussed in more detail in our companion volume (Naidoo and Wills, 2010).

8.8 Reflection on one's interventions to promote health may reveal alternatives that were not considered at the time, as well as identifying one's priorities. Such reflection is important to clarify one's underlying values, ethics and concerns, and to identify to what extent these are shared with other workers and organizations.

8.9

Incentive	Advantages	Disadvantages
• Develop campaigns which focus on top public health priorities, seeking to educate the population to behave differently	Easy to implement	Expensive and largely ineffective
• Health education as part of the core remit of community nurses, to be documented and monitored	Could reach large numbers of people	• Difficult to monitor • Practice may not be health promoting
• Pay primary care doctors an incentive fee to call in 'at-risk' patients such as 25–40-year-old men	Early identification means more effective management	Low take-up
• Pay primary care doctors to screen all 'high-risk' patients for specific diseases such as diabetes, kidney disease, stroke	Early identification means more effective management	Low take-up
• Financial incentives for individuals if they can show they are leading healthy lives by subsidizing insurance schemes	Can aid behaviour change	Expensive and difficult to monitor

Continued

8.10 Identifying who promotes health depends on how it is defined. If you adopt a fairly narrow medical model of health, you may have included a range of health-sector professionals such as GPs and health visitors. If, however, your definition is wider and health is seen as socially and economically determined, then a much wider range of partners (e.g. local authorities, businesses) can be seen to promote health.

8.11 **The roles of the district nurse include the following.**

1. Building community intelligence:
   a. sharing information about older patients and their needs

   b. broad public health approach to health needs assessment, e.g. transport to shops, street safety
   c. access to private accounts of health.
2. User participation strategies:
   a. access to the most vulnerable and least heard
   b. access to a large population, both well and ill.
3. Working in partnership with individual patients:
   a. the expert patient and the contribution of district nurses to patients managing their own conditions and educating others.

References

Arnold, P., Topping, A., Honey, S., et al., 2004. Exploring the contribution of district nurses to public health. British Journal of Community Nursing 9, 216–223.

Bowden, J., 2006. Health promotion and the midwife. In: Bowden, J., Manning, V. (Eds.), Health Promotion in Midwifery, second ed. Hodder Arnold, London, pp. 13–24.

Bunton, R., Wills, J., 2005. War and public health. Critical Public Health 15, 79–81.

Coote, A., 2002. Claiming the Health Dividend: Unlocking the Benefits of NHS Spending. Kings Fund, London. Available online at: http://www.kingsfund.org.uk/sites/files/kf/field/field_publication_file/claiming-health-dividend-unlocking-benefits-nhs-spending-summary-anna-coote-kings-fund-1-may-2002_0.pdf (accessed 25.02.15).

Darzi, A., 2007. Healthcare for London: A Framework for Action. NHS London, London. Available online at: http://www.nhshistory.net/darzilondon.pdf (accessed 25.02.15).

Department of Health, 2001. The Report of the Chief Medical Officer's Project to Strengthen the Public Health Function. Department of Health, London. Available online at: http://webarchive.nationalarchives.gov.uk/+/www.dh.gov.uk/en/Publicationsandstatistics/Publications/PublicationsPolicyAndGuidance/DH_4062358 (accessed 25.02.15).

Department of Health, 2004. Choosing Health: making healthy choices easier. Department of Health, London. Available online at: http://webarchive.nationalarchives.gov.uk/+/dh.gov.uk/en/publicationsandstatistics/publications/publicationspolicyandguidance/dh_4094550 (accessed 14.09.15).

Department of Health, 2008. Pharmacy in England: Building on Strengths – Delivering the Future Cm 7341. TSO, London. Available online at: www.gov.uk/government/uploads/system/uploads/attachment_data/file/228858/7341.pdf (accessed 25.02.15).

Department of Health, 2012. The Public Health Outcomes Framework for England 2013-2016. Available online at: https://www.gov.uk/government/uploads/system/uploads/attachment_data/file/216159/dh_132362.pdf (accessed 20/01/16).

HSCIS, 2013. Monthly Hospital Episode Statistics for Admitted Patient Care, Outpatients and Accident and Emergency Data April 2012–March 2013. Information Centre, London.

Krogsboll, L.T., Jorgensen, K.J., Gronhoj Larsen, C., Gotzsche, P.C., 2012. General health checks in adults for reducing morbidity and mortality from disease. Cochrane Database of Systematic Reviews 10, CD009009.

Levy, S.B., Sidel, W., 2002. The health and social consequences of diversion of economic resources to war and preparation for war. In: Taipale, I. (Ed.), War or Health? a Reader. Zed Books, London.

MacAuley, D., 2012. The value of conducting periodic health checks. BMJ 345, e7775.

Maryon-Davis, A., 2005. Weight management in primary care: how can it be made more effective? Proceedings of the Nutrition Society 64, 97–103.

Matthews, P., Fletcher, J., 2001. Sexually transmitted infections in primary care: a need for education. British Journal of General Practice 51, 52–56. Available online at: bjgp.org/content/bjgp/51/462/52.full.pdf (accessed 14.09.15).

McNeil, J., Lyn, F., Alderdyce, F., 2012. Public health interventions in midwifery: a systematic review of systematic reviews. BMC Public Health 12, 955. Available online at: http://www.biomed-central.com/1471-2458/12/955 (accessed 25.02.15).

Murray, C.J., Lopez, A.D., 1997. Mortality by cause for eight regions of the world: Global Burden of Disease study. Lancet 349, 1269–1276.

Naidoo, J., Wills, J., 2010. Public Health and Health Promotion: Developing Practice, third ed. Baillière Tindall, London.

Needle, J., Petchey, R., Benson, J., Scriven, A., Lawrenson, J., Hilari, K., 2011. The Allied Health Professions and Health Promotion: A Systematic Literature Review and Narrative Synthesis. Final report NIHR Service Delivery and Organisation programme. Available online at: http://www.nets.nihr.ac.uk/__data/assets/pdf_file/0004/82399/ES-08-1716-205.pdf (accessed 25.02.15).

Popay, J., Kowarzik, U., Mallinson, S., et al., 2007. Social problems, primary care and pathways to help and support: addressing health inequalities at the individual level: the GP perspective. Journal of Epidemiology and Community Health 61, 966–971.

Wanless, D., 2002. Securing Our Future Health. Taking a Long Term View. HM Treasury, London. Available online at: http://webarchive.nationalarchives.gov.uk/+/http://www.hm-treasury.gov.uk/consult_wanless_final.htm (accessed 25.02.15).

Wanless, D., Appleby, J., Harrison, A., et al., 2007. Our Future Health Secured? Kings Fund, London.

Wise, M., Nutbeam, D., 2007. Enabling health systems transformation: what progress has been made to re-orienting health services? Promotion & Education (Suppl 2), 23–28.

World Health Organization, 1946. Constitution. WHO, Geneva. Available online at: http://www.who.int/governance/eb/who_constitution_en.pdf (accessed 25.02.15).

World Health Organization, 1978. In: Declaration of Alma Ata, International Conference on Primary Health Care, Alma Ata, 6–12 September. World Health Organization, Geneva. Available online at: http://www.who.int/publications/almaata_declaration_en.pdf (accessed 25.02.15).

World Health Organization, 1986. Ottawa Charter for Health Promotion. Journal of Health Promotion 1, 1–4. Available online at: http://www.who.int/healthpromotion/conferences/previous/ottawa/en/ (accessed 25.02.15).

World Health Organization, 2000. The World Health Report 2000 Health Systems: Improving Performance. WHO, Geneva. Available online at: http://www.who.int/whr/2000/en/ (accessed 27.02.15).

World Health Organization, 2007. Challenging Inequity through Health Systems. Final report. Knowledge network on health systems. WHO, Geneva. Available online at: http://www.who.int/social_determinants/resources/csdh_media/hskn_final_2007_en.pdf (accessed 25 02 15).

Ziglio, E., Simpson, S., Tsouros, A., 2011. Health promotion and health systems: some unfinished business. Health Promotion International 26 (Suppl 2), ii216–ii225.

Chapter **Nine**

9

Developing personal skills

Learning Outcomes

By the end of this chapter you will be able to:
- discuss the relative roles of knowledge, attitudes and skills in behaviour change
- discuss the influence of social norms on health behaviour
- understand a range of models that can be applied to understanding influences on health-related decision-making and behaviour.

Key Concepts and Definitions

Behaviour change involves actions to change health-related behaviour, for example, smoking. Action may be at the individual, household, community or population level.

Health psychology is a discipline that seeks to understand the psychological and behavioural processes in health, illness and healthcare.

Attitudes involves how a person feels about something, including affective and cognitive components.

Self-efficacy is a person's belief in his or her ability to succeed.

Social norms are the behaviours and beliefs appropriate for a social group.

Locus of control is a person's belief in the control she or he has over her or his life.

Empowerment is a process through which people gain greater control over their lives and health.

Motivational interviewing is a counselling technique used to assess motivation to change.

Brief intervention is a short, time-limited intervention to raise awareness of a lifestyle issue, and assess a person's willingness to address it.

Importance of the Topic

People's health behaviours or lifestyles have been regarded as the cause of many modern diseases, thus a main focus of health promotion has been on modifying those aspects of behaviour which are known to have an impact on health. In previous chapters we have argued that such an approach is unlikely to be effective unless it acknowledges how people's behaviour may be a response to, and maintained by, the environment in which they live. Many health promoters, however, see their role as helping people to live their lives to their best potential, which may involve some change in their health behaviour.

This chapter is concerned with those aspects of health behaviour that people can control. Understanding why people behave in certain ways and how they can be helped to maintain chosen behaviours is central to self-empowerment. The chapter explores the usefulness of social psychology, which offers several theoretical models that identify the determinants of behaviour change. These can contribute to if not the prediction then at least an understanding of how people make decisions about their health, and can be a useful tool in planning health promotion interventions. The influence of specific factors such as individual self-esteem or people's perceptions of control over their lives needs to be taken into account by the health promoter in order to offer practical support and positive experiences in making choices.

Empowerment is a term much used in health promotion. It is a complex concept that encompasses various levels of working for change:

- individual, working *with* people to develop confidence and control
- community (see Chapter 10)
- organizational (see Part Three), to create supportive environments.

Enabling people to change is often assumed by health promoters simply to mean health education covering those things the clinician or health promoter regards as important, with compliance as the goal. Client-centred health promotion, by contrast, is concerned with a person's agency in decision-making. Such an approach acknowledges that people can take some control over their lives through knowledge, skills and confidence, and it may enable people to identify structural barriers and facilitators to their health. This kind of empowering education was described by Paolo Freire in his approach to radical adult literacy pedagogy (see Chapter 10). Frequently, however, developing personal skills is equated with helping people to change, drawing on psychological theories of behaviour change, motivation and self-efficacy. Increasingly, techniques such as motivational interviewing, which draw upon such theories, are used.

Several theories have attempted to explain the influence of different variables on an individual's health-related behaviour:

- the health belief model (Becker, 1974)
- the theory of reasoned action (Ajzen and Fishbein, 1980)
- the stages of change model (Prochaska and DiClemente, 1984).

This chapter explores the application of these models of behaviour change to health, and considers how an understanding of cognition and decision-making can be incorporated into empowerment and education strategies.

Definitions

According to social psychology theories of behaviour change, people's behaviour is partly determined by their attitude to that behaviour. An individual's *attitude* to a specific action and the intention to adopt it are influenced by *beliefs*, motivation which comes from the person's *values*, *attitudes* and *drives* or instincts, and the influences from social norms.

Beliefs

A belief is based on the information a person has about an object or action. It links the object to some attribute. For example, a person believes that potatoes (object) are fattening (an attribute). Theories of health-related behaviour change are based on the idea that an individual's behaviour will be based on his or her beliefs. In this example, the person will cut down on potatoes if he or she wishes to lose weight. If this person is encouraged to believe that potatoes are not fattening but a useful bulk food, then he or she may include them in the diet. In other words, information can influence attitudes and beliefs, which will in turn influence behaviour. This simple model is sometimes referred to as the knowledge–attitudes–behaviour model. Of course, behaviour change is never quite as simple as that. Information alone is neither necessary nor sufficient for behaviour change. The health risks of smoking are well known, and yet nearly 30% of the UK population continue to smoke.

Values

Values are acquired through socialization, and are those emotionally charged beliefs which make up what a person thinks is important. A person's values will influence a whole range of feelings about family, friendships, career and so on. For example, values relating to sex and gender give rise to a number of attitudes towards motherhood, employment of women, body image, breastfeeding and sexuality.

Attitudes

These are more specific than values, and describe relatively stable feelings towards particular issues. There is no clear association between people's attitudes and their behaviour. Sometimes changing attitudes may stimulate a change in behaviour, and sometimes behaviour change may influence attitudes. For example, many people continue to smoke despite a negative attitude to smoking; yet once the behaviour is stopped, they may develop vehement anti-smoking views.

People's attitudes are made up of two components.
1. Cognitive – the knowledge and information they possess.
2. Affective – their feelings and emotions and evaluation of what is important.

Attitudes are very hard to change, but may be changed by providing more or different information or by increasing a person's skills. For example, providing information about different types of physical activity and their effects on the body might influence a person's attitude towards the benefits of exercise. It might also be influenced by improved performance, which motivates the person and encourages him or her to think of exercise as enjoyable.

Festinger (1957) used the term *cognitive dissonance* to describe a person's mental state when new information is given which is counter to that already held. This prompts the person either to reject the new information (as unreliable or inappropriate) or to adopt attitudes and behaviour which would fit with it.

 Learning Activity 9.1 Health risks and behaviour

How do people respond to information about the risks to their health from particular behaviours?

Drives

The term 'drive' is used in the health action model (Green et al., 2015) to describe strong motivating factors such as hunger, thirst, sex and pain. It is also used to describe motivations which can become drives, such as addiction. Addiction can be seen as a consequence of frequently repeated acts which become a habit, and its base is a psychological fear of withdrawal. Social learning theory (Bandura, 1977) uses the term *instinct* to describe behaviours which are not learned but are present at birth. Instincts can override attitudes and beliefs. Hunger, for example, can easily override a person's favourable attitude and intention to diet.

Understanding the impact of people's beliefs in their behaviour is key to addressing those issues. Take the example of smoking.

- If you regard smoking as an addiction (50% of smokers have a cigarette within 30 minutes of waking), then the aim is to help the individual gain control.
- If you regard smoking as a learned behaviour which smokers associate with specific actions and rewards (confidence, less stress), then the aim is to restructure thinking and activities to avoid potentially stressful situations.
- If you regard smoking as having a social meaning (e.g. young women see smoking as providing status), then the aim is to clarify such associations.

 Learning Activity 9.2 Skills and behaviour change

What personal skills are needed to take greater control over one's health? Consider this in relation to a change of behaviour you have made.

Practitioners need to understand what contributes to people's decision-making about health and what makes some people more amenable to change than others. The social cognition models that we shall now consider highlight the following as important.

- People's views about the cause and prevention of ill health.
- The extent to which people feel they can control their life and make changes.

- Whether they believe change is necessary.
- Whether change is perceived to be beneficial in the long term, outweighing any difficulties and problems which may be involved.

 Learning Activity 9.3 The gap between knowledge and behaviour

How do you explain consistent findings in many studies that show a gap between knowledge and behaviour change? For example, there is a high awareness of the impact of transport on climate change, yet only a small minority act on this knowledge by, for instance, giving up their cars.

The following theoretical models try to unpack the relative importance of these factors, recognizing that what people say is not necessarily a guide to what they will do, and that there are numerous antecedent and situational variables.

The health belief model

The health belief model is probably the best-known theoretical model highlighting the function of beliefs in decision-making (Fig. 9.1).

This model, originally proposed by Rosenstock (1966) and modified by Becker (1974), has been used to predict protective health behaviour, such as screening or vaccination uptake and compliance with medical advice (e.g. Gillam, 1991). The model suggests that whether or not people change their behaviour will be influenced by an evaluation of the change's feasibility and its benefits weighed against its costs. In other words, people considering changing their behaviour engage in a cost–benefit or utility analysis. This may include their beliefs concerning the likelihood of the illness or injury happening to them (their susceptibility); the severity of the illness or injury; and the efficacy of the action and whether it will have some personal benefit, or how likely it is to protect the person from the illness or injury.

For a behaviour change to take place, individuals:
- must have an incentive to change
- feel threatened by their current behaviour

- feel a change would be beneficial in some way and have few adverse consequences
- must feel competent to carry out the change.

 Learning Activity 9.4 Applying the health belief model to immunization intentions

Consider the following situation, and then try to apply the health belief model to see if you can predict how the woman might respond.

A mother of three children under five receives a card from her GP informing her that her oldest child should receive a pre-school booster against diphtheria, tetanus, whooping cough and polio. The woman works full time at a local factory as an hourly paid packer. Her mother cares for the children while she is at work, but has no transport.

Most learning theories are based on the premise that people's behaviour is guided by consequences. If these are positive or deemed to be positive, the person is more likely to engage in that behaviour. These explanations, which see behaviour as a simple response to positive or negative rewards, do not seem to account for the persistence of health behaviours which have apparently negative consequences, such as smoking or drinking and driving. However, it is frequently the case that short-term gratification is a greater incentive than possible long-term harm.

Becker (1974) suggests that individuals are influenced by how vulnerable they perceive themselves to be to an illness, injury or danger (their *susceptibility*) and how serious they consider it to be (*severity*). People's perception and assessment of risk are central to the application of this model. Most people make a rough assessment about whether they are at risk. This seems to be influenced by four factors.

1. Personal experience.
2. Ability to control the situation.
3. A feeling that the illness or danger is rare.
4. Any outcomes are in the distant future.

Where a situation is not well known, however, people have an unrealistic optimism that 'it won't happen to me' (Weinstein, 1984).

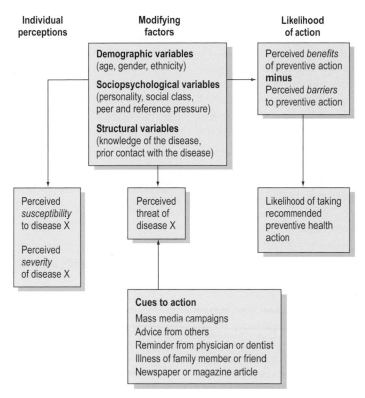

Fig. 9.1 ● The health belief model. (From Becker, M.H. (Ed.), 1974. The Health Belief Model and Personal Health Behaviour. Slack, Thorofare, New Jersey.)

Learning Activity 9.5 Applying behaviour change theory

There are over 250,000 traffic accidents each year with 30,000 casualties, of which 3400 are fatalities. Excess speed is a contributory factor in a significant number of road accidents. In one survey (Scottish Office, 1998) 88% of drivers admitted to driving at 40 mph in a 30 mph zone at least sometimes. The current response to speeding is:

- traffic calming
- police enforcement
- media campaigns, for example, 'speed kills'.

How might an understanding of social cognitions help to target a strategy for safer driving?

Since beliefs may be affected by experience, direct contact with those who have a condition can powerfully affect attitudes, exposing stereotypes and preju-dice. For example, contact with a person who is human immunodeficiency virus (HIV) positive or who is living with acquired immunodeficiency syndrome (AIDS) can change beliefs about the fatality of the disease, and about who is affected and how. Those who work with young people find perceptions of risk are very differ-ent. Risk taking is an important task of adolescence and part of separation from the family. It is hard for young people to appreciate the long-term effects of, for example, smoking when 25 can seem old.

Many health education campaigns have attempted to motivate people to change their behaviour through fear or guilt. Drink-drive campaigns at Christmas show the devastating effects on families of road accident fatalities; smoking-prevention posters urge parents not to 'teach your children how to smoke'. Increas-ingly hard-hitting campaigns are used to raise aware-ness of the consequences of binge drinking, smoking and drug use. Whether such campaigns do succeed in shocking people to change their behaviour is the subject of ongoing debate (see e.g. Hill et al., 1998). Although fear can encourage a negative attitude and even an intention to change, such feelings tend to disappear over time and when faced with a real decision-making situation. Being very frightened can also lead to denial and an avoidance of the message. Protection motivation theory (Rogers, 1975) suggests that fear only works if the threat is perceived as serious and likely to occur if the person does not follow the recommended advice (see also Chapter 12).

The health belief model suggests that people need to have some kind of cue to take action to change a behaviour or make a health-related decision. The issue needs to become salient or relevant. The cue could be noticing a change in one's internal state or appearance. For example, a pregnant woman stops smoking when she feels the baby move. It could be an external trigger, such as altered circumstances from a change in job or income, or the death or illness of someone close. It could be a comment from a 'significant other' or a newspaper article. Healthcare workers can be significant others. For example, GPs' advice is taken seriously. The GP has expertise, is trustworthy and has authority, leading the patient to wish to comply. The effects of persuasive communications on attitudes are discussed more fully in Chapter 12 on mass media.

 Learning Activity 9.6 Applying the health belief model to sexual health behaviour

According to the 2014 Gay Men's Sexual Health Survey in Scotland (Sigma Research, 2014 – http://gaymensurvey.sphsu.mrc.ac.uk/home.html), 50% of sexually active gay men had unprotected anal sex in the previous year. A total of 40% of gay men were unaware of their own HIV status.

- Consider how the health belief model could be used to explain this health behaviour.
- What reasons could you offer for individuals not carrying out their intentions to act in ways that are perceived as beneficial?

The health belief model has been widely criticized. Some of these criticisms relate to its lack of weighting for different factors – all cues to preventive action, for example, are seen as equally salient. It may appear that complex behaviour and actions are informed and chosen via analysis of a set of conceptual components that are isolated from one another. What we have seen so far is that behaviour is far more nuanced, with many different interwoven arguments and scripts. The model may not be particularly helpful in predicting behaviour or identifying those elements that are important in influencing people to change, but it does highlight the range and complexity of factors involved.

Theory of reasoned action and theory of planned behaviour

According to the theory of reasoned action (Ajzen and Fishbein, 1980), behaviour is dependent on two variables.

1. Attitudes – beliefs about the consequences of the behaviour, and an appraisal of the positive and negative aspects of making a change.
2. Subjective norms – what 'significant others' do and expect, and the degree to which the person wants to conform and be like others.

These two influences combine to form an intention.

Ajzen and Fishbein (1980) acknowledge that people do not necessarily behave consistently with their intentions. The ability to predict behaviour will be influenced by the stability of a person's belief. Stability is determined by strength of belief, how long it has been held, whether it is reinforced by other groups to which the individual belongs, whether it is related to and integrated with other attitudes and beliefs and how clear or structured it is. The theory of reasoned action differs from the health belief model in that it places importance on social norms as a major influence on behaviour.

Figure 9.2 shows the significance of this factor in the theory of reasoned action. Social pressure may be exerted through societal norms (such as those relating to weight and body image), community norms, the peer group and the beliefs of 'significant others' (such as parents or partners).

The motivation to comply with perceived social pressure from 'significant others' could cause individuals to behave in a way that they believe these other people or groups would think is right. The influence

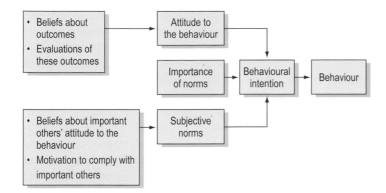

Fig. 9.2 ● The theory of reasoned action. (From Ajzen, I., Fishbein, M., 1980. Understanding Attitudes and Predicting Social Behaviour. Prentice Hall, Englewood Cliffs.)

of so-called peer-group pressure (even if it does not amount to pressure) can be very powerful within a small group if the individual values membership of that group or wants to belong to it. Young people have many potential social pressures and increased social competition due to internet websites such as Facebook, and are exposed to marketing and advertising that may encourage early adoption of a teen lifestyle.

The role of modelling has been particularly important in health promotion. Concern has been expressed that there is indirect modelling of behaviour depicted in the media. For example, people on television are able to drink heavily without any apparent ill effects (Hansen, 2003). Direct modelling is sometimes assumed to be less influential, but models who have status and credibility, such as musicians and people in sport, have been used to present health promotion messages. If people are influenced by role models, then health promoters may themselves be taken as exemplars.

Learning Activity 9.7 Health promoters as role models

- Should health promoters 'practise what they preach'?
- Think of some examples where practitioners' behaviour may be at odds with the health improvement they wish to promote.

Some health promotion programmes use the influence of the peer group to promote positive health.

The rationale is that peers may be seen as having more credibility, are able to communicate in appropriate ways and are models to follow, although doubts may be expressed about the skills and information that peer educators possess (Wilton et al., 1995; Harden et al., 1999).

Social norms are the beliefs that people hold about how health behaviours are practised or how common they are in society or among family and friends, for example, the consumption of fruit, vegetables and sweets among pre-school children. What is important is what the individual believes other people do, not the actual extent of the activity.

Research Example 9.1 Non-suicidal self-injury

Non-suicidal self-injury (NSSI), or self-harm, is an increasingly prevalent health behaviour among adolescents. Considerable research has been conducted to understand potential risk factors that may motivate or reinforce adolescents' engagement in NSSI. This research refers to 'peer contagion' effects on a variety of other health-risk behaviours, and suggests that given the salience of peer relationships in adolescence, peer influence may be implicated in the emergence and maintenance of NSSI. Discussions of NSSI and methods and feelings are popular on the internet, and serve as an information source. Social learning theory predicts that individuals may conform to behaviours that they believe will earn them high levels of peer status. NSSI is seen as a means of emotional regulation and, if associated with high-status peers, may be adopted (Heilbron and Prinstein, 2008).

Group techniques, such as those used by Alcoholics Anonymous, appear to have some success by getting clients to identify with the group through personal testimony and a public commitment, which encourages the group members to provide support for each other.

Bandura's (1977) social learning theory suggests that the health choices people make are related to:

- outcome expectancies (whether an action will lead to a particular outcome)
- self-efficacy (whether people believe they can change).

Perceptions of self-efficacy are based on people's assessment of themselves – whether they have the knowledge and skills to make changes in their behaviour, and whether external factors such as time and money will allow that change.

 Learning Activity 9.8 Self-efficacy

How might observing others' behaviour influence our own? To what extent does believing we can do something enable us to do it?

Self-efficacy is determined by:

- our previous experiences of success and failure (e.g. having lost weight before)
- relevant vicarious experiences (e.g. seeing someone else lose weight)
- verbal/social persuasion (e.g. being told you can do it)
- emotional arousal (e.g. being scared).

Personal judgement of worth, expressed in the attitudes people hold towards themselves, is also part of a sense of self-efficacy. We talk of high or low self-esteem in the sense of feeling more or less worthwhile and valued. Self-concept is a global term which refers to all those beliefs which people have about themselves and their abilities and attributes. It includes ideas about appearance, intelligence and physical skills. It is built and modified through our perceptions of the way other people behave towards us, how we are accepted and affirmed or rejected and criticized. It will thus also derive from having a network of social support.

The development of self-concept and self-esteem has been at the centre of work in health education and promotion. It is assumed that people with high self-esteem are likely to feel confident about themselves and have social and life skills which will enhance their feelings of personal efficacy. Because of these feelings of personal effectiveness, the person's self-esteem is enhanced. Many health education programmes, particularly those targeted at young people, have been based on the premise that there is a relationship between low self-esteem and harmful health behaviours.

 Research Example 9.2 Drug use and young people

A review of research studies (Frisher et al., 2007) found that the key predictors of drug use are parental discipline and family cohesion, rather than psychological factors. Male gender and older age are associated with higher levels of drug use. Pupils' school behaviour (e.g. truancy, poor attendance) is linked to drug use. What is clear from the many studies included in the review is the diversity of factors influencing drug use, reflecting the complexity of the social environment and the situational determinants. There appears to be little consensus on the value of drug education.

As shown in the research studies on drug use among young people, personal or 'micro' factors are played out in many issues of choice, and real-life decision-making is often not a rational process. A study of HIV-positive people and sex (Ridge et al., 2007) found that although they may have the intention to use a condom, 'irrational feelings' such as intimacy, trust and desire could all influence perceptions of risk.

Ajzen (1991) further developed the theory of reasoned action, and recast it as the theory of planned behaviour (Fig. 9.3). This model incorporated another variable – that people's behaviour is a consequence of their perceived control. People differ in the extent to which they think they can make changes in their lives. Social learning theory suggests that the ways in which people explain the things that happen to them are a product of their childhood experiences. Those

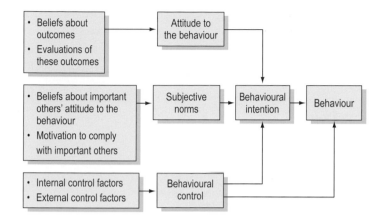

Fig. 9.3 ● The theory of planned behaviour. (From Ajzen, I., 1991. The theory of planned behaviour. Organisational Behaviour and Human Decision Processes 50, 179–211.)

who are rewarded for their successes and punished consistently and fairly will come to believe that they are in control of their lives. Those who have inconsistent rewards or punishments irrespective of their behaviour are more likely to see events as a consequence of chance and their own role as irrelevant (Rotter, 1954).

Control in the context of health can be understood in terms of:

- internal locus of control (the extent to which individuals believe that they are responsible for their own health)
- external locus of control (people who believe that their actions are influenced by powerful others, chance, fate or luck).

Research has focused on categorizing attitudes to health by using a locus of control measure such as a multiple-choice inventory. It has been assumed that those who have a strong internal locus of control will see themselves as more coping and more able to act decisively and capably, and will be those people who undertake preventive health actions or change to more healthy behaviours. So far it has generally been found that there is only a weak relationship between feelings of control and specific behaviours, although associations have been found with smoking cessation and weight loss and the propensity to use preventive medical services (Wallston et al., 1978). Indeed, a lifestyle survey of 9000 adults found that 'unhealthy' kinds of behaviour are more likely to be associated with an internal locus of control (Blaxter, 1990). At the

same time, those who recorded positive or responsible attitudes to health were also more likely to have a high internal locus of control. This confirms the argument earlier in this chapter that specific behaviour cannot necessarily be predicted from attitudes.

People who register as 'externals' on the multidimensional health locus of control scale are those with lower levels of education and of lower socioeconomic class – in other words, people who have every reason to believe that they do not have much control over their lives or health status.

Figure 9.4 is a diagrammatic representation of some of the influences on a person's decision to take up an exercise programme. It shows how confidence to participate in physical activity could be built through positive attributions such as fitness, weight loss and successful performance. Social support networks will also be crucial in maintaining commitment.

The stages of change model

So far in this chapter we have discussed the factors influencing the decisions people make in relation to their health.

Prochaska and DiClemente's (1984, 1986; Prochaska et al., 1992) transtheoretical model is important in describing the process of change. The model derived from their work on encouraging change in people with addictive behaviours, although it can be

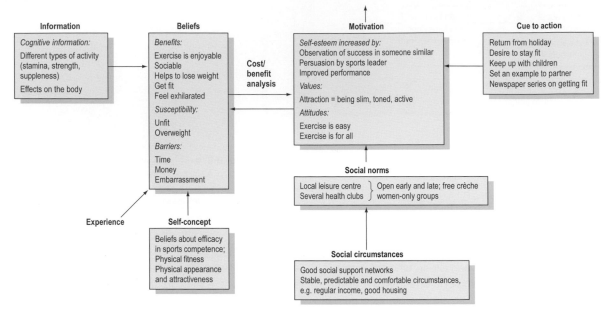

Fig. 9.4 ● Health-related behaviour change: the example of exercise in women.

used to show that most people go through stages when trying to change or acquire behaviours.

Figure 9.5 illustrates this process and identifies the following stages.

Pre-contemplation

Those in the pre-contemplation stage have not considered changing their lifestyle or become aware of any potential risks in their health behaviour. When they become aware of a problem, they may progress to the next stage. Assessing a client's readiness to change is a key first step.

Contemplation

Although individuals are aware of the benefits of change, they are not yet ready and may be seeking information or help to make that decision. This stage may last a short while or several years. Some people never progress beyond this stage.

Preparing to change

When the perceived benefits seem to outweigh the costs and when the change seems possible as well as worthwhile, the individual may be ready to change, perhaps seeking some extra support.

Making the change

The early days of change require positive decisions by the individual to do things differently. A clear goal, a realistic plan, support and rewards are features of this stage.

Maintenance

The new behaviour is sustained and the person moves into a healthier lifestyle. For some people maintaining

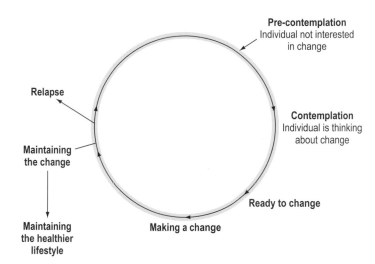

Pre-contemplation
Individual not interested
in change

Contemplation
Individual is thinking
about change

Relapse

**Maintaining
the change**

Ready to change

**Maintaining
the healthier
lifestyle**

Making a change

Fig. 9.5 ● The stages of change model. (Adapted from Prochaska, J.O., DiClemente, C., 1984. The Transtheoretical Approach: Crossing Traditional Foundations of Change. Don Jones/Irwin, Harnewood, IL.)

the new behaviour is difficult, and they may revert or relapse back to any of the previous stages.

Change is not a smooth process. While few people go through each stage in an orderly way, they will go through each stage if they make a change. This has proved helpful for many healthcare workers, who find it reassuring that a relapse on the part of a client is not a failure, but that the individual can go both backwards and forwards through a series of cycles of change – like a revolving door. Thus a smoker may stop smoking many times before finally giving up completely. Nevertheless, the client is still aware of the benefits of giving up smoking and healthcare workers may be able to focus on such small changes, which can give both them and their clients a sense of achievement and identifiable progress. While individuals may not have an awareness of contemplating, actioning and maintaining change, their intention will be based on deciding that it is in their best interests to change. The key to successful interventions is thus for a client to be motivated. Health promoters must bear in mind that their clients may not share their perceptions about the worth of a particular behaviour.

The Com B model (Michie et al., 2011; Fig. 9.6) is a simple model to understand behaviour which identifies the following.

- Capability: the psychological or physical ability to enact the behaviour. Capability can be encouraged by education or modelling.

- Motivation: the reflective or automatic mechanisms that activate or inhibit the behaviour. Motivation can be encouraged by incentives, persuasion and training.
- Opportunity: the physical and social environment that enables the behaviour. Opportunity can be provided by fiscal measures, regulations or service provision.

Helping people to change

Health promoters may use a range of methods to support people in changing:
- information giving
- education
- counselling.
  The aim of all these methods is to discuss:
- any concerns people may have with their health
- what needs they have, whether for information or for support
- what other influences there may be on their health that may be a barrier to change
- what changes they may wish to make.

If people feel more in control of their lives, they are more likely to feel enabled to make health choices and empowered to take part in their own health decision-making. Poor information giving is a common source of patient dissatisfaction. A health promoter has to be able to give information in a manner that is acceptable, understandable, coherent, contemporaneous

157

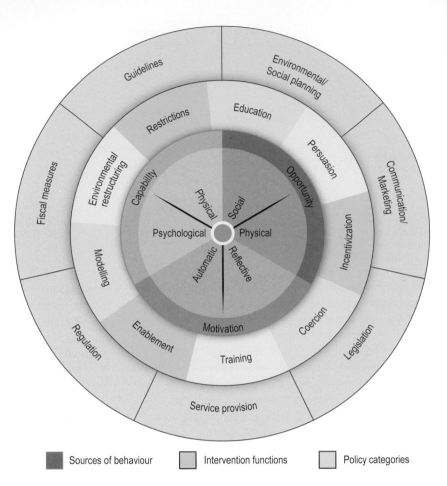

Fig. 9.6 ● The behaviour change wheel. (Michie, S., Van Stralen, M., West, R., 2011. The behaviour change wheel: A new method for characterizing and designing behaviour change interventions. Implementation Science 6, 42. Available online at: www.implementationscience. com/content/pdf/1748-5908-6-42.pdf. © 2011 Michie et al; licensee BioMed Central Ltd. This is an Open Access article distributed under the terms of the Creative Commons Attribution License [http://creativeco mmons.org/licenses/by/2.0], which permits unrestricted use, distribution, and reproduction in any medium, provided the original work is properly cited.)

and evidence-based. Written information may be used to reinforce verbal information. The presentation of health information should be understandable, accurate, acceptable (as much as possible), visually appealing, clear and precise.

Ewles et al. (2010) devised a checklist to help health promoters to appraise health promotion leaflets.

- Is the leaflet brief and to the point?
- Does the leaflet emphasize the key points?
- Does the leaflet use language that is easy to understand?
- Are the words and images easy to see?
- Is the design of the leaflet visually appealing, for example, colour, images and size?
- How could you use the leaflet to make an effective display?

Educational approaches to health promotion are important (see Chapter 4) because they aim not merely to give people information but to give them an informed choice and help them to acquire knowledge and skills in order to make that choice. Counselling approaches aim to work with a person in relation to his or her own health agenda. They place the individual at the centre of the intervention, and the health promoter takes on the role of facilitator and empowerer. They will enable patients to decide on their own course of health action and support them in this, rather than setting the health agenda.

Motivational interviewing is a specific technique, originally developed for use with addictive behaviours, with a non-directive counselling style. It starts with an exploration of the clients' readiness to change (in keeping with the transtheoretical model of

Table 9.1 Using client-directed counselling techniques

Do	Don't
• Summarize your understanding of the client's thoughts and feelings	• Interrupt or finish sentences
• Look and sound interested	• Advise or tell the client what to do
• Keep eye contact and use positive body language	• Disagree or contradict (raise alternatives)
• See things from the client's point of view	• Project your own beliefs or feelings onto the client
• Ask open questions to get more information	• Assume your experiences are the same as the client's
• Be curious rather than intrusive	• Constantly repeat the same paraphrases, e.g. 'it sounds like' or 'you feel like'
• Give the client time to think as well as talk	• Pretend you understand if you don't – ask for more explanation
• Respond to what the client is saying rather than trying to lead the conversation	

From Michie et al. (2006).

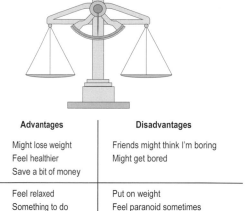

	Advantages	Disadvantages
Changing my behaviour	Might lose weight Feel healthier Save a bit of money	Friends might think I'm boring Might get bored
Not changing my behaviour	Feel relaxed Something to do Be with my friends Sleep well	Put on weight Feel paranoid sometimes Argue with friends and family Smoker's cough

Fig. 9.7 ● Exploring ambivalence about cannabis use.

change) and how important change or the behaviour is to the person (Miller and Rollnick, 2002). Central to this technique is the view that motivation is enhanced if the person articulates for himself/herself the costs and benefits of change. The person's confidence that change can happen is bolstered by support, discussion of barriers and negotiated action plans.

The health promoter uses open questions and interventions borrowed from counselling techniques to encourage the person to develop these elements, often in brief interventions of 5 to 10 minutes. Table 9.1 illustrates some of the core techniques that should be adopted.

The intervention follows a series of stages.
● Establishing rapport

The health promoter uses questions to encourage patients to examine their knowledge about their health behaviour and the extent to which they want to change. There may be a discrepancy between what is happening at present and what the person values for the future, and the importance of a change can then be emphasized.
● Exploring ambivalence

One of the principles of motivational interviewing is that people feel some ambivalence about their health behaviour. There is a common and natural experience of feeling torn between wanting and not wanting to do something, for example, the desire to give up smoking but the desire not to put on weight. Resolving ambivalence can be a key to change. Attempts to force a person in a particular direction through direct persuasion, or by making her or him frightened of the consequences, can lead to a paradoxical response and even strengthen the behaviour. One way of helping a person to become clearer is to use a decision-balance matrix in which the person works out for himself/herself the costs and benefits of changing or not changing his or her behaviour. Figure 9.7 illustrates this in relation to cannabis use.
● Assessing the patient's readiness to change

This assessment is based on the cost-benefit analysis and how important a change seems to the person and his/her confidence in being able to make the change, for example, do the advantages outweigh the disadvantages? A scaling question might be used: 'On a scale of one to ten how able do you feel to make a change?' Sometimes the person may be willing but not feel able to make a change.
● Developing an action plan

Even when the person may see the importance of a change and has the confidence to do so, it may not be top of his or her priorities: 'I want to, but not now'. Relative priorities are part of normal functioning: low readiness can be viewed as the person needing information about what the next step is towards change. Motivational interviewing is about negotiation and working with people to devise a health action plan if they are ready to change.

- Setting goals

Motivational interviewing is about goal setting, which should be realistic, specific and measurable, and not too ambitious or have unrealistic outcomes. For example, a person's aim may be to drink sensibly; his/her objectives may be that he/she reduces the number of times a week that he/she consumes alcohol and the amount of alcohol he/she drinks.

Such client-centred approaches arguably need specific characteristics, which Carl Rogers (1951) called core qualities, on the part of the health promoter. These core qualities help clients to have a therapeutic relationship with the health promoter, and include the following.

- Unconditional positive regard – acceptance of people irrespective of their condition, age, gender, culture, ethnicity, socio-economic background, expressed thoughts, behaviours or beliefs. The person should not be judged by any set of rules or standards. Health promoters must set aside their own values and beliefs, biases and prejudices in order to help their patients. This acceptance should not be confused with liking or approval.
- Genuineness or congruence – this means being oneself or being true and sincere, being non-defensive and free in behaviour and being real. The health promoter would therefore use his/her own language and own behaviour and be genuine.
- Empathy – this means being able to appreciate meanings and understand the world as seen through the eyes of the patient or client.

Thus the focus of the intervention is to take on board the person's 'frame of reference', endeavour to understand her/him and her/his circumstances, and enable and encourage the patient to take responsibility for her/his own health decisions and actions. Self-empowerment approaches have at their centre the principle of participation. These techniques allow people to examine their own values and beliefs;

explore the factors that affect the choices they make; and develop the skills to act upon their intentions. Rogers (1951) argues that if all this is in place then behaviour change is more likely to happen.

Case Study 9.1 Making Every Contact Count

Making Every Contact Count (MECC) is an English national initiative originally developed in 2009 by NHS Yorkshire and Humber to extend radically the delivery of public health advice to the public. MECC works by training non-specialist staff from a wide range of service organizations in the basic skills of health promotion and prevention, thus creating an 'extended sales force for healthier living' (Ion, 2011). In Wigan, for example, a 'Making Health Everyone's Business' workstream has been embedded within key organizations, including Bridgewater community healthcare, children's centre and nursery provision, Greater Manchester Fire & Rescue, Greater Manchester Police, Wigan Council's Adult Social Care, Economic Regeneration and Environmental Services departments, and a range of voluntary sector partners.

A range of training materials is available for those wishing to develop skills to practise MECC. They enable participants to:

- recognize opportunities to deliver key messages about adopting a healthy lifestyle, and overcome any personal barriers to MECC
- provide appropriate lifestyle advice confidently
- understand the relevance of MECC to their role
- understand where to find additional information. Freely available education resources include:
- Royal College of Nurses behaviour change e-learning tool which supports delivery of MECC, http://www.rcn.org.uk/development/practice/cpd_online_learning/support_behaviour_change.
- Yorkshire and Humber e-learning tool, http://www.makingeverycontactcount.co.uk/Training%20and%20Resources/eLearning.html.
- local authority e-learning module, developed with Warwickshire County Council and available to local authorities through the learning pool platform, http://warwickshire.learningpool.com/.
- NHS West Midlands e-learning module, available at HEE West Midlands Website: http://learning.wm.hee.nhs.uk/resource/making-every-contact-count.

www.makingeverycontactcount.com.

The prerequisites of change

All the models of behaviour change discussed in this chapter suggest that people are involved in a rational processing of information when they make a decision. People are not usually so consciously rational, as a study of the health beliefs of working-class mothers in south Wales illustrates:

> In the subjects we studied there was little evidence of a rational approach to the personal decision-making process, i.e. a weighing up of the advantages and disadvantages of a particular change followed by a decision to act. Instead any change was a consequence not just of thought but also a mix of emotion, habit, impulse, social influences and bolshie lack of forethought, which is so typically human.
>
> Pill and Stott (1990)

Pill and Stott's study of self-initiated change shows the importance of precipitating life events and the minor part played by health concerns. For example, women who gave up smoking did so to save money, and those who took up exercise did so to join in with their children.

The importance of considering the social context and everyday life is brought out clearly by this study, which showed that eventually most women reverted to their original behaviours because of the influence of partners or children, or because it was too difficult to juggle personal and family priorities.

The evidence from people who have changed their health behaviour suggests that there are certain minimum conditions required for that change to take place.

The change must be self-initiated

Some people react adversely or wish to contain any attempt to look at their 'unhealthy behaviour'. To some people their behaviour may not seem unhealthy at all, but may constitute a clear source of well-being, its benefits far outweighing its risks. There is a clear message here for those health promoters who work with individual clients and are sometimes accused of 'telling people what to do' – people will only change if they want to.

The behaviour must become salient

Most health-related behaviours, including smoking, alcohol use, eating and exercise (or lack of it), are habitual, and built into the flow of everyday life such that the individual does not give them much thought. For a change to occur, that behaviour or habit must be called into question by some other activity or event so the behaviour becomes salient. For example, a smoker going to live with a non-smoker causes the smoking behaviour to be reappraised. The death of a relative from breast cancer may similarly prompt a woman to go for screening.

The salience of the behaviour must appear over a period of time

The habitual behaviour needs to become difficult to maintain. The new behaviour must, in turn, become part of everyday life. For example, one reason why people on diets often resume their previous eating pattern is because they are made constantly aware of the diet and it is never allowed to become a habit. Similarly, exercise is often not maintained because it requires effort; hence the advice to reluctant 'couch potatoes' to build physical activity into their daily life by walking to work or running up stairs rather than going out to exercise at a pool or gym.

The behaviour is not part of the individual's coping strategies

People have various sources of comfort and solace, and will resist change to these behaviours. It is sometimes possible to enable clients to identify alternative coping strategies. For example, a person who eats chocolate when depressed may be encouraged to become physiologically aroused by taking up jogging.

The individual's life should not be problematic or uncertain

There is a limit to a person's capacity to adapt and change. For example, those living on low incomes will be stretched by coping with poverty and its uncertainties. Having to make changes in their health behaviour may be too much to expect for people whose lives are already problematic.

Social support is available

The presence and interest of other people provides reinforcement and keeps the behaviour salient. Changing one's behaviour can be stressful, and individuals need support. The influence of peer-group pressure and support is not given sufficient weight in the various psychological theories of change.

 Learning Activity 9.10 Individual behaviour change

Think about an attempt you have made to enhance your health, for example, giving up smoking, losing weight.
- Were you successful in the change?
- What influenced you to make the change?
- Can you identify any specific triggers that prompted you to make the change?
- How do your family and friends regard the behaviour?
- What were the costs and benefits of making the change?

Look at the list of minimum conditions above. Do any of these factors help to explain your success or failure in making the health-related behaviour change?

Conclusion

What is clear from this outline of psychological theories of behaviour change is that none provides a full explanation. However, the variables identified by these models do appear in people's accounts of their health behaviour:
- perceptions of risk and vulnerability
- perceptions of the severity of the disease
- perceived effectiveness of the behaviour in contributing to better health
- perception of own ability to make a change
- perception of how 'significant others' evaluate the behaviour.

While these models may not help to predict who will adopt preventive or protective health practices,

they can help to plan programmes of education by making clear those factors which influence decisions.

Elsewhere in this book we argue that a focus on people's health lifestyles can minimize the structural barriers such as poverty or discrimination that may make choices more difficult for some groups. The client-centred approaches described reflect a shift away from traditional didactic and persuasive methods. Their aim is to enable clients to have the understanding and skills to translate intention into practice. Those most likely to benefit, however, are people with good education and literacy, social support and personal and economic resources. For this reason such approaches must be accompanied by broader programmes that make the healthier choice the easier choice.

Questions for further discussion

- Do social psychology theories help you to understand the reasons why people may or may not change their health behaviour?
- What factors should health promoters take into account when helping clients to change their health behaviour?

Summary

This chapter has reviewed the role of psychosocial factors in health behaviour and discussed three theoretical models. These models have been used to explain and predict health-related decisions, such as screening or compliance with a medical regimen. All the models identify some common variables which influence the likelihood of people adopting 'healthy' behaviours: beliefs about the efficacy of the new behaviour; motivation and whether they value their health enough to change; and normative pressures and the influence of significant people around them. The limitations of the role of social psychology in health promotion are outlined, but it is concluded that an understanding of those factors influencing individual behaviour can help in planning appropriate health promotion interventions.

Further reading and resources

Dixon, A., 2008. Motivation and Confidence: What Does It Take to Change Behaviour? Kings Fund, London. Available online at: www.kingfund.org.uk/sites/files/kf/field/field_document/motivation-confidence-health-behaviours-kicking-bad-habits-supporting-papers-anna-dixon.pdf (accessed 21.02.15)

Mason, P., Butler, C., 2010. Health Behaviour Change: A Guide for Practitioners, second ed. Churchill Livingstone, Edinburgh. *A really useful guide for practitioners using brief interventions with clients. It describes techniques and includes case study material.*

Nice, 2006. Behaviour Change: The Principles of Effective Interventions PH6. Available online at: www.nice.org.uk/guidance/ph6. *Current guidance on behaviour change approaches and the evidence on what works.*

Nice, 2014. Behaviour Change: Individual Approaches. NICE, London. Available online at: www.nice.org.uk/guidance/ph49.

Ogden, J., 2012. Health Psychology: A Textbook, fifth ed. Open University, Buckingham. *An accessible textbook on psychological theory integrating case studies and examples of research studies.*

Payne, S., Walker, J., 2007. Psychology for Nurses and the Caring Professions, third ed. Open University, Buckingham. *A clear and comprehensive introduction to social psychology.*

Feedback to learning activities

9.1 Some people may become concerned and change when presented with information about health risks. Others may make some change, such as switching to a lower-risk substitute (e.g. low-fat spread). Others may deny their risk, perhaps by underestimating the frequency or amount of their current potentially health-damaging behaviour.

9.2 Practitioners often prioritize knowledge and information as necessary to take control over one's health. You probably also mentioned self-confidence and a belief that change is possible, as well as a willingness and motivation to make a change.

9.3 Such findings illustrate that knowledge of health benefits is only loosely associated with behaviour change. Equally, self-reported motivation is often unrelated to propensity to change. Although opportunities to change are greatest in most affluent areas, little action is taken. Understanding the wider cultural frameworks such as pleasure, comfort and convenience underpinning decision-making is essential to motivating individuals and groups.

9.4 If we use the health belief model for predicting health behaviour, we would see the mother as a rational problem-solver who would be aware of not only the causes of childhood diseases but also the risks of contracting them (the child's susceptibility and severity). We would assume that the mother would have been made aware of the efficacy of the vaccine and its role in increasing the child's protection following his routine vaccination as a baby. She would also be aware of any possible side-effects or contraindications. If the mother has had this child or other children immunized against other diseases, with no adverse effects, then she is more likely to view this vaccination favourably and have confidence in its effectiveness. In using this model as a predictor of behaviour, we need to take into account the perceived barriers and costs to taking this action. The mother would need to ask her own mother to take the child to the doctor. The child's grandmother may be unwilling or unable to take three children on public transport; or the mother would have to take time off work with consequent loss of earnings.

9.5 Although responses to road traffic accidents and speed tend to focus on adaptation of the environment or enforcement through speed cameras, driver-offender training is becoming more common (Wood et al., 2012). In relation to changing people's attitudes, you may have considered people's beliefs about:
- the consequences of accidents
- likelihood of being stopped by police
- likelihood of putting people at risk
- social disapproval
- perceived control over driving.

9.6 Factors associated with HIV-positive men having unprotected sex were:
- being in a serodiscordant (only one partner HIV-positive) or unknown-status relationship.
- having 30 or more sexual partners
- having a high self-rating for attractiveness
- drug or alcohol use.

9.7 Being a role model usually refers to an individual who engages in positive health behaviours, for example someone who is a healthy weight and a non-smoker. It is often assumed that nurses in particular, can better encourage behaviour change

Continued

in their patients if they themselves embody the desired behaviours. A counter-argument suggests that an idealized role model may be off-putting for patients.

9.8 Observing others who are similar to ourselves doing something can act vicariously as encouragement. For example, if a friend quits smoking, this may well encourage you to quit. One's own experience of success with previous attempts to change behaviour can also build self-belief and self-efficacy.

9.9 There are many reasons why people are unable to change a health-related behaviour, for example:
- a lack of motivation
- a lack of support
- a social environment that encourages the unhealthy behaviour
- a lack of time or other resources
- a psychological inability to enact a change.

Overcoming any of these barriers can trigger a behaviour change.

9.10 Reflection on whether all the minimum conditions for behaviour change were met, and the relative weighting of each of the conditions, will help clarify the importance of these factors for you. It might be helpful to do this exercise with a friend or colleague and then compare notes, especially regarding the relative importance of different factors and triggers for behaviour change.

References

Ajzen, I., 1991. The theory of planned behaviour. Organisational Behaviour and Human Decision Processes 50, 179–211.

Ajzen, I., Fishbein, M., 1980. Understanding Attitudes and Predicting Social Behaviour. Prentice Hall, Englewood Cliffs, New Jersey.

Bandura, A., 1977. Social Learning Theory. Prentice Hall, Englewood Cliffs, New Jersey.

Becker, M.H. (Ed.), 1974. The Health Belief Model and Personal Health Behaviour. Slack, Thorofare, New Jersey.

Blaxter, M., 1990. Health and Lifestyles. Tavistock/Routledge, London.

Ewles, L., Simnett, I., Scriven, A., 2010. Promoting Health: A Practical Guide, sixth ed. Elsevier, London.

Festinger, L., 1957. A Theory of Cognitive Dissonance. University Press, Stanford.

Frisher, M., Crome, I., Macleod, J., Bloor, R., Hickman, M., 2007. Predictive Factors for Illicit Drug Use Among Young People: A Literature Review. Home Office, London. Available online at: dera.ioe.ac.uk/6903/1/rdsolr0507.pdf.

Gillam, S., 1991. Understanding the uptake of cervical cancer screening: the contribution of Health Belief Model. British Journal of General Practice 41, 510–513.

Green, J., Tones, K., Cross, R., Woodall, J., 2015. Health Promotion. Planning and Strategies, third ed. Sage, London.

Hansen, A., 2003. The Portrayal of Alcohol and Alcohol Consumption in Television News and Drama Programmes. Alcohol Concern, London.

Harden, A., Weston, R., Oakley, A., 1999. A review of the appropriateness of peer delivered health promotion interventions for young people. EPPI Centre Social Science Research Unit, Institute of Education, University of London, London. Available online at: https://eppi.ioe.ac.uk/cms/LinkClick. aspx?fileticket=bCmFZQRwu-o%3D&tabid=255&mid=1071 (accessed 15.09.15).

Heilbron, N., Prinstein, M.J., 2008. Peer influence and adolescent nonsuicidal self-injury. A Theoretical Review of Mechanisms and Moderators Applied and Preventive Psychology 12, 169–177. Available online at: http://mitch.web.unc.edu/files/2013/10/Heilbron-Prinstein-2008-APP.pdf (accessed 15.09.15).

Hill, D., Chapman, S., Donavan, R., 1998. The return of scare tactics. Tobacco Control 7, 5–8. Available online at: http://m.tobaccocontrol.bmj.com/content/7/1/5.full.pdf (accessed 15.09.15).

Ion, V., 2011. Making every contact count: a simple but effective idea. Perspectives in Public Health 131 (2).

Michie, S., Rumsey, N., Fussell, A., et al., 2006. Improving Health: Changing Behaviour. NHS Health Trainer Handbook Available online at: http://www.nsms.org.uk/public/CSDDownload.aspx ?casestudy=53&document+29.

Michie, S., Van Stralen, M., West, R., 2011. The behaviour change wheel: a new method for characterizing and designing behaviour change interventions. Implementation Science 6, 42. Available online at: www.implementationscience.com/content/pdf/1748-5908-6-42.pdf.

Miller, W., Rollnick, S., 2002. Motivational Interviewing: Preparing People to Change, second ed. Guildford Press, London.

Pill, R.M., Stott, N.C.H., 1990. Making Changes: A Study of Working Class Mothers and the Changes Made in Their Health Related Behaviour over Five Years. University of Wales College of Medicine, Cardiff.

Prochaska, J.O., DiClemente, C., 1984. The Transtheoretical Approach: Crossing Traditional Foundations of Change. Don Jones/Irwin, Harnewood, IL.

Prochaska, J.O., DiClemente, C.C., 1986. Towards a comprehensive model of change. In: Miller, W.R., Heather, N. (Eds.), Treating Addictive Behaviours: Processes of Change. Plenum, New York.

Prochaska, J.O., DiClemente, C., Norcross, J.C., 1992. In search of how people change. American Psychologist 47, 1102–1114.

Ridge, D., Ziebland, S., Williams, J., et al., 2007. Positive prevention: contemporary issues facing HIV positive people negotiating sex in the UK. Social Science and Medicine 65, 755–770.

Rogers, C., 1951. Client Centred Therapy. Houghton Mifflin, Boston.

Rogers, R.W., 1975. A protection motivation theory of fear appeals and attitude change. Journal of Psychology 91, 93–114.

Rosenstock, I., 1966. Why people use health services. Millbank Memorial Fund Quarterly 44, 94–121.

Rotter, J.B., 1954. Social Learning and Clinical Psychology. Prentice Hall, Englewood Cliffs.

Scottish Office, 1998. The Speeding Driver. Scottish Office, Edinburgh.

Wallston, K.A., Wallston, B.S., DeVellis, R.F., 1978. Locus of control and health: a review of the literature. Health Education Monographs 6, 107–117.

Weinstein, N., 1984. Why it won't happen to me; perceptions of risk factors and susceptibility. Health Psychology 3, 431–457.

Wilton, T., Keeble, S., Doyal, L., et al., 1995. The Effectiveness of Peer Education in Health Promotion: Theory and Practice. HEA, London.

Wood, S., Bellis, M., Watkins, S., 2012. Road Traffic Accidents: A Review of Evidence for Prevention. Available online at: http://www.cph.org.uk/wp-content/uploads/2012/08/road-traffic-accidents-a-review-of-evidence-for-prevention.pdf (accessed 19.03.15).

Chapter Ten

Strengthening community action

Learning Outcomes

By the end of this chapter you will be able to:
- define community/communities
- understand theories of empowerment and social action
- understand the different processes of a community development approach
- discuss the challenges presented by a community development approach.

Key Concepts and Definitions

Community means the identification and sense of belonging attached to a group of people who may be defined by geography, culture, faith or interests.

Community development is a process whereby members of a community get together to address common problems and take collective action. Community development often leads to community well-being (material and social).

Community action involves campaigns and activities taken collectively by people who identify themselves as a community, in terms of geography or shared interests.

Social capital is the networks and relationships of people who have something in common (typically living in the same area, working for the same employer or sharing the same interests and beliefs).

Empowerment is individual or community action to gain control over life choices and the determinants of health.

Importance of the Topic

We have seen in previous chapters how there are many different ways of working for health. Strengthening community action is one of the key action areas identified in the Ottawa Charter (World Health Organization, 1986), and community development has been seen as the central defining strategy for health promotion which aims to empower people to gain control over the factors influencing their health (Green and Raeburn, 1990).

There has been an increased focus on working with communities in recent years, for different reasons. The policy context in the last couple of decades has been on devolved services and seeing individuals as consumers; as such, consumers are expected to participate in deciding the nature of services to be provided by government. The community is also seen as where needs are both defined and met. There is a recognition that some groups, such as migrants or older people, may be marginalized, harder to reach or excluded from mainstream services. The public health white paper *Healthy Lives, Healthy People* (Department of Health, 2011) asserts the need to address health needs at different stages of life and in different settings, rather than tackling individual risk factors in isolation. Laverack and Mohammadi (2011) argue that strengthening community action is a key area for health promotion, and that particular attention should be given to engaging with socially marginalized and excluded minorities.

 Learning Activity 10.1 Belonging to a community

- Which communities do you belong to?
- Are these the same communities as those to which your parents belonged?
- What are the key characteristics of these communities?

Defining community

The concept of community is frequently used in discussions about health and healthcare. In general, the context of the community is taken to be desirable; thus we have care in the community, community policing and community education, all of which are seen as preferable to alternative (non-community) practice. In contrast to the state or the bureaucratic organization, services provided by and in the community are viewed as being more appropriate and sensitive. But what is the community that is referred to in these ways?

There are different ways of defining a community, but the most commonly cited factors are geography, culture and social stratification. These factors are viewed as being linked to the subjective feeling of belonging or identity which characterizes the concept of 'community'. Other characteristics of communities are social networks or systems of contact, and the existence of potential resources such as people's skills or knowledge.

Geography

A community may be defined on a geographical or neighbourhood basis (see Chapter 15). A well-known example is the East End of London, but this use of community is not restricted to working-class or urban areas. It is this notion of community which gives rise to 'patch'-based work, where people such as social

workers, police officers or health visitors are assigned a geographically bounded area. The assumption is that people living in the same area have the same concerns, owing to their geographical proximity. This in turn rests on an assumption that the physical environment is a key factor in influencing health and social identity.

Culture

Community may be defined in cultural terms, as in 'the Chinese community' or 'the Jewish community'. Here the assumption is that common cultural traditions may transcend geographical or other barriers, and unite otherwise scattered and disparate groups of people. There is an expectation that members of a cultural community will assist each other and share resources. The most commonly cited elements of a common cultural heritage are ethnic origin, language, religion and customs.

Social stratification

A community may be based on common interests, which are usually the product of social stratification. Thus we have 'the working-class community' and 'the gay community'. This definition implies that members of a community share networks of support, knowledge and resources which may transcend other boundaries, even national ones.

Most definitions of community tend to suggest that it is a homogeneous entity. However, it is obvious that any geographical community will include people whose primary identity is based on different factors, for example, class, race, gender or sexual orientation. People who feel united by a shared interest, for example, pensioners or the unemployed, will also be members of other communities, geographical and otherwise. People may belong to several different communities, some of which may have more salience for the individual than others. In practice, people may find their allegiance to different communities shifting at different points in their life span.

The meaning and significance of community vary enormously. How one defines community is important, because it influences how practitioners understand the dynamics within communities and the potential challenges that may arise when working with them.

Some communities may be easier to work with than others, and practitioners may feel more comfortable working with some communities than with others.

Why work with communities?

Community participation – the active involvement of people in formal or informal activities to bring about a planned change or improvements in community life, services and/or resources – has long been a central tenet of health promotion. Communities, both place-based and where people share a common identity or affinity, have a vital contribution to make to health and well-being. South (2015) gives several reasons for working with communities.

- Participatory approaches directly address the marginalization and powerlessness caused by entrenched health inequalities.
- The assets within communities, such as skills and knowledge, social networks, local groups and community organizations, are building blocks for good health.
- Social connectedness and engagement with community life are not only good for mental health but also offer protection in times of adversity.
- The National Health Service (NHS), local government and their partners can create safe and supportive places, fostering resilience of local communities.

Approaches to strengthening community action

A distinction needs to be made about ways of working with communities. Many practitioners are community-based, i.e. they work in the community, organizing projects to meet people's health needs or doing outreach work where a professional service such as screening is extended into the community to make it more accessible. The Sure Start programme is an example of a community project providing early educational interventions in specific areas. Community development work seeks to build capacity within communities, to enable self-sufficiency. Table 10.1 illustrates some of the differences between community-based work and community development work.

UK community health practice is rich and diverse, encompassing both national programmes and small local projects. This chapter discusses the long and productive, if marginalized, history of community development. A recent report for Public Health England introduces a 'family of community-centred approaches' (South, 2015). A systematic review of studies of the impact of community engagement approaches on reducing inequalities in health grouped interventions into three types (O'Mara Eves et al., 2013).

1. *Patient/consumer involvement in development.* This involves engagement with communities, or members of communities, in strategies for

Table 10.1 Characteristics of community-based versus community development models

Community-based	Community development
• Problem, targets and action defined by sponsoring body	• Problem, targets and action defined by community
• Community seen as medium, venue or setting for intervention	• Community itself the target of intervention in respect to capacity building and empowerment
• Notion of 'community' relatively unproblematic	• Community recognized as complex, changing, subject to power imbalances and conflict
• Target is largely individuals within either a geographic area or a specific subgroup in a geographic area defined by sponsoring body	• Target may be community structures or services and policies that impact on the health of the community
• Activities largely health-oriented	• Activities may be quite broad-based, targeting wider factors with an impact on health, but with indirect health outcomes (empowerment, social capital)

After Labonte (1998).

service development, including consultation or collaboration with the community about the intervention design or local plans (see Chapter 18).

2. *Peer-/lay-delivered interventions.* This involves services engaging communities, or individuals within communities, to deliver interventions. In this model, change is believed to be facilitated by the credibility, expertise or empathy that the community member can bring to the delivery of the intervention. Examples are health trainer services, befriending schemes and breastfeeding support workers.

3. *Empowerment of the community.* Empowerment models require that the health need is identified by the community and the people mobilize themselves into action. These models have the underlying belief that when people are engaged in a programme of community development, the result is an empowered community – the product of mutual support and collective action to mobilize resources to make changes within the community.

 Research Example 10.1 Community engagement approaches and evidence of outcomes

A systematic review of community engagement approaches (O'Mara-Eves et al., 2013) found that these interventions are effective in improving health behaviours, health consequences, participant self-efficacy and perceived social support for disadvantaged groups. There also appear to be gains to human and social capital, and there is evidence of benefits for those engaged in community activities, including skills acquisition and future employment. The review did not find one approach to be more effective than another, although it did suggest that there is greater effectiveness of peer-/lay-delivered interventions than interventions taking an empowerment approach or those that involve community members in the design of the intervention. The review concluded by suggesting that community engagement in public health is more likely to require a 'fit-for-purpose' rather than a 'one-size-fits-all' approach.

There is a substantial body of evidence on the benefits of community participation and empowerment. Table 10.2, from a report by South (2015), summarizes the possible outcomes and the levels at which they may be evident.

Defining community development

Community development has been defined as:

Building active and sustainable communities based on social justice and mutual respect. It is about changing power structures to remove the barriers that prevent people from participating in the issues that affect their lives. Community workers support individuals, groups and organisations in this process.
Standing Conference for Community Development (2001)

Community development is thus both a philosophy and a method. As a philosophy its key features are:

- a commitment to equality, and the challenging of attitudes and practices which discriminate against and marginalize people
- an emphasis on participation and enabling all communities to be heard
- an emphasis on lay knowledge and the valuing of people's own experience
- the collectivizing of experience and seeing problems as shared, and working together to identify and implement action
- recognizing the skills, knowledge and expertise that people contribute
- the empowerment of individuals and communities through education, skills development, sharing and joint action.

The community development approach has been influenced by the work of Paulo Freire, a Brazilian educationalist who worked on literacy programmes with poor peasants in Peru and Brazil during the 1970s. Freire saw education as a way to liberate people from cycles of oppression. He aimed to engage the people in critical consciousness-raising

Table 10.2 The outcomes of community-centred approaches

Individual	Community level	Community process	Organisational
• Health literacy – increased knowledge, awareness, skills, capabilities • Behaviour change – healthy lifestyles, reduction of risky behaviours • Self-efficacy, self-esteem, confidence • Self-management • Social relationships – social support, reduction of social isolation • Well-being – quality of life, subjective and objective well-being • Health status, physical and mental • Personal development – life skills, employment, education	• Social capital – social networks, community cohesion, sense of belonging, trust • Community resilience • Changes in physical, social and economic environment • Increased community resources – including funding	• Community leadership – collaborative working, community mobilization/coalitions • Representation and advocacy • Civic engagement – volunteering, voting, civic associations, participation of groups at risk of exclusion	• Public health intelligence • Changes in policy • Redesigned services • Service use – reach, uptake of screening and preventive services • Improved access to health and care services, appropriate use of services, culturally relevant services

or 'conscientization', helping them to understand their circumstances and why they have been oppressed. The process of 'conscientization' begins with problem-posing groups which seek to break down barriers and establish a dialogue between individuals and between individuals and the facilitator. Eventually a state of praxis is reached, in which there is a common understanding and development of action and practice whereby people collectively can transform their circumstances. The process is summarized as:

• reflection on aspects of reality
• search and collective identification of the root causes of that reality
• an examination of their implications
• development of a plan of action to change reality (Freire, 1972).

Community development is a recognized way of working which has given rise to a specific profession – community development workers, who are generally employed by local authorities to support, facilitate and empower communities. Community development workers have their own training courses, qualifications and professional associations.

Community development and health promotion

Community development is a recurring theme in health promotion, but its role as a strategy reflects a changing political environment. In the 1960s the women's movement emphasized the need for women to reclaim knowledge about their bodies and control over their lives. Shared personal experience led to a new understanding of health issues as well as providing positive effects and social cohesion for participants. Black and minority ethnic groups also addressed health issues, particularly the effect of racism within the health services (Jones, 1991).

In the 1970s and early 1980s numerous community development projects were set up, mostly funded and located outside the NHS. Inner-city decline prompted youth work, neighbourhood centres and planning groups which drew attention to the relationship between poverty, health and inequalities in service provision (Rosenthal, 1983).

 Learning Activity 10.2 Participation, involvement and community development

Consider the following statements from the World Health Organization on the importance of participation, involvement and community development. What do you think contributed to this emphasis on working with 'the community'?

The people have a right and a duty to participate individually and collectively in the planning and implementation of their health care.

World Health Organization (1978)

Health for all will be achieved by people themselves. A well-informed, well-motivated and actively participating community *is a key element for the attainment of the common goal.*

World Health Organization (1985), p. 5, original emphasis.

Health promotion works through concrete and effective community action in setting priorities, making decisions, planning strategies and implementing them to achieve better health. At the heart of this process is the empowerment of communities, their ownership and control of their own endeavours and destinies.

World Health Organization (1986)

Community action is central to the fostering of health public policy.

World Health Organization (1988)

Health promotion is carried out by and with people, not on or to people. It improves the ability of individuals to take action, and the capacity of groups, organizations or communities to influence the determinants of health. Improving the capacity of communities for health promotion requires practical education, leadership training and access to resources.

World Health Organization (1997)

By the mid-1980s the UK Community Health Initiatives Resource Unit (1987) estimated that there were 10,000 local projects in existence. By the 1990s the lead health promotion agencies for developing strategies were under pressure, as community development was seen as too radical. Its focus on structural causes of inequality, such as class, race and gender, was not acceptable to New Right political ideology (see Chapter 7 for more discussion of this). The Community and Professional Development Division of the Health Education Authority was disbanded, the National Community Health Resource lost its funding from the Health Education Authority and Community Health UK lost its funding from the Department of Health.

Yet the 1990s also saw an emphasis on the concept of 'community'. Strategies for service delivery were linked to the notion of community. This focus on the community needs to be seen in relation to the developing crisis in the role of welfare state provision and broader debates around accountability. Chapter 7 showed how neoliberal concerns to retreat from welfare have been linked to a focus on individuals as consumers of services. Devolved services and an emphasis on participation and 'consumer involvement' were all strategies designed to achieve these aims. By the turn of the century the focus was on action aimed to bolster social capital (see Chapter 15 for a discussion of how neighbourhoods and the community became a focus for policy and analysis). In England a new government department of communities and local government was set up, and there was a new emphasis on civil society – that domain between the state and individuals, households or communities where people volunteer (there are an estimated 3 million volunteers in England), may be carers (there are an estimated 6 million informal carers) or belong to a charity or community group.

The tradition of community development has radical roots and is closely associated with work to challenge the status quo, redistribute resources and address power imbalances across society. Although many have welcomed the adoption of once-radical terms such as empowerment and participation into mainstream policy language, there are those who suggest this mainstreaming of community development has diluted its aims and processes and resulted in a gulf between theory and practice (Berner and Philips, 2005). There have been warnings that such 'state-commissioned' community development results in 'not government by communities but government through communities' (Shaw, 2005). The policy focus on communities to bring about change (e.g. in neighbourhood renewal or antisocial behaviour) leads to communities, rather than society, being seen as responsible for the problems they face. This may be viewed as an extension, from individuals to communities, of the 'victim-blaming' principle.

Case Study 10.1 The Troubled Families programme

The Troubled Families programme was introduced in England in December 2011 as a means to improve outcomes for an estimated 120,000 families who were identified as having the greatest need, who place a significant burden on public services and are claimed to cost £9 billion a year. According to the government's national criteria, troubled families are defined as those in which there is crime and/or antisocial behaviour, children absent from school or with high levels of truancy, a parent out of work on benefits, domestic violence, 'children who need help' and 'parents and children with a range of health problems'. The programme is based on financial incentives and a payment-by-results scheme, with local councils having to demonstrate successful outcomes to qualify for funding.

There is an active social and political critique of how recent governments have framed these families as 'antisocial' or indeed 'troubling', moving away from a previous discourse which saw people as vulnerable, disadvantaged or having needs (Bond-Taylor, 2014). The 'lumping together' of a number of different problems under the umbrella of 'troubled families' echoes a longstanding discourse from the 1970s that described 'cycles of deprivation' and the 1980s' discourse of the challenging underclass.

Working with a community-centred approach

The ways in which community-centred approaches are carried out vary enormously. However, there are a number of core principles which overlap and link together:
- participation
- community empowerment
- community led

- social justice
- asset based.

Participation

Participation, engagement and involvement are terms that are frequently used in the health sector. While these terms have different meanings, increasing people's involvement in decisions, service design and delivery has been identified as a discrete approach to community engagement (O'Mara-Eves et al., 2013; South, 2015). The emphasis is on increasing people's power, control and participation in decision-making. Participation may be thought of as a ladder which includes many different activities. The National Institute of Health and Care Excellence (NICE) model (Popay, 2010) shows a range extending from services through to health and social outcomes, and demonstrates how the more penetrating health and social outcomes are only achievable through higher levels of participation. Table 10.3 shows a hierarchical ladder with different levels of power, and what this might imply about ways of working.

A distinction can be made between the amount of power sharing involved and the degree of influence

Table 10.3 Ladder of participation

Level	Typical process	Stance
• Supporting local initiatives • Acting together • Deciding together • Consultation • Information	• Community development • Partnership building • Consensus building • Communication and feedback • Presentation and promotion	• 'We can help you achieve what you want, within guidelines' • 'We want to carry out joint decisions together' • 'We want to develop options and decide together' • 'These are the options: what do you think?' • 'Here's what we are going to do…'

Adapted by South (2015) from Wilcox (1994).

over decisions. At the low or weak end it may mean consultation to 'rubber stamp' plans already drawn up by official agencies. At the high or strong end of the spectrum it may mean control over the setting of priorities and implementation of programmes.

 Learning Activity 10.3 A ladder of participation

Consider the following examples of participation. Where would you place them on a ladder of participation?
- A public forum to discuss local health needs.
- The attendance of a mother at a court hearing about the care of her child.
- A service user group to discuss services and give feedback to service providers.

Community empowerment

Empowerment as a health promotion approach is discussed in Chapter 5, and the distinction is made between empowerment of individuals and empowerment of communities. Empowering communities is a core principle of community development and identified as one of the 'family' of community-centred approaches. It has been defined as:

a process by which communities gain more control over the decisions and resources that influence their lives, including the determinants of health. Community empowerment builds from the individual to the group to the wider collective and embodies the intention to bring about social and political change.

Laverack (2007), p. 29

Community empowerment starts with a process of critical consciousness-raising in which individuals and communities begin to question and challenge the social justice of their situation (Ledwith, 2005) (see the earlier section on defining community development for a more detailed discussion of critical consciousness-raising). Woodall et al. (2012) argue that empowerment has lost its links with its original and radical self, and is now more associated with individual self-empowerment. There is evidence that these

approaches can have a positive impact on individuals' self-esteem and sense of control. The evidence that empowerment approaches make a difference to community well-being is less clear cut (Woodall et al., 2011).

Community led

The term *community led* requires us to make a commitment to learning from communities, being accountable to communities and working in partnership. This is not without its tensions, for example, when needs and priorities identified by communities are not compatible with those identified by statutory and funding bodies. An important aspect of community-centred approaches is legitimizing people's knowledge about health and well-being and giving them a voice. Not only does this pose a challenge to medical dominance, but it is also very different from systematic research into needs (see Chapter 18). Establishing the needs of the community also means a shift towards more participatory and locality-based involvement.

 Learning Activity 10.4 Community development and health promotion

How important do you think community development is as a health promotion strategy?

Social justice

Inequalities exist within society, and some communities are more privileged and better resourced – and consequently healthier – than others. Community development sees these inequalities as having been created by society and therefore amenable to change by society. Community development seeks to strengthen civil society in a democratic and participatory way by giving a voice to communities that are disadvantaged or oppressed (Craig et al., 2004). In so doing, it focuses on the determinants of health rather than on individual lifestyles. This may mean:
- working to promote the health of disadvantaged groups

- increasing the accessibility of services
- influencing the commissioning of services
- acting as an advocate and representing the interests of disadvantaged groups
- building a social profile of the community, highlighting the relationship to health status

Asset based

Asset-based ways of thinking are very different from traditional ways of viewing communities, typified in the case study on the Troubled Families programme. Asset-based principles are to identify what works well in an area and what has the potential to improve and support individuals' health and well-being through self-esteem, coping strategies, resilience skills, relationships, friendships, knowledge and personal resources. The approach is exemplified in a statement by Michelle Obama:

> We can't do well serving communities… if we believe that we, the givers, are the only ones that are half-full, and that everybody we're serving is half-empty… there are assets and gifts out there in communities, and our job as good servants and as good leaders… [is] having the ability to recognize those gifts in others, and help them put those gifts into action.
>
> www.abcdinstitute.org/faculty/obama.

An asset is any of the following (Foot and Hopkins, 2011):

- the practical skills, capacity and knowledge of local residents
- the passions and interests of local residents that give them energy for change
- the networks and connections – known as 'social capital' – in a community, including friendships and neighbourliness
- the effectiveness of local community and voluntary associations
- the resources of public, private and third-sector organizations that are available to support a community
- the physical and economic resources of a place that enhance well-being.

Case Study 10.2 Asset-based community development

Asset-based community development has emerged as a counter to approaches that identify the deficits or needs in a community and then provide services (or not). Instead, the asset-based community development approach works from a salutogenic perspective, identifying the factors that keep people well and resilient within the community. Asset mapping is a process that makes explicit the knowledge, skills and capacities that already exist. This can be 'any factor (or resource) which enhances the ability of individuals, groups, communities, populations to maintain and sustain health and wellbeing. These assets can operate at the level of the individual, family or community as protective and promoting factors to buffer against life stresses'. Morgan and Ziglio (2007), p. 18.

Types of activities involved in strengthening community action

A large number of activities may be included as part of a community development approach:

- profiling
- capacity building
- organizing
- networking
- negotiating.

Profiling

Chapter 18 discusses the process of undertaking a community profile and how it differs from a needs assessment. The role of the community worker is to build on initial research and any baseline data and contact with people living and working in the community, so that the needs they identify can be explored and solutions developed (see Chapter 18). Asset mapping is an activity that has gained much importance. Because public services have traditionally been focused on problems and needs, there is an absence of information about the wealth of experience, practical skills, knowledge, capacity and passion of local people and associations, and the potential for communities to become equal partners.

Capacity building

Capacity building is working with individuals and groups within communities to recognize and develop the skills and resources they have (their assets) to identify and meet their own needs. This may mean:

- providing opportunities for people to learn through experience – opportunities that would not otherwise be available to them
- involving people in collective effort so that they gain confidence in their own abilities and their ability to influence decisions that affect them.

 Case Study 10.3 Time banking

Time banking works by facilitating the exchange of skills and experience within a community. It aims to build the 'core economy' of family and community by valuing and rewarding both the people (and their skills) and the work done in it. Time banking values everyone's time as equal: one hour equals one hour, or one credit. For every hour spent helping someone in the community, a person is entitled to an hour of help in return. One of the first time banks in the UK, Rushey Green in south-east London, describes it in very positive terms as 'a chain reaction caused by healthy and productive relationships that bind us together and provide a strong incentive to care for our planet'

See www.rgtb.org.uk and www.timebanking.org.uk.

Organizing

An important area that community workers are engaged in is the process of helping to organize the community to work together effectively. This may include helping to establish small self-help groups or organizing community events such as health forums.

Networking

Networks are the ties that link people together within a community. Gilchrist (2009) identifies two different types of networks: those linked by strong ties

and those linked by weak ties. Networks linked by strong ties are based on bonds of friendship or family relations, and are those we are most likely to turn to for daily support and companionship. Networks based on weak ties link different clusters of networks together. They have been described as the links that operate over the whole network, forming bridges between sections of the community or between organizations. Both types of network are an important asset within a community and an indicator of levels of social capital. Strong networks create opportunities for skills, information and learning to be shared across the community, to create synergy and lead to more effective community action.

Building such networks by making the links between individuals, groups and local organizations is therefore an important part of the community development worker's role. As one refugee advocate puts it:

Community development can be quite an invisible job, but the relationships you build with groups over the months or years is vital. By getting to know different groups, you can identify the issues they face and where they can work together. We have strategic bodies at one level, and the communities and grassroots activity at another level, and community development somewhere in the middle. If you take that out, the structures will collapse; the issues which need to be addressed by policy makers just won't reach them… one of the things I have done is to help set up a Refugee Forum. The refugee community organisations now come together in a group and talk about their issues, what action they want to take and how to make a strong voice

Mani Thapa, community development officer, Refugee Action, quoted in Community Development Exchange (undated)

Negotiating

Community work recognizes the diversity and division that may exist within communities. Communities are not homogeneous entities but include hierarchies, imbalances in power and differences. Such diversity must be negotiated and managed in order to achieve a consensus, particularly in relation to prioritizing needs and agreeing actions to meet needs. As well as negotiating and managing conflict within communities, the community worker must negotiate and advocate on behalf of the community. This may involve negotiating with funding or statutory bodies to ensure that the needs and views of the community are heard and considered.

 Learning Activity 10.5 Community development in practice

Read the following excerpt. What positive outcomes are attributed to community development working?

Carol Osgerby, community health development worker for West Hull Primary Care Trust, describes community development work.

Question: Please explain your job as simply as possible.

Answer: When people want their community to get more healthy and prevent illness, I help them to set up groups and keep them going, by encouraging them and helping sort out problems.

Question: Please describe a typical week.

Answer:

Monday: Work on an evaluation of the health impact of community groups. Later, I join a local walking group to talk to them about raising funds and developing the group.

Tuesday: Prepare display materials for Thursday's event. Attend a committee meeting of a local community orchard. Discuss insurance, tenancy agreement and annual budget. Agree to work with the secretary to draft a funding application and help them make contacts with other similar groups so they can share information.

Wednesday: Catch up with paperwork and e-mails. Team meeting in the afternoon. We are a team of four community health development workers, trying to cover a city of 250,000 people.

Thursday: More paperwork, and reading the latest on the reorganization of public health in Hull. Later I attend a health event at a community centre where I run a quiz about food labelling and offer tasters of fruit smoothies. Get into discussion with many of the residents and workers there about nutrition, exercise, slimming and assorted queries about healthcare and illness. My real aim is to publicize community groups, and maybe make some links that could lead to new projects. In the evening I attend a neighbourhood management meeting. Good turnout of residents, as well as council staff, Community Empowerment Network, youth workers, etc. I help to get residents' ideas on to paper.

Friday: Meet with the community orchard secretary to help draft a budget and fill in grant application form. We discuss how we can encourage local residents to get involved in winter, when there is less physical work to do. Later, I work on our community group's newsletter.

Question: Please describe what you feel makes your work specifically 'community development'.

Answer: Community development develops and leaves behind structures that were not there before, and those structures are managed by members of the community. A vital part of community development is to support individuals to develop skills which they can use to develop community groups, organizations and networks. When I'm asked to take on a new piece of work, I ask myself: 'Is there potential to produce a project which is truly led by the community it's meant to serve?' If not, to me it's not community development. You have to respect the ability of the communities you work with to make their own decisions.

Community Development Exchange information sheet.

Dilemmas and challenges in community-centred practice

Community-centred practice is challenging. It offers the prospect of improving health and well-being, but there are many practical difficulties to overcome. Table 10.4 illustrates some of the advantages and disadvantages of these approaches.

The question of whether the community worker is engaged in radical practice or supporting the status quo is at the root of much of the ambiguity surrounding practice. Common dilemmas facing the community development worker relate to funding, accountability, acceptability, the role of the professional and evaluation.

Funding

Most community development projects are funded by statutory agencies, such as health and education

Table 10.4 Advantages and disadvantages of a community-centred approach

Advantages	Disadvantages
• Starts with people's concerns, so it is more likely to gain support • Focuses on root causes of ill health, not symptoms • Creates awareness of the social causes of ill health • The process of involvement is enabling and leads to greater confidence • The process includes acquiring skills which are transferable, for example, communication and lobbying skills • If health promoter and people meet as equals, it extends the principle of democratic accountability	• Time-consuming • Results are often not tangible or quantifiable • Evaluation is difficult • Without evaluation, gaining funding is difficult • Health promoters may find their role contradictory; to whom are they ultimately accountable – employer or community? • Work is usually with small groups of people • Draws attention away from macro issues and may focus on local neighbourhoods

authorities, sometimes in partnership through joint funding. Other projects which might come under the label 'community development' belong in the voluntary sector, and are funded from a variety of sources, including direct government grants and independent fundraising. Most community development work is funded in the short term only. Lack of security and the impossibility of guaranteeing an input in the long term increase the problems of planning and evaluating such work. Insecure funding arrangements can also subvert a project's focus, leading workers to spend time fundraising instead of working around defined issues.

Accountability

Community workers have a dual accountability: to their employers and to their communities. Funding agencies naturally require projects to be accountable, and this can lead to problems where the priorities of the community and the agency are not

the same. Organizational objectives, such as service take-up, may become incorporated into the community worker's role.

Community and worker responses to issues may also differ. For example, both may identify safety as a priority, but whereas the worker may respond by advocating structural changes such as better lighting and common responsibility for shared areas, the community might respond by advocating increased vigilance or the exclusion of specific groups, families or individuals.

Community development workers may feel themselves to be trapped in the role of mediator, informing statutory services about community needs and informing the community about how services work so that people can participate.

Acceptability

Employing authorities often view community development as not quite respectable. Community development and other community-centred approaches may be seen as absorbing unacceptably large amounts of time and resources for dubious results. Community development tends to focus on small numbers of people, whereas employers tend to be responsible for large populations. The long-term nature and diffuse outcomes of community development and community-centred approaches are at odds with the organizational need to allocate resources on the basis of demonstrable results. While there may be a commitment to addressing inequalities, issues raised through a community-centred approach may be unacceptable to employing authorities. Community workers may also find that they need to establish and negotiate their role before they are accepted by a community. The role of these workers is ambiguous. Their status and employment set them apart from the community in which they are working. Relationships of trust may need to be created before any other work can take place.

Role of the professional

Community-centred work also poses problems for workers whose primary training lies in other areas.

Problems may arise from the different kind of client–worker relationship envisaged in professional training and community work. Professional workers are taught a particular area of expertise and tend to assume that they know what is best for their clients. They may be sensitive to individual circumstances, but the secondary socialization encountered during professional training reinforces the notion of expertise.

Learning Activity 10.6 Adopting a community development approach

A health visitor wishes to adopt a community development approach in her work. She has identified setting up a postnatal mothers' group as an appropriate project.
- What arguments might she use in favour of this kind of work?
- What arguments might her manager use against it?

By contrast, community development workers see their role as that of catalyst and facilitator rather than expert. Their task is to enable a community to express its needs, and support the community in meeting those needs themselves. This requires a different worker–client relationship, based on egalitarianism and the sharing of knowledge. For professionals, whose identity is bound up in their work role, this can be a difficult switch to make.

The skills involved in community work also tend to be different from those acquired in professional training (unless this includes community development). Key skills concern process rather than content and include:
- organizational skills, for example, developing appropriate management structures such as management committees or steering groups
- communication skills, for example, consultation and communication with a variety of groups, including community groups, funding agencies and co-workers
- evaluation skills, for example, monitoring the impact of interventions and self-evaluation.

Learning Activity 10.7 Skills in community development

One of the key areas in the National Occupational Standards for the Practice of Public Health PHP22 is 'working in partnership with communities' to assess health and well-being and related needs (see www.skillsforhealth.org.uk). Its standards include:
- facilitate the development of people and learning in communities
- create opportunities for learning from practice
- support communities to plan and take collective action
- facilitate the development of community groups/networks.
- Which of these skills are covered in your professional training?
- How much time is devoted to these areas compared to other areas in the curriculum?
- Do you think your professional training has equipped you to practice community development?

Evaluation

Community development has often been described as difficult to evaluate because it works on so many levels, is a long-term strategy and encompasses so many strands of work. However, many of the principles used for evaluating health promotion work discussed in Chapter 20, particularly around assessing process, impact and outcomes, are relevant. Barr (2002) provides a useful checklist of questions to consider when evaluating community development work which reflect the principles and goals of this approach.
- Are we gaining a new understanding of community issues and needs?
- Are we being effective in tackling them?
- Are we being inclusive?
- Are the participants achieving their personal goals?
- Are we building community assets and resources?
- Is our work empowering people?
- Are we building a culture of collaboration, participation and sustainable change?
- Are we learning from our experience?

- Are we contributing to health and well-being?
- Are we making the best possible use of the resources we have?
- Do we have the evidence we need to influence future decisions?

As part of the drive to build an evidence base in community development work as well as to support the work of practitioners, a number of evaluation models that provide frameworks for assessing work have been developed. The ABCD model was developed by the Scottish Community Development Centre to support both the planning and the evaluation of projects, and provides a framework for measuring participation and empowerment (Barr and Hashagen, 2000). This model was used as the basis for the learning evaluation and planning (LEAP) model. LEAP provides a strategy through which community representatives and professionals jointly consider a number of question.

- What needs to change?
- How will we know it has changed?
- How will we change it?
- How will we monitor what we do?
- How will we learn from our experience?

The answers to these questions are used to devise a framework against which community activity is planned, monitored and evaluated.

 Learning Activity 10.8 What is community development?

Consider the following statements describing what community development is about.
- Trying to create a 'better' community.
- Getting the community to do what the authorities want it to do.
- Promoting equal access to resources.
- Getting the community to take responsibility for its own problems.
- A political process.
- Controlling social unrest by providing diversionary activities.
- Helping people to see the root causes of problems.
- Providing people with opportunities to become involved in decision-making.

Which of these statements would you say were true? What issues or dilemmas were raised when you were thinking about these statements?

Conclusion

Community development and community-centred approaches do not fit tidily into most health promoters' working lives, but strengthening community action is an increasing expectation. There are many reasons why community engagement is now seen as desirable, few of which are based on a body of evidence and most of which derive from an ideological view of society in which the community/volunteer workforce are the agents of change in creating health and well-being, and service users and people with lived experience of deprivation co-design services so that they are more appropriate and better used.

In contrast to how most health promotion workers have been trained, community-centred approaches rely upon a different set of assumptions about the nature of health and a different set of skills. This can make it a problematic activity to undertake. However, practitioners who have espoused community development are enthusiastic about its potential and outcomes. It is claimed to be the most ethical and effective form of health promotion, and one which makes a real impact on people's lives. Community-centred approaches appear to address many of the problems inherent in more traditional forms of health promotion: they avoid victim blaming, address structural causes of inequalities in health and seek to empower people. This goes some way to explaining their popularity with health promoters and why they are regarded as a central strategy.

Questions for further discussion

- Would you consider adopting a community development approach in your work?
- Do you think community development has advantages over other health promotion strategies?

Summary

This chapter has examined the history and theoretical underpinnings of community development as an approach to health promotion alongside other community-centred approaches. We have seen that community-centred approaches are often viewed by workers as the most ethical and effective means of promoting health. At the same time, practice poses dilemmas for the health promoter, and evaluation is fraught with problems. However, we would argue that the reasons put forward for the privileged position of community development and other approaches to strengthening community action are sound. Practical difficulties should not obstruct the continuing development and spread of this health promotion strategy. On the contrary, what is needed is a more open outlook from statutory organizations, and a willingness to experiment with this kind of strategy.

Further reading and resources

Gilchrist, A., Taylor, M., 2011. A Short Guide to Community Development. Policy Press, Bristol. *This book provides an introduction to community development and its origins and current challenges. The book explores how community development can achieve a range of policy objectives.*

Henderson, P., Thomas, D., 2012. Skills in Neighbourhood Work, fourth ed. Routledge, London. *Describes the skills and techniques for working with communities.*

Jones, L., Douglas, 2012. Public Health. Building Innovative Practice. Sage, London. *Part Three of this interesting textbook explores working at local level and the challenges of building partnerships.*

Laverack, G., 2007. Health Promotion Practice; Building Empowered Communities. Open University Press, Buckingham. *Combines theory with practice in discussing how to build community empowerment using experiences from the UK, Asia and Africa.*

South, J., 2015. A Guide to Community-centred Approaches for Health and Wellbeing. Public Health England, London. Available online at: https://www.gov.uk/government/uploads/system/uploads/attachment_data/file/402887/A_guide_to_community-centred_approaches_for_health_and_wellbeing.pdf (accessed 21.02.15). *Provides an invaluable evidence-based guide to place-based approaches that develop local solutions, drawing on all the assets and resources of an area, integrating public services and also building resilience of communities in order to improve health and well-being for all and to reduce health inequalities.*

Useful websites include:

Community Development Foundation: www.cdf.org.uk.

Scottish Community Development Centre. www.scdc.org.uk.

 ## Feedback to learning activities

10.1 You might have identified communities based on geographic location, professional identity, interests, religious faith or culture. These may be the same communities your parents belonged to; this is more likely if you have not relocated away from your family origins. Key characteristics of communities are mutual interests and beliefs, a sense of belonging and identity, and a willingness to help in times of need.

10.2 Participation is one of the core principles of health promotion, and is a vital component of empowerment. Working with the community helps demarcate health promotion as distinct from healthcare and medicine (where services are provided by medical experts for the community). Working with the community ensures that the right priorities are addressed, and builds expertise and knowledge within the community. It is intended that this will lead in the long term to an empowered, health promoting community and a reduction in health needs.

10.3 The public meeting involves consultation, but no decisions are made.

The child protection hearing involves information and the parent has little power.

The service user group involves consultation and placation. Service users are invited to be involved but decision-making is likely to be done by the service provider.

10.4 Marking the 25th anniversary of the Ottawa Charter, Laverack and Mohammadi (2011) suggested that strengthening community action has not become part of health promotion's day-to-day work. Actively engaging with communities demands a long-term commitment and dialogue, and remains a challenge.

10.5 The outcomes of community development are:
- community members learning
- building social capital, with people feeling more connected
- networking and bringing together people with common interests
- an increase in the number of people who feel they can influence decisions, and a democratic renewal
- co-production of service design that meets needs.

10.6 The health visitor might argue that such work is important for health because it increases self-esteem, autonomy, confidence and a sense of belonging. She could argue that such work is effective. For example, postnatal networking among mothers could prove effective in reducing mental illness among this client group. The health visitor might also argue that time spent on setting up the group will reduce claims on her time in future, and it is therefore a cost-effective option.

The health visitor's manager might respond that there is not enough time to carry out such work. Full caseloads and many other priority claims (such as visiting all new mothers and carrying out child development check-ups) mean there is no spare time available for other activities. The manager might also argue that such activities need to be thoroughly evaluated and of proven effectiveness before resources can be committed.

10.7 Community development is not a core subject within health workers' courses, although specialist community public health nurses may have community development as part of their training (Department of Health, 2011). Some postgraduate courses in public health may also include working with communities. As public health is now located within local government, there are increased opportunities for working with local communities.

10.8 Community development is about the community engaging in decision-making and tackling the root causes of problems. As such, it is a political process which empowers people. Community development is not a panacea designed by local authorities to control people or get them to conform to some ideal template. Dilemmas may arise for local authority staff engaged in community development if communities are in direct opposition to local authority policies or plans.

References

Barr, A., 2002. Learning Evaluation and Planning. A Handbook for Partners in Community Learning. Scottish Community Development Centre. Available online at: http://www.gov.scot/Publications/2007/12/05101807/1 (accessed 19.03.15).

Barr, A., Hashagen, S., 2000. ABCD Handbook. A Framework for Evaluating Community Development. Community Development Foundation, London.

Berner, E., Philips, B., 2005. Left to their own devices? Community self help between alternative development and neo-liberalism. Community Development Journal 40, 17–29.

Bond-Taylor, S., 2014. The politics of 'anti-social' behaviour within the 'Troubled Families' programme. In: Pickard, S. (Ed.), Anti-Social Behaviour in Britain: Victorian and Contemporary Perspectives. Palgrave, Basingstoke.

Community Development Exchange, undated. CDX Information Sheet: Community Development in Action. CDX, Sheffield. Available online at: http://www.iacdglobal.org/files/what_is_cd.pdf (accessed 19.03.15).

Community Health Initiatives Resource Unit/London Community Health Resource, 1987. Guide to Community Health Projects. NCVO, London.

Craig, G., Gorman, M., Vercseg, I., 2004. The Budapest Declaration; Building European Civil Society through Community Development. Available online at: http://www.iacdglobal.org/files/budapestdeclaration4683d.pdf.

Department of Health, 2011. Educating Health Visitors for a Transformed Service. DH, London. Available online at: https://www.gov.uk/government/publications/educating-health-visitors-for-a-transformed-service (accessed 19.03.15).

Foot, J., Hopkins, T., 2011. A Glass Half Full: How an Asset Approach Can Improve Community Health and Wellbeing. Improvement and Development Agency, London. Available online at: http://janefoot.com/downloads/files/Glass%20half%20full.pdf (accessed 19.03.15).

Freire, P., 1972. Pedagogy of the Oppressed. Penguin, Harmondsworth.

Gilchrist, A., 2009. The Well Connected Community. A Networking Approach to Community, second ed. Policy Press, Bristol.

Green, L.W., Raeburn, J., 1990. Community wide change: theory and practice. In: Bracht, N. (Ed.), Health Promotion at the Community Level. Sage, California.

Jones, J., 1991. Community development and health education: concepts and philosophy. In: Community Development and Health Education, vol. 1. Open University Press, Milton Keynes.

Labonte, R., 1998. A Community Development Approach to Health Promotion: A Background Paper on Practice Tensions, Strategic Models and Accountability Requirements for Health Authority Work in the Broad Determinants of Health. Prepared for Health Education Board of Scotland, Research Unit on Health and Behaviour Change. University of Edinburgh.

Laverack, G., 2007. Health Promotion Practice: Building Empowered Communities. Open University Press, Buckingham.

Laverack, G., Mohammadi, N.W., 2011. What remains for the future: strengthening community action to become an integral part of health promotion practice. Health Promotion International 26 (Suppl. 2), 258–262.

Ledwith, M., 2005. Community Development: A Critical Approach. Policy Press, Bristol.

Morgan, A., Ziglio, E., 2007. Revitalising the evidence base for public health: an assets model. Global Health Promotion (Suppl. 2), 17–22.

Popay, J., 2010. Community Engagement PH 9. NICE, London. Available online at: http://guidance.nice.org.uk/PH9/Guidance/pdf/English (accessed 19.03.15).

O'Mara-Eves, A., Brunton, G., McDaid, D., Oliver, S., Kavanagh, J., Jamal, F., Matosevic, T., Harden, A., Thomas, J., 2013. Community engagement to reduce inequalities in health: a systematic review, meta-analysis and economic analysis. Public Health Research 1 (4). Available online at: http://www.journalslibrary.nihr.ac.uk/phr/volume-1/issue-4#abstract (accessed 19.03.15).

Rosenthal, H., 1983. Neighbourhood health projects – some new approaches to health and community work in some parts of the United Kingdom. Community Development Journal 18, 120–130.

Shaw, M., 2005. Political, professional, powerful: understanding community development. In: Transcript of Introductory Presentation – Community Development Exchange Annual Conference, 23–25 September, 2005, Leeds.

South, J., 2015. A Guide to Community-centred Approaches for Health and Wellbeing. Public Health England, London. Available online at: https://www.gov.uk/government/uploads/system/uploads/attachment_data/file/402887/A_guide_to_community-centred_approaches_for_health_and_wellbeing.pdf (accessed 21.02.15).

Standing Conference for Community Development, 2001. Strategic Framework for Community Development. SCCD, Sheffield. Available online at: http://www.iacdglobal.org/files/stramepdf.pdf (accessed 19.03.15).

Wilcox, D., 1994. The Guide to Effective Participation. Partnership Books, Brighton.

Woodall, J., Raine, G., South, J., Warwick-Booth, L., 2011. Empowerment and Health and Wellbeing: Evidence Review. Available online at: www.altogetherbetter.org.uk.

Woodall, J., Warwick-Booth, L., Cross, R., 2012. Has empowerment lost its power? Health Education Research 27 (4), 742–745.

World Health Organization, 1978. Alma Ata 1978: Primary Health Care. WHO, Geneva. Available online at: http://www.who.int/publications/almaata_declaration_en.pdf (accessed 19.03.15).

World Health Organization, 1985. Targets for Health for All. WHO Regional Office for Europe, Copenhagen. Available online at: http://www.euro.who.int/__data/assets/pdf_file/0006/109779/WA_540_GA1_85TA.pdf (accessed 19.03.15).

World Health Organization, 1986. The Ottawa Charter for Health Promotion. Health Promotion 1, iii–v. Available online at: http://www.euro.who.int/en/publications/policy-documents/ottawa-charter-for-health-promotion-1986 (accessed 19.03.15).

World Health Organization, 1988. Adelaide Recommendation on Health Public Policy. WHO, Adelaide. Available online at: http://www.who.int/healthpromotion/conferences/previous/adelaide/en/ (accessed 19.03.15).

World Health Organization, 1997. New players for a new era: leading health promotion into the 21st century. In: 4th International Conference on Health Promotion, Jakarta, Indonesia, 21–25 July, 1997. Conference Report. World Health Organization, Geneva/Ministry of Health, Indonesia. Available online at: http://www.who.int/healthpromotion/conferences/previous/jakarta/declaration/en/index1.html (accessed 19.03.15).

11

Developing healthy public policy

Learning Outcomes

By the end of this chapter you will be able to:
* understand what is meant by healthy public policy
* discuss the development of, and challenges associated with, getting health issues to be considered in all policies
* understand the contribution of health impact assessments to predicting the consequences of a policy or programme
* discuss how to work across sectors so that the policies of all sectors and agencies are health promoting.

Key Concepts and Definitions

Health in all policies (HiAP) A commitment since 2006 that all policies across different sectors will systematically take into account the health implications of decisions.

Healthy public policy (HPP) A policy that has a clear concern for health, well-being and equity. Also used to describe the role of government in creating the conditions that support health.

Health impact assessment (HIA) A method used to judge the potential effects of a policy or programme on the health of a population.

Importance of the Topic

Healthy public policy was identified in the Ottawa Charter (WHO, 1986) as one of the five key strategies for promoting health and the means of creating supportive environments for health. HPP focuses on changing the environment in order to make the healthy choice easier. The Adelaide Charter (WHO, 1988, p. 1) describes HPP as 'having an explicit concern for health and equity in all areas of policy and by an accountability for health impact'. Health is affected by many different policy areas:

Everyone has the right to a standard of living adequate for the health and well-being of himself and of his family, including food, clothing, housing and medical care and necessary social services, and the right to security in the event of unemployment, sickness, disability, widowhood, old age or other lack of livelihood in circumstances beyond his control

United Nations Universal Declaration of Human Rights, Article 25(1).

HPP therefore includes all the major areas of policy that are the responsibility of democratic governments – employment, welfare, education, transport, food, health and social services. Relevant policies may also be instigated by private commercial organizations or devolved government agencies. Promoting HPP across this range of agencies and issues appears to be a daunting task. How to make inroads into this aspect of health promotion is the subject of this chapter, which examines the infrastructure required to facilitate HPP, the role of the practitioner and the potential of this approach to promote health. Readers are referred to Chapter 4 of our companion volume (Naidoo and Wills, 2010) for a more detailed discussion of the policy process. Understanding the policy process is crucial for health promoters, enabling them to debate what is shaping policy and how it effects change.

Defining HPP

Policy is a contested term, with meanings ranging from intentions to decisions and strategies. Milio (2001, p. 622), in a glossary of definitions, describes it as 'a guide to action to change what would otherwise occur, a decision about amounts and allocations of resources: the overall amount is a statement of commitment to certain areas of concern; the distribution of the amount shows the priorities of decision makers. Policy sets priorities and guides resource allocation.' We shall adopt a broad definition of policy as a plan of action to guide decisions and actions. Policy can be developed and implemented at many different levels, from organizational to national to international. While policy may be allocated to a specific sphere, such as health, education or transport, in practice its effects are often wide-ranging and extend beyond the sphere originally targeted. Figure 8.3 in Chapter 8 illustrates the many agencies and organizations that promote health in some way. At government level the Treasury, for example, tries to influence individual behaviour through taxation of unhealthy products, while the Department of Education tries to do this through school-based health education. Joined-up policymaking is the term used to refer to integrated

policymaking across different spheres. The determinants of health are multiple and interconnected, so in order to be effective, policy also needs to be holistic. It is often assumed that policy, once made and adopted by the relevant agency, translates smoothly into the intended action and anticipated outcomes. However, this is the exception rather than the rule. Policy is (re)interpreted at all levels and its practical application may diverge from the original intention. It is therefore not enough to make policy; it must be followed through, monitored and supported by appropriate training and resources.

The World Health Organization (WHO) defined HPP as 'placing health on the agenda of policy makers in all sectors and at all levels, directing them to be aware of the health consequences of their decisions and to accept their responsibilities for health' (WHO, 1986, p. 2). This is a very broad definition, as is the Ottawa Charter's definition of HPP as a central plank for health promotion (WHO, 1986). The Ottawa Charter cited the following fundamental resources for health: peace, shelter, education, food, income, a stable ecosystem, sustainable resources, social justice and equity. This embraces all governmental activities, except, ironically enough, the provision of health services, although they might be counted as part of the social justice and equity resources. HPP has remained a consistent commitment of the WHO. The second International Conference on Health Promotion in Adelaide, Australia, in 1988 (WHO, 1988) explored HPP. It called for a political commitment to health by all sectors and an explicit accountability for health impacts. The eighth conference in Helsinki in 2013 took the theme of 'health in all policies' (HiAP).

 Learning Activity 11.1 Healthy public policy values

Are there any core values that should underpin HPP? If so, what are they?

This focus on HPP underpins many governments' commitment to promoting behaviour change. Its importance can be seen in relation to an issue such as the 'obesity crisis' in many countries. While developing personal skills such as dietary know-how (see Chapter 9), and health services to support weight management (see Chapter 10) are important, so too is tackling the obesogenic environment through, for example, transport policy, food policy and food advertising.

Health in all policies (HiAP)

By the twenty-first century the language and vision of HPP had evolved into 'health in all policies'. This broad strategy focuses on addressing health challenges through an integrated policy response across different sectors of government, such as transport, agriculture, housing, education and public safety (Kickbusch, 2010). HiAP was the theme of Finland's 2006 presidency of the European Union, but although there was little disagreement about its importance, its operationalization has been limited. Governments are divided into departments or ministries responsible for particular areas and with a designated budget. While health is often the biggest ministry, its budget is largely spent on healthcare rather than the prevention of ill health. HiAP requires intersectoral collaboration, and yet this rarely happens at government level when each department has its own goals. Electoral cycles are also not conducive to long-term strategies. A specific impetus can foreground health, for example when a city hosts the Olympics.

 ### Case Study 11.1 The Public Health Responsibility Deal

The Public Health Responsibility Deal set up by the UK government in 2011 is a public-private partnership organized around a series of voluntary agreements to undertake actions for a public health benefit. The deal covers food, alcohol, physical activity and health at work. While many large corporations signed up, many voluntary sector organizations refused to take part, criticizing the deal for prioritizing the needs of industry for sales and profit over potential benefits to public health. There is little evidence that voluntary

approaches work (Mackenbach and McKee, 2013; Panjwani and Caraher, 2014). Legislation and fiscal measures which impact on the three main commercial determinants of consumption (price, availability and marketing) have been the most effective in tackling tobacco and harmful drinking. Current campaigns call for restrictions on advertising food high in sugar, salt and fat to children, as well as for minimum unit pricing for alcohol and standardized packaging of cigarettes.

No policy would claim to have adverse health effects and most would claim to increase well-being in some way, albeit indirectly. Yet many policies may have apparently contradictory effects. For example, it has been argued that the overall economic effect of a reduction in smoking would be negative, due to the loss of tobacco tax revenue to the exchequer and the extra demand on services due to people living longer. Economic policies that increase the income of the wealthiest have been defended on the grounds that there would be a 'trickle-down' effect, despite evidence that increases in relative inequality are detrimental to health (Wilkinson, 1996). The application of stringent animal and environmental welfare regulations in the UK has resulted in an increase in meat imports from other countries where the same regulations do not apply. The consequences of policy programmes therefore need to be thought through in some detail.

Health impact assessment (HIA)

HIA is an approach that does just this. HIA enables the identification, prediction and evaluation of likely changes to health, both now and in the future, as a consequence of a policy programme or plan. HIA recognizes that health is affected by a broad range of determinants linked by various pathways. For example, an HIA of a policy to extend licensing hours would weigh up the benefits and disadvantages of the proposal's impact on individuals, the local community, the environment and the economy. While the proposal may benefit the local economy, disadvantages for health, law and safety, and community cohesion are likely. HIA as an approach is becoming more widespread as various international agreements require an assessment be made of the likely impact of policy. For example, the European Union (EU) requires the establishment of mechanisms to ensure a high level of human health protection in the definition and implementation of all EU policies and activities (Article 152 of the Treaty of Rome). Thailand has made HIA mandatory at all levels of government to identify and address health problems caused by environmental hazards such as pesticides and coal-fired power plants. In the UK there have been several HIAs that assess transport plans, housing strategy and the siting of new airports or runways and waste management landfill sites.

Cycling,Strategy,Health,Impact,Assessment,,2013.pdf) identified its impact in three domains.

1. Personal
   - quality of life (positive impact)
   - social inclusion (positive impact)
   - physical and mental well-being (positive impact)
   - prevention of disease (positive impact).
2. Environmental
   - air quality (positive impact)
   - noise quality (positive impact)
   - connectivity (positive and negative impacts).
3. Societal
   - road traffic accidents (negative impact)
   - community cohesion (positive impact)
   - accessibility (positive impact).

 Case Study 11.2 Health impact assessment

HIAs are often used to evaluate the impact of policies that focus on factors other than health. An HIA includes qualitative and quantitative methodologies and collaboration with interested partners, including workers, clients and other stakeholders. This allows for a multidisciplinary definition of health to evolve. Some examples may be found at:

- HIA Gateway, www.hiagateway.org.uk
- Welsh Health Impact Assessment Support Unit network, WHIASU at http://www.wales.nhs.uk/sites3/home.cfm?OrgID=522
- Scottish Health Impact and Inequalities Assessment Network, SHIIAN at http://www.healthscotland.com/resources/networks/shian.aspx.

There are numerous examples of HIAs on topics as varied as building on green space, fast-food outlets and the siting of airports. A rapid HIA of the proposed Olympic Games was conducted for London (www.londonshealth.gov.uk/PDF/Olympic_HIA.pdf). It concluded that hosting the Olympics would provide net benefits to local communities due to increased employment, greater physical activity and enhanced community cohesion. An assessment of Liverpool as a cycling city (http://www.liv.ac.uk/media/livacuk/instituteofpsychology/impactpdfs/hiaimpactdocs/

Conducting an HIA can appear to be a simple matter of collecting epidemiological evidence using models of exposure and outcomes defined primarily in relation to mortality and morbidity. But HIAs do differ from traditional research primarily because they engage with the local community and stakeholders and draw on local knowledge and informed opinion about the potential impact.

There are many different models and guidance, but generally it is agreed that there are several stages to an HIA.

1. Screening: this is to see whether a project or policy is likely to pose significant health questions and therefore whether it is worth doing an HIA.
2. Scoping: this stage will outline the possible hazards and benefits and the questions that should be asked in the HIA.
3. Risk assessment: this stage will identify the nature and magnitude of the harmful and beneficial factors; how many and which population groups will be affected by them; how they will be affected; and what might enhance or mitigate the impact. This stage will include an evaluation of the level of confidence or certainty in the effects' prediction.
4. Decision-making.
5. Implementation and monitoring.

The history of HPP

Public policies to promote or protect health have a long history in the UK, dating back to the nineteenth century and the rise of the sanitary reform movement prompted by concerns about the spread of disease in overcrowded industrial slums. Edwin Chadwick's *Report from the Poor Law Commissioners on an Inquiry into the Sanitary Conditions of the Labouring Population of Great Britain* (1842) made it clear that poor people did not have the power to change their conditions, and that protecting and promoting their health were tasks of local government. The nineteenth century saw a plethora of legislation and regulations to protect and promote health – a trend that was carried on into the twentieth and twenty-first centuries.

Case Study 11.3 Landmarks in Healthy Public Policy (HPP) in the UK during the nineteenth, twentieth and twenty-first centuries

1842 Edwin Chadwick's Report from the Poor Law Commissioners on an Inquiry into the Sanitary Conditions of the Labouring Population of Great Britain is published.

1845 Final report from the Royal Commission on the Health of Towns is published.

1848 Public Health Act for England and Wales requires local authorities to provide clean water supplies and hygienic sewage disposal systems, and introduces the appointment of medical officers of health for towns.

1854 John Snow controls a cholera outbreak in London by removing a contaminated local water supply.

1866 Sanitary Act – local authorities have to inspect their districts.

1868 Housing Act – local authorities can ensure owners keep their properties in good repair.

1871 Local Government Board (which becomes the Ministry of Health in 1919) is established.

1872 Public Health Act makes medical officers of health mandatory for each district.

1875 Public Health Act consolidates earlier legislation, and the tone changes from allowing to requiring local authorities to take public health measures.

1906 Education Act establishes the provision of school dinners.

1907 Education Act establishes the school medical service. Notification of Births Act is passed and the development of health visiting is encouraged.

1930 Housing Act (known as the Greenwood Act after Arthur Greenwood, the Labour Minister of Health) introduces, for the first time, a state subsidy specifically for slum clearance.

1944 Education Act makes secondary education compulsory until the age of 15 years and provides meals, milk and medical services in every school.

1946 National Insurance Act provides sickness and unemployment benefit, retirement pension and widows' and maternity benefits. It is claimed that social provision was made for citizens from the 'cradle to the grave'.

1956 Clean Air Act to reduce air pollution and respiratory diseases.

1967 Road Safety Act sets a legal limit of 80 mg of alcohol per 100 ml of blood and imposes a 70 miles per hour maximum speed limit.

1973 Wearing of helmets for motorcyclists becomes compulsory.

1974 National Health Service (NHS) reorganization – community and public health services are transferred from local authorities to the NHS.

1974 Heath and Safety at Work Act requires all employers to secure the health, safety and welfare at work of all employees.

1977 Housing (Homeless Persons) Act places a duty on local authorities to house homeless persons.

1983 Seat-belt legislation. Wearing of seat belts in front seats becomes law in 1991. Children are legally required to be restrained in car seats in 2006.

1988 Water Bill requires privatized water suppliers to conform to health standards.

1989 Tax subsidy on unleaded petrol is introduced.

2000 The Food Standards Agency, an independent body, is established to protect the public's health and consumer interests in relation to food.

2004 Smoking ban in all public places is introduced in the Republic of Ireland.

2005 Pubs and clubs are able to apply for unlimited extension to their opening hours.

2005 Civil Partnership Act allows same-sex couples to enter a civil partnership, giving them the same next-of-kin rights in relation to healthcare as married couples.

Continued

2006 Smoking ban introduced in all public places in Scotland.

2006 Work and Families Act extends maternity and adoption leave from 6 to 9 months' paid leave, to be taken by the father or the mother.

2007 Smoking ban in all enclosed workplaces and public places introduced in England, Northern Ireland and Wales.

2007 Junk-food advertising banned from television programmes aimed at young children (aged four to nine).

2012 Minimum pricing for alcohol introduced in Scotland.

2012 Displays promoting tobacco banned from supermarkets.

2013 Marriage for same-sex couples becomes legal.

2014 Free school meals introduced for children in reception and years one and two in state-funded schools in England (https://www.gov.uk/government/policies/giving-all-children-a-healthy-start-in-life/supporting-pages/universal-free-school-meals-for-infants).

2015 Proposal to introduce plain packaging for cigarettes.

2015 Displays promoting tobacco banned from all shops.

The inevitably selective list of some HPPs in Case Study 11.3 shows how the effects of the physical environment on health dominated the nineteenth-century view of public health. The twenty-first-century view of public health, by contrast, is ecological, whereby economic, environmental and social factors interconnect and impact on health. Current health concerns that have prompted public policy include ensuring that everyone has clean and safe environments at work and in the neighbourhood, safe and clean transport, and clean and safe land and water. The regulation of unhealthy products, for example alcohol and tobacco, has been the focus of much discussion.

Single-issue pressure groups or non-governmental organizations (e.g. Age UK, Greenpeace) may also act as champions, lobbying and advocating for specific policies. An example is Oxfam's lobbying to change trade-related aspects of intellectual property rights regulations in relation to patented medicines. The new Trans-Atlantic Trade and Investment Partnership between the EU and the USA continues to raise concerns about companies owning monopolies on pharmaceuticals, and the subsequent reduction in access to affordable medicines. An HIA on the Trans-Pacific Partnership Agreement in 2015 found not only a potential impact on the cost of medicines, but also a risk to the ability of governments to regulate in relation to tobacco advertising, food labelling or alcohol-outlet density (http://hiaconnect.edu.au/wp-content/uploads/2015/03/TPP_HIA.pdf).

Regulation is just one way in which policy can support health. Governments may also use fiscal or monetary means, such as taxing unhealthy products or hypothecation (a dedicated tax to support a specific purpose, e.g. funding cycling routes through a congestion charge on motor vehicles). Examples of hypothecation are the use of the TV licence to fund the BBC in the UK and the use of tobacco taxation to fund health promotion in some Australian states.

Evidence for the effectiveness of HPP, given the long timescales and complexity of interrelated factors, has proved to be problematic. Policymakers and researchers have long commented on the lack of a robust evidence base for HPP, despite it being adopted as a WHO strategy (Petticrew et al., 2004). The Marmot Review into Health Inequalities (2010) gathered evidence on health inequalities and lobbied to spell out the implications for health. Some of its recommendations were incorporated into subsequent policies, for example early-years education, active transport, sustainable food production and zero-carbon houses.

Globalization is having a huge impact on public health and poses new challenges for public policy. The changes in trade, travel, communication and migration mean that many factors impacting on health operate on a global scale that transcends national boundaries, for example infectious diseases, poverty and food shortages, war and civil conflict and climate change. The focus of HPP can be summarized as follows.

- Health as security: addressing issues that are not global risks but are perceived as security threats, for example HIV/AIDS or avian flu.
- Health as development: policies and programmes that invest in developing the economies and infrastructure of low-income countries.
- Health as a public good: policies that promote collective benefits, for example tackling climate change.
- Health as a human right: embodied in treaties and covenants.

 Learning Activity 11.2 Global healthy public policy

What challenges are posed by addressing global health in public policy?

At the global level, international organizations such as the United Nations (UN), the WHO, the World Trade Organization, the World Bank and the International Monetary Fund (IMF) are all hugely influential in affecting the socio-economic determinants of health (see Chapter 8). Examples of global health promoting policymaking are the WHO's establishment of the Commission on Social Determinants of Health in 2005 and the UN Millennium Development Goals (MDGs), which include targets to reduce poverty, hunger, child and maternal mortality, and infectious diseases, and to promote universal primary education, gender equality and environmental sustainability (United Nations Development Programme, 2006). The impact of global players is not always beneficial, however. For example, financial bodies such as the World Trade Organization support free-trade policies which often benefit middle- and high-income countries rather than low-income countries. The IMF has imposed structural adjustment programmes in low-income countries, which has had the effect of reducing their public spending, including spending on health. There is a 'brain drain' of skilled health professionals from low-income countries to

middle- and high-income countries, which leads to a spiral of reduced service delivery and further migration of professionals. The issue has become so acute that the WHO has a code of practice on the international recruitment of health personnel. The World Health Report (2006) demonstrates that a minimum of 2.3 health workers per 1000 population is required to meet the health-related MDGs. The recent outbreak of ebola highlighted the fragility of health systems – Liberia, for example, had only 150 doctors for a population of 4 million people.

The role of states is usually emphasized in HPP, but policy is also made at other levels. In Part Three we discuss how settings such as schools and hospitals can be supportive environments for health. Organizational policies, for example those relating to cultural competence, may have an impact on working practices.

Key characteristics of HPP: advantages and barriers

HPP is a vehicle for tackling structural and environmental barriers to health by making health improvement choices easier and protecting the public from risks.

 Learning Activity 11.3 The pros and cons of HPP

Take a topic, for example obesity, sexual health or drug use. What might be the advantages of an HPP approach to health promotion? And what might be the disadvantages?

HPP has the potential to make clear inroads into the state of the health of the public. While issues relating to healthcare systems are visible and challenging for governments, HPP requires that all sectors, including those that traditionally do not see health as part of their remit, for example housing, must appreciate the social determinants of health and see linkages between their policy area and health and well-being. Attempts to increase cycling in the UK for reasons of health and to reduce carbon emissions have found municipal policies do have an influence on individuals' transport choices, by reducing transport costs and making competing modes more expensive (e.g. increasing car-parking costs), and improving infrastructure and safety.

 Learning Activity 11.4 The use of HPP as a strategy in health improvement

Why, given the benefits outlined above, has HPP such a low profile?

Opponents of an HPP approach might argue that it removes personal responsibility and supports a 'nanny state' that dictates to its citizens their opportunities and behaviours. Indeed, Beattie (1993) described legislative action in his model of approaches to health promotion as authoritative and 'top-down' (see Chapter 5). Those who subscribe to conservative and individualistic political beliefs and ideology might be particularly likely to hold this view. This criticism has been met by the proposal that governments should act as stewards, guiding and protecting the health of the public, but not replacing the need for individual responsibility. Stewardship is about collective responsibility, which requires agreement about what needs to be done. The WHO ranks stewardship as more important than health service delivery or funding, because 'the ultimate responsibility for the overall performance of a country's health system must always lie with government' (WHO, 2000).

Intervention can be seen as paternalistic, especially when the behaviour (e.g. smoking in one's own space) is considered private. Where there are evidence-based risks to health, for example not wearing seat-belts, intervention is often deemed more acceptable. The intervention ladder developed by the Nuffield Council on Bioethics (2007) points to the acceptability and justification for public health policies. The least intrusive policies to the most intrusive legislation are debated, balancing the loss of liberty against health gains. Figure 11.1 shows the ladder of intervention, which has been discussed in relation to numerous issues including food labelling and cutting carbon emissions from car ownership. Many current governments favour enabling choice following provision of better information and education or 'nudging' (see Chapter 6).

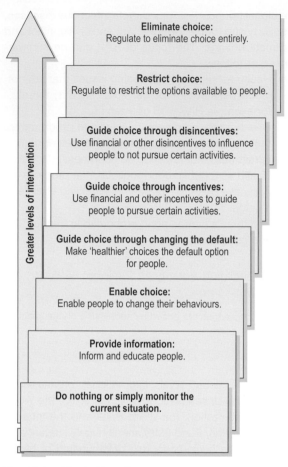

Fig. 11.1 ● The ladder of intervention. (Nuffield Council on Bioethics, 2007. Public Health: Ethical Issues. Nuffield Council, London. Available online at: http://nuffieldbioethics. org/project/public-health/ [accessed 03.03.15].)

Joffe and Mindell (2004) argue that the focus should shift from telling people what to do to making healthy choices easier, and the state should shift from being a 'nanny state' to a 'canny state' – one 'that is clever, prudent, capable, and shrewd' (Joffe and Mindell, 2004, p. 967). There are therefore several roles that governments may adopt in order to pursue HPPs. Some, such as the 'nanny state', appear old-fashioned and deeply unpopular; others, such as stewardship or the 'canny state', appear more contemporary and in tune with a range of current values and ideologies in which the people in a civic society determine direction and government 'steers' but does not 'row' (Giddens, 1998). Any form of legislative action requires agreement by the public. Tones has argued that without health education, HPP would not be possible. Health education can not only set an agenda, such as environmental concern, but can also help 'to create a climate of opinion that will enable government, for example, to institute and claim the credit for change without risking electoral unpopularity' (Tones, 2001, p. 14). Chapter 5 includes a representation of Tones's model of health promotion which illustrates the importance of agenda setting and consciousness raising in moves towards HPP.

 Case Study 11.4 The ethics of legislating about obesity

In Japan the 'Metabo Law' refers to a set of guidelines, officially called the Standards Concerning Implementation of Special Health Examinations and Special Public Health Guidance, which call for local governments and employers to conduct mandatory annual examinations including measurement of waistlines for people between the ages of 40 and 74 – representing 56 million or 44% of the entire population. Individuals should not exceed a maximum waistline of 33.5 inches (85 cm) for men and 35.4 inches (90 cm) for women. People in the highest measurement category are required to attend counselling sessions over the next 3 months. The individual's insurers and employers can face penalties that will go on to fund elderly care if the person does not lose weight.

In 2011 Denmark passed a 'fat tax' that implemented an across-the-board tax on all foods with saturated-fat content above 2.3%. Instead of causing consumers to make healthier food choices, people bought their fatty foods online or in neighbouring Germany. In 2012 the Danish government announced that it would abolish the tax.

In America the so-called Safeway Amendment allows employers to offer insurance incentives and discounts to people who take steps towards better health. Employers can increase premiums for all employees by, for example, $500. The employer will pay back $500 if a person meets certain targets, for example if body mass index is below 25. Those already at a healthy weight get lower premiums, and those who want to change their behaviour may be incentivized; but those for whom the change is difficult get a financial penalty.

 Learning Activity 11.5 HPP in practice

Identify an example of HPP, for example smoking ban, food-labelling regulations, transport policy to promote walking and cycling, or neighbourhood regeneration. What kind of skills and resources are necessary to formulate and implement the HPP?

The Public Health Skills and Knowledge Framework outlines the standards for those working in public health (see www.skillsforhealth.org.uk or www.phorcast.org.uk). The framework identifies a core area in policy and strategy development, and expects practitioners to know of methods to assess the impact of policies, to understand the policymaking process and different methods of HIA, to have the ability to compare the health consequences of different policy options and to understand interagency working. These methods have been described elsewhere, and the Ottawa Charter (WHO, 1986) noted three key skills which are necessary for effective action: mediation, advocacy and enablement.

Yet 'health in all policies' is far from being enacted. Organizations and local governments lack champions of public health. In addition the policymaking process is complex, as described elsewhere (Naidoo and Wills, 2010, Chapter 4). The four key stages are as follows (Walt, 1994).

1. Problem identification and issue recognition.
2. Policy formulation.
3. Policy implementation.
4. Policy evaluation.

Various different skills are needed at each stage of the policymaking process. For example, stage 1, problem identification and issue recognition, may require research, lobbying and advocacy to prompt awareness of a particular issue. An HIA can raise awareness of health impacts in stage 2. Partnership working is an important element within the policy process during formulation and implementation. The benefits and statutory requirements for collaboration are outlined in Chapter 5 of our companion volume (Naidoo and Wills, 2010). Identifying key stakeholders, clarifying their interests in the proposed policy and making links with others to present a united agenda for change is all part of the wider policy process. Chapter 8 outlines the roles of some agencies. An awareness of different organizational cultures and their interests is vital for partnership working. Key skills are how to influence, negotiate, facilitate and manage in a multiagency environment to bring about change.

Public health advocacy has been described as the process of influencing and then expressing public opinion to influence policymakers' judgements about what is politically desirable and acceptable (Kemm, 2001). It may also involve generating support and a climate of opinion among the public, the media and interest groups. Presenting the case for a policy might mean finding areas of overlap or congruence between the interests of the people you are representing and the key people with influence. It may mean encouraging informed debate by conveying usable translations of a message (Laverack, 2013). Advocacy may also be used to present the case against a policy. The use of the mass media in advocacy is discussed further in Chapter 12.

It cannot be assumed that once a policy has been approved that the implementation stage is straightforward. This stage may be particularly problematic for policies that affect organizational working. Implementation involves getting the agreement of those who are affected by a policy, and their commitment to its operationalization. There is often resistance to the imposition of change from above. Frontline workers or 'street-level bureaucrats' (Lipsky, 1979) have been identified as playing a key role in the implementation and delivery of policy changes, with the capacity to progress or impede the policy process.

Although in an ideal world HPP would be a rational process, in reality policymaking is not rational but incremental, or what has been labelled 'muddling through' (Lindblom, 1959; Green et al., 2015). Ideally policymaking would be driven by clarity about the problem, desired goals and outcomes and the best means of achieving these. This in turn would require an objective assessment of all alternatives at each stage of the policy process. The outcome would be the best possible choice, and there would

be consensus about this. In reality, policymaking is incremental and typically considers a restricted range of options, blurs the distinction between goals and implementation, and achieves consensus about small changes rather than radical overhauls. In the twenty-first century policymaking has become even more complex as it seeks to address 'wicked' problems and evidence on different options grows. One of the strategies advocated for HiAP is to adopt a 'health lens' that examines all policies, as has occurred in South Australia (http://sahealth.sa.gov.au).

Case Study 11.5 The Framework Convention on Tobacco Control WHO (2003)

The Framework Convention on Tobacco Control (FCTC) is an attempt to challenge the powerful economic interests of the tobacco industry and tobacco growers, and protect individual nations and populations from their power. The treaty establishes measures to reduce demand for tobacco through price and tax, controls the supply, for example in sales to minors and illicit trade, and agrees measures to control the promotion of tobacco. The FCTC was agreed by the member states of the WHO in 2003, following almost 4 years of negotiation. Lobbying from anti-tobacco pressure groups and the tobacco lobby's persistent manoeuvring from the inside made the creation of the FCTC a difficult task. By 2004, 131 countries had signed the treaty and 21 had ratified it. The USA was a notable omission to those ratifying the convention, which illustrates the influence that interest groups can have on HPP. The FCTC is the first global health treaty, and came into force in 2005.

The practitioner's role in HPP

Although many practitioners might not think of HPP as being part of their work remit, there are a number of ways in which they might become involved. Depending on job role and employing organization or service, practitioners may take on various roles in relation to HPP, ranging from leading the process, sharing the vision and promoting the benefits of the

HPP approach to active involvement in the process of lobbying, advocacy and partnership working.

Learning Activity 11.6 The practitioner and the policy process

Your local council is proposing a new transport plan to encourage cycling and walking. The plan includes congestion charging, the introduction of cycling lanes and dedicated lanes for cars carrying more than one person. Proponents argue that this will encourage people to integrate exercise into their personal travel plans. Opponents argue the scheme will lead to more congestion and longer travel times due to reduced road space and more speed restrictions. The council is inviting consultation with all interested parties. What, if anything, would you see as your role as a practitioner? How, if at all, would this differ from your role as a member of the public?

The policy context, process and implementation, as well as specific skills helpful for those engaging with policy, tend to be neglected areas within professional training. This is the current situation despite the fact that practitioners are often crucial in determining whether or not a policy achieves its goals. Policies need to be implemented in order to have an impact. This will usually involve a change in working practices, and there is a tendency to resist change within organizations. Change is often stressful and time-consuming, and unless people are convinced of its merits, there may well be resistance. Inertia or misinterpretation of what is required may also mean policies get no further than the paper they are written on. To be effective, practitioners need to be 'on board' and committed partners in implementing policies. This in turn depends on whether and how their organizations have engaged them in the policymaking process.

Within the health services there is a long history of continual change and reorganization. This can lead to a degree of cynicism and lack of engagement with the policymaking process. For many, policy implementation in the past has been experienced as increased levels of micro-management, leading to a negative stance towards policy. However, policymaking is a powerful professional tool, and the skills for effective engagement in the policy process need to be embedded in professional training.

Evaluating an HPP approach

Evaluating the impact of policies is often difficult, due to the long timescale involved, the lack of controlled comparisons and the complexity of factors and relationships affected by policy changes. The benefits of HiAP are descriptive and rest on assumptions. Areas that are commonly researched to assess the impact of policy changes are:

- knowledge of the policy change
- attitudes towards the policy change – for or against
- self-assessed behaviour change following the policy change
- independently assessed behaviour change, for example monitoring before and after sales of products or use of services
- media coverage of the policy change – amount; positive or negative
- economic analysis to demonstrate whether or not the policy change is cost-effective.

More details of the evaluation process are given in Chapter 20.

Conclusion

HPP is a vital cornerstone of health promotion. Policy is a complex phenomenon that exists at many different levels. HPP has a sound rationale and some notable successes, but remains rather underused as a strategy. This is probably due to its complexity and the feeling that addressing the many determinants of health together seems too enormous. Addressing the social determinants of health calls into question politics, values and ideologies about the willingness of governments to intervene and to acknowledge their role in tackling issues such as poverty. The potential of HPP to be an effective and efficient means of promoting health and preventing ill health suggests that the policymaking process should be embedded in professional training. The ability to understand and engage effectively in the policy process should be part of every practitioner's professional skills base.

Questions for further discussion

- To what extent do you engage with policy issues as a practitioner? Would you like to increase or decrease your level of engagement?
- Select a controversial new policy, for example plain paper packaging for cigarettes, and search the newspapers for reporting about this issue. What issues are highlighted in media coverage about this issue?

Summary

This chapter has outlined the history of public policy for health. It discusses the new strategy of attempting to put HiAP in place and why this poses challenges. HPP is one of the action areas of the Ottawa Charter and, despite political ideologies that have moved away from state intervention, acceptance has grown of the need to legislate and regulate to tackle a range of issues. The practitioner's role in HPP and the importance of developing an understanding of the policy process are discussed.

Further reading and resources

Baggott, R., 2011. Public Health: Policy and Politics, third ed. Palgrave Macmillan, Basingstoke. *A comprehensive account of British, European and international policy and public health.*

Buck, D., Gregory, S., 2013. Improving the Public's Health. A Resource for Local Authorities. Kings Fund, London. Available online at: https://www.rsph.org.uk/filemanager/root/site_assets/about_us/latest_news/improving_the_public_s_health_print_version_final.pdf (accessed 06.03.15). *A useful guide and case studies about the ways in which local government can contribute to health improvement.*

Coles, L., Porter, E. (Eds.), 2011. Policy and Strategy for Improving Health and Wellbeing. Learning Matters, Exeter. *A useful textbook on national policies, with case studies from the UK.*

Douglas, J., Earle, S., Handsley, S., Jones, L., Lloyd, C.E., Spurr, S. (Eds.), 2007. A Reader in Promoting Public Health. Sage, London. *Part Three discusses promoting health through public policy, with many interesting examples.*

Lloyd, C.E., Handsley, S., Douglas, J., et al. (Eds.), 2007. Policy and Practice in Promoting Public Health. Sage and Open University Press, London. *A comprehensive discussion of public health policy at different levels (global, national, local) and within different settings. Policy principles such as partnership working and collaboration are also discussed in depth.*

Naidoo, J., Wills, J., 2010. Public Health and Health Promotion: Developing Practice, third ed. Baillière Tindall, London. *Chapter 4 on the policy context gives a detailed account of the policy process and the realities of engaging with policy.*

Pitt, B., Lloyd, L., 2015. Social policy and health. In: Naidoo, J., Wills, J. (Eds.), Health Studies: An Introduction, third ed. Palgrave Macmillan, Hampshire. Chapter 7. *A concise overview of the discipline of social policy, with a focus on health. The chapter includes a historical account and a discussion of methodological issues, including policy analysis and the policy process.*

Several toolkits for conducting a Health Impact Assessment can be found at the World Health Organization site, at http://www.who.int/hia/tools/toolkit/en/.

 Feedback to learning activities

11.1 Some core values underpinning HPP may be inferred from the conferences and charters outlined above and also discussed in Chapter 4. These include:
- equity – an active redistribution of the material resources required for healthy living, for example income, housing
- upstream focus – concentrating on the socio-economic determinants of health rather than individual lifestyles

- participation – the involvement of all interested partners, including governments, practitioners and the public
- collaboration – working across organizational and national boundaries to meet agreed goals
- sustainability – meeting existing needs without compromising the ability of future generations to meet their own needs.

11.2 While there is acknowledgement of the need for global public health policy, it is often challenging. Promoting health can become repressive, for example when people's movements are restricted to prevent the transmission of disease. Development can be steered by global economic forces. Some issues, for example food policy, have been very difficult to change (Lee, 2010). The voice of the WHO has often not been heard against that of the World Trade Organization, where considerations of trade and profit predominate.

11.3 HPP as an approach to health promotion has many strengths. Perhaps most important is its recognition of the multiple socio-economic environmental determinants of health, and the necessity to change these determinants in order to promote health. Alongside this recognition and 'upstream' focus goes a commitment to reducing inequalities in health and promoting equity. An upstream approach also has economic benefits. A positive impact on determinants of health will prevent much ill health and disease, thus averting the need to spend money on services and treatment. Prevention is typically far more cost-effective than treatment.

11.4 There are many barriers to achieving HPP. Hunter (2003) identifies several, including the tendency of both the government and the public to focus on health services instead of public health, and the silo mentality of government departments that means cross-departmental working to promote public health remains an aspiration rather than a reality. Public health issues tend to be 'wicked issues' (Rittel and Webber, 1973), meaning they are complex issues that are not well understood and not amenable to easy manipulation or solution.

Public health issues, such as sustainability or reducing health inequalities, are multidisciplinary in nature, and effective action is likely to require a long timescale, well beyond political parties' terms of office. As Hunter (2003, p. 17) puts it, 'Almost by definition public health issues are wicked issues.'

11.5 Influencing, planning for and operationalizing HPP calls for a variety of skills. The required skills include health education, partnership working, lobbying, advocacy, managing, leadership and public relations.

11.6 As a practitioner faced with a proposed new policy affecting your clients, you would probably consider it your duty to assess the plan in terms of its likely impact on the health of your clients. This might include initiating discussions and forums with clients to gauge their reaction to the proposal, or a more *ad hoc* process of sounding things out with individuals as and when you deem it appropriate. Perhaps you would take it upon yourself to translate research findings into plain English, or to spell out the likely effects of the proposed policy. You might propose that a rapid HIA is undertaken which would ensure the views of community groups are heard. You might also take the issue up with your professional association, and get it involved in the issues.

As a member of the public, you might be involved in the same spectrum of activities (apart from working with professional associations). However your role and expertise would be different, and you would engage as an interested member of the public rather than as a practitioner with a duty of care. This might give you more freedom to voice your opinions and make your principles and values known.

References

Beattie, A., 1993. The changing boundaries of health. In: Beattie, A., Gott, M., Jones, L., et al. (Eds.), Health and Wellbeing: A Reader. Macmillan/Open University, London, pp. 260–272.

Chadwick, E., 1842. Report from the Poor Law Commissioners on an Inquiry into the Sanitary Conditions of the Labouring Population of Great Britain. Poor Law Commission, Home Office, London.

Giddens, A., 1998. The Third Way. The Renewal of Social Democracy. Polity Press, Cambridge.

Green, J., Tones, K., Cross, R., Woodall, J., 2015. Health Promotion: Planning and Strategies, third ed. Sage, London.

Hunter, D.J., 2003. Public Health Policy. Polity Press, Cambridge.

Joffe, M., Mindell, J., 2004. A tentative step towards healthy public policy. Journal of Epidemiology and Community Health 58, 966–968. Available online at: http://m.jech.bmj.com/content/58/12/996.full.pdf (accessed 16.09.15).

Kemm, J., 2001. Health Impact Assessment: a tool for healthy public policy. Health Promotion International 16, 79–85. Available online at: http://m.heapro.oxfordjournals.org/content/16/1/79.full.pdf (accessed 16.09.15).

Kickbusch, I., 2010. Health in all policies: where to from here? Health Promotion International 25 (3), 261–264. Available online at: http://m.heapro.oxfordjournals.org/content/25/3/261.full.pdf (accessed 16.09.15).

Laverack, G., 2013. Health Activism: Foundations and Strategies. Sage, London.

Lee, K., 2010. Global health promotion: how can we strengthen governance and build effective strategies? In: Douglas, J., Earle, S., Handsley, S., Jones, L., Lloyd, C.E., Spurr, S. (Eds.), A Reader in Promoting Public Health. Sage, London, pp. 171–176.

Lindblom, C., 1959. The science of muddling through. Public Administration Review 19, 79–88.

Lipsky, M., 1979. Street Level Bureaucracy. Russell Sage, New York.

Mackenbach, J.P., McKee, M. (Eds.), 2013. Successes and Failures of Health Policy in Europe: Four Decades of Diverging Trends and Converging Challenges. Open University Press, Buckingham.

Marmot, M., 2010. Fair Society, Healthy Lives. Institute of Health Equity, London. Available online at: http://www.instituteofhealthequity.org/projects/fair-society-healthy-lives-the-marmot-review (accessed 19.03.15).

Milio, N., 2001. Glossary: healthy public policy. Journal of Epidemiology and Community Health 55, 622–623. Available online at: http://m.jech.bmj.com/content/55/9/622.full.pdf (accessed 16.09.15).

Naidoo, J., Wills, J., 2010. Developing Practice for Public Health and Health Promotion, third ed. Baillière Tindall, London.

Nuffield Council on Bioethics, 2007. Public Health: Ethical Issues. Nuffield Council, London. Available online at: http://nuffieldbioethics.org/project/public-health/ (accessed 03.03.15).

Panjwani, C., Caraher, M., 2014. The Public Health Responsibility Deal: brokering a deal for public health, but on whose terms? Health Policy 114, 163–173. Available online at: http://www.adph.org.uk/wp-content/uploads/2014/08/Panjwani-and-Caraher1.pdf (accessed 16.09.15).

Petticrew, M., Whitehead, M., Macintyre, S.J., et al., 2004. Evidence for public health policy on inequalities: 1: the reality according to policymakers. Journal of Epidemiology and Community Health 58, 811–816. Available online at: http://www.ncbi.nlm.nih.gov/pmc/articles/PMC1763325/pdf/v058p00811.pdf (accessed 16.09.15).

Rittel, H., Webber, M., 1973. Dilemmas in a general theory of planning. Policy Science 4, 155–169. Available online at: http://www.ask-force.org/web/Discourse/Rittel-Dilemmas-General-Theory-Planning-1973.pdf (accessed 16.09.15).

Tones, K., 2001. Health promotion: the empowerment imperative. In: Scriven, A., Orme, J. (Eds.), Health Promotion Professional Perspectives, second ed. Palgrave Macmillan, Hampshire, pp. 3–18.

United Nations. Universal Declaration of Human Rights, article 25(1). United Nations, Geneva. Available online at: http://www.un.org/en/documents/udhr/ (accessed 16.09.25).

United Nations Development Programme, 2006. Millennium Development Goals. Available online at: http://www.undp.org/mdg/goallist.shtml.

Walt, G., 1994. Health Policy: An Introduction to Process and Power. Zed Books, London.

Wilkinson, R., 1996. Unhealthy Societies: The Afflictions of Inequality. Routledge, London.

World Health Organization, 1986. Ottawa Charter for Health Promotion: An International Conference on Health Promotion. November 17–21. WHO, Copenhagen. Available online at: http://www.who.int/healthpromotion/conferences/previous/ottawa/en/ (accessed 03.03.15).

World Health Organization, 1988. In: Second International Conference on Health Promotion. WHO, Adelaide, Australia. Available online at: http://www.who.int/healthpromotion/conferences/previous/adelaide/en/ (accessed 02.03.15).

World Health Organization, 2000. The World Health Report 2000 – Health Systems: Improving Performance. WHO, Geneva. Available online at: http://www.who.int/whr/2000/en/ (accessed 03.03.15).

World Health Organization, 2003. Framework Convention on Tobacco Control. WHO, Geneva. Available online at: http://www.who.int/fctc/about/en/ (accessed 03.03.15).

World Health Organization, 2006. World Health Report 2006, Working Together for Health. WHO, Geneva. Available online at: http://www.who.int/whr/2006/en/ (accessed 03.03.15).

Chapter Twelve

Using media in health promotion

By the end of this chapter you will be able to:
* understand how information is used to promote behaviour change
* discuss the contribution of mass media and public information to behaviour change
* assess critically the differences between social marketing and health promotion
* consider the potential contribution of social media and new technologies to health communication.

Key Concepts and Definitions

Medium/media is/are the channel of communication, for example, social media.

Media advocacy is the use of media to promote a policy change.

Message is what is being communicated.

Social marketing is an approach used to develop activities aimed at changing people's behaviour, borrowing ideas from commercial marketing.

Behaviour change communication involves communication strategies to promote positive behaviours. Strategies follow a systematic process from formative research through planning, implementation and evaluation.

Importance of the Topic

Communication of information and advice is central to health promotion strategies. A knowledge of how communication between the sender and receiver of messages takes place and an understanding of the medium through which communication occurs are therefore important tools for the health promoter. Mass media are a powerful agent of communication, reaching large numbers of people. In addition to the traditional media (radio, television, press) social media, most notably the internet, have changed communication patterns and coverage. The mass media now combine the capacity to reach large numbers of people with the capacity to be accessed individually as and when people choose. Mass media have a long history of persuading people to buy a vast array of products and lifestyles which create ill health, such as tobacco, alcohol and fast cars, through both paid advertising and current affairs coverage. Paid advertising and campaigns, unpaid news coverage, social media, social marketing and media advocacy are all used to promote health. Practitioners also use posters, leaflets and other tools to enhance communication with service users. This chapter looks at the potential and limitations of using various media in these different ways to promote health. Readers can find a more detailed discussion of health communication and social marketing in Chapter 8 of our companion volume (Naidoo and Wills, 2010).

Introduction

The term mass media includes any communication which reaches large sections of the population. Examples of mass media are television and radio broadcasting, print media such as newspapers, posters and leaflets, and social media such as Facebook. The mass media are a 'broad-spectrum' intervention, as distinct from 'narrow-gauge' personalized interventions tailored to individuals and small groups. The use of public announcements to promote health has a long history.

In 1953 John Burton, the editor of the *Health Education Journal*, stated that:

> *The first 10 years of our existence could well be called the era of propaganda. Health education has been realised mainly in terms of mass publicity on all fronts. Ad hoc exhortations have been directed at the public following closely the patterns of commercial advertising.*
>
> Burton, cited in Tones (1993), p. 128

However, by this time concern had already developed that such a strategy was not working and that the role of the mass media in health promotion needed to be redefined:

> *Many [have come] to feel that mass publicity methods were expensive and relatively ineffective in changing people's health habits and beliefs, and that health education would have to be planned on a more personal basis.*
>
> Burton, cited in Tones (1993), p. 128

The relationship between the media and the public is complex. In addition to their primary function of informing and entertaining, the media play a pivotal role in social cohesion, or keeping people connected, defining what is normal and desirable and what is not. McQuail (2010) identifies several different roles played by the media:

- the main source of essential information
- the arena where public-life affairs are played out
- the source of definitions and images of social reality
- where values are constructed and expressed
- a benchmark for what is normal.

The mass media are important to health promotion because they are so widely used. Many public health issues, for example, human immunodeficiency virus/acquired immunodeficiency syndrome (HIV/AIDS), alcohol misuse and smoking, have been the subject of extensive mass-media campaigns. The aim of such campaigns is usually to raise awareness or present a message advocating healthy lifestyles, as shown in the example in Figure 12.1.

Beattie et al. (1993) describe the use of the media as 'health persuasion', by which they mean a top-down conservative method designed to infuse an audience with information (see Chapter 5).

The media may also be an unhealthy influence, advertising unhealthy products, for example, fast food, or transmitting unhealthy messages, for example, that drinking excessively is fun and fashionable. The media also play a major role in constructing society's views on health issues and services. What health issues are covered and the slant the reporting takes are powerful forces in public discourse around health. Social media have emerged in the last decade, and Twitter, Facebook and YouTube have enabled the sharing of information and opinions. It is estimated that nearly one in four people use social networks and in the USA 75% of adults are online (www.pewinternet.org).

Case Study 12.1 Ebola and social media

In 2014 an outbreak of Ebola spread across West Africa, killing over 10,000 people in Liberia, Guinea, Sierra Leone, Nigeria and Mali. Targeted social media campaigns in Nigeria during 2014 helped to disseminate accurate information quickly. Nigeria has 114 million mobile phone subscribers and 56 million Nigerians use the internet regularly. A Twitter campaign, Ebola Alert, recruited volunteers and disseminated public health advice on hygiene and how to conduct a safe burial. Within a few weeks it had 76,000 followers. The BBC launched a WhatsApp service (online chat) in English and French to offer information on identifying symptoms and effective handwashing (Carter, 2014).

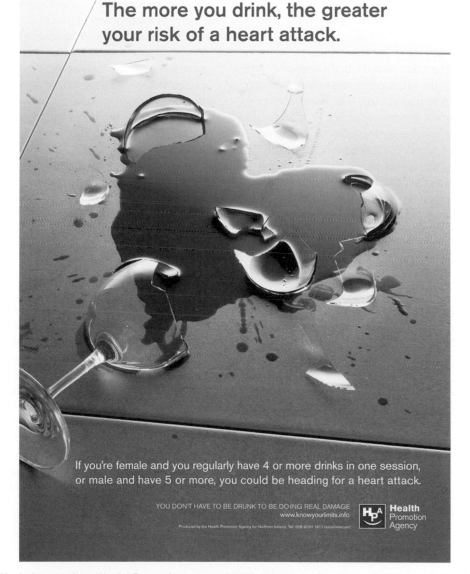

Fig. 12.1 ● Alcohol poster from Health Promotion Agency Northern Ireland. (Reproduced with permission from the Health Promotion Agency for Northern Ireland: photography, David Gill.)

The nature of media effects

The mass media are a distinctive form of communication with specific properties, including:

- large scale
- standardized content
- one-directional flow
- impersonal
- based on a market relationship (McQuail, 2010).

These characteristics include both strengths and weaknesses when the aim is to promote health. Although a mass audience is guaranteed, with favourable cost implications, 'correct' reading, understanding and recall of the intended message by the target audience is by no means certain. A great deal of research is needed to develop suitable messages that will appeal to the target audience and evaluate their real-life impact. Chapter 8 in our companion volume (Naidoo and Wills, 2010) discusses the nature of health promotion messages.

 Learning Activity 12.1 The portrayal of drinking alcohol in television programmes

Some people argue that representations of people drinking alcohol in television programmes encourages viewers to do the same. What do you think?

Views on the effects of the mass media shifted from an early belief that they could produce dramatic changes in attitudes and behaviour to the opposite view that the media have negligible effects (Gatherer et al., 1979). Today there is a more tempered view, which regards the media as influential in certain circumstances and in specific ways.

Lasswell (1948) recommended that when analysing mass communication, the following issues should be examined.

- *Who* says *what*, in *which channel*, to *whom* and with *what effect*?

This framework is useful in flagging up all the key elements of the process of mass communication.

- *Who*? The credibility of the source of the message.
- *What?* The message and how it is presented, for example, fear, arousal, positively.
- *Which channel?* Television, radio, poster, internet, mobile phone.
- *Whom?* Who is the target audience in terms of, for example, age, gender, socio-economic class, ethnic group, personality?
- *What effect?* Changes in knowledge, attitudes, beliefs, behavioural intentions, actual behaviour.

The framework is represented simply in Figure 12.2.

The framework, which was developed into the Hovland-Yale model of persuasion, was designed with traditional forms of mass media in mind, which may limit its applicability to newer forms of instant and overlapping communication and technologies such as social media. The new technologies, such as text messaging or social network sites, are particularly relevant if young people are the target group. Young people are media literate, i.e. they can access, understand and create communications using a variety of new technologies, including the internet and mobile phones. These new forms of communication may be used to promote health. Text messaging has been successfully used to improve self-management of diabetes (Franklin et al., 2006), and has also been used to engage young people in health messages (Dobkin et al., 2007). Atkin and Rice (2014) argued

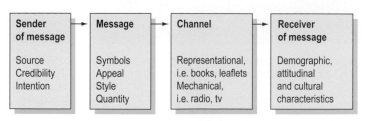

Fig. 12.2 ● Analysing mass communication.

that the new interactive and individually tailored communication technologies empower users. Benefits of these new means of communication include relative anonymity, avoidance of stigmatization and marginalization and immediate access wherever people are.

 Research Example 12.1 The effectiveness of mass-media campaigns for smoking cessation

Mass-media campaigns have been shown to increase smoking cessation and reduce smoking prevalence and uptake in adults, but have been less successful in preventing smoking uptake in young people. Campaigns tend to convey messages about the negative health consequences of smoking or information about how to quit (Bala et al., 2008; Brinn et al., 2010; Durkin et al., 2012), although a counter-marketing campaign in Florida called 'Truth' was very successful. This campaign used the techniques of traditional marketing satirically. One poster promoted a spoof cigarette called 'True' (Hicks, 2001), with the strapline 'No other cigarette can make this statement: US government tests show True is lowest in both tar and nicotine of the 20 best selling cigarettes.'

Two-step or diffusion of innovation model

This model suggests that mass communication influences key opinion leaders who are active members of the mass-media audience. These opinion leaders then spread ideas to other people through interpersonal means of communication (Katz and Lazarsfeld, 1955). The process of diffusing innovation or new ideas through a population is based on the finding that the adoption of new behaviours typically follows an S-shaped trajectory (Rogers and Scott, 1997). There is usually a slow initial uptake followed by rapid acceptance, as opinion leaders or early adopters (who are usually from higher socio-economic groups) communicate the benefits, and then a final slowing as a minority (who tend to be from isolated traditional communities) resist acceptance or change. This suggests that the mass media may be important in raising awareness and communicating basic information, but interpersonal sources,

such as friends, peers and known 'experts', are most influential in persuading people to make changes. The mass media are influential in disseminating new ideas, for example, the use of folic acid during pregnancy. However, factors such as education level and income continue to influence uptake.

Uses and gratifications

This model tends to see the audience as more active in selecting and interpreting communications. It suggests that people use the media to meet their own needs, reinforcing existing beliefs and rejecting or reinterpreting communications that do not fit their existing values or beliefs.

Cultural effects

This model sees the media as having a key role in creating beliefs and values about health, medicine, disease and illness. The ways in which these are presented, from the kindly doctor in soap operas to news bulletins on miracle cures and high-tech interventions, all contribute to people's understanding of health (see e.g. Lupton, 2012). Many studies use discourse analysis to reveal the underlying values, concepts and messages implicit in media portrayals of health and ill health. Public health's long timescale and basis in numerical data make it unattractive to the mass media. Instead, 'shock-horror' stories of crisis within the National Health Service (NHS) or the appearance of rare diseases tend to dominate the news headlines.

 Learning Activity 12.2 Media coverage of public health

Monitor media coverage on television, in magazines, on radio and in broadsheet and tabloid newspapers for items about health over a 1-week period. Use the following categories to allocate coverage by type:
- medical dominance, for example, medical breakthroughs, high-technology interventions
- crisis or scare stories, for example, failures in services or outbreaks of unusual diseases or illnesses

Continued

- individual consumerism and lifestyles, for example, stories about how to choose and access healthier lifestyles and health services
- celebrities illustrating how health or anti-health behaviours can be perceived as attractive
- social, economic or political health determinants, for example, policy changes and how these might affect health
- environmental or global determinants of health, for example, the loss of agriculture and the ability to grow food due to climate change.

Does the media coverage you monitored fit into these categories?

Which categories were least/most common? What are the implications of this?

How much of the coverage was in entertainment programmes?

Think about and find some examples of how the following are represented in popular media culture:

- doctors
- hospitals and healthcare services
- chronic illnesses, for example, coronary heart disease, cancer
- acute illnesses, for example, flu
- social and environmental health
- individual state of positive health and well-being
- prevention of ill health
- protection of health.

Communication is concerned with the transmission of messages from a sender to a receiver. Messages are coded into signs and symbols which have meaning within specific codes. The message is encoded by the sender and decoded by the receiver (as shown in Fig. 12.2). The intention is that messages should be decoded and understood according to the intentions of the sender, but this can be problematic when using the mass media. This is because the mass media target large audiences simultaneously and, unlike direct personal communication, there is typically no feedback loop from the receiver back to the sender of the message. This means messages may be interpreted in ways that were not anticipated or intended by the sender. This is one reason why researching the target audience and piloting messages are an important stage in the planned use of the mass media for health promotion.

The role of mass media

Mass communication has been used in health promotion in the following ways.
- To raise public awareness through:
  - providing information
  - reminding the population of the effects of their health-damaging behaviour and the benefits of adopting healthy behaviours and lifestyles.
- Media advocacy – creating a climate of opinion conducive to policy change through maintaining the salience of an issue and making sure it is thought about.
- Social marketing – using the 'marketing mix' to achieve behaviour change.
- Direct communication – using social media, usually to support behaviour change.

There are two main ways in which mass media is used.

1. Planned campaigns and advertising. This has the advantage of reaching large numbers of people from all social classes and population groups quickly. Messages can be developed and targeted to meet specific objectives. A downside is the necessity for adequate funding in order to make an impact.
2. Unpaid publicity and media advocacy. This has the advantage of low cost and greater credibility, as messages are not seen as being directly promoted by health organizations. A downside is the lack of control over what appears in the media, which means messages may be misinterpreted or refuted.

Planned campaigns

Mass-media campaigns have been used by national health promotion agencies in the UK and worldwide to promote various health messages. Different media, including billboards, press advertisements and radio announcements, have been used, but television is the principal medium because, although it is expensive, it reaches much larger audiences and recall has been shown to be better. The end goal of most media campaigns is to achieve a specific behaviour change, although their ability to achieve such aims is disputed. Figure 12.3 is an example of a poster to promote the wearing of a helmet, targeted especially at young people, as over 40% of road traffic deaths involve people aged 0 to 25 years.

The examples below of mass-media campaigns suggest that, on their own, they are unreliable in achieving behaviour change. However, used in combination with other strategies, such as personal reinforcement from trusted peers or experts, or policy changes affecting the environment, mass-media campaigns can be effective.

 Research Example 12.2 Evaluation of mass-media campaigns

1. Sun safety – evaluation of repeated campaigns in Australia using the mass media to promote sun protection measures among children concluded that using the message 'slip, slap, slop' was linked to a decrease in the incidence of melanoma in young people since the 1990s. However, health promotion campaigns are competing against a range of commercial messages, for example, about the safety of sunscreens and vitamin D deficiency (www.sunsmart.com.au).

2. Change for Life – a social marketing campaign to reframe childhood obesity as a health issue. Mass media were effective in raising awareness in the targeted group, but there was little impact on behaviour (Croker et al., 2012). However, other campaigns, for example, VERB in the USA (www.cdc.gov/youth-campaign/) and ParticipACTION (Craig et al., 2009) in Canada, which both focused on physical activity, showed behavioural effects.

3. Weight gain – a repeated campaign aimed at preventing weight gain in the Netherlands resulted, after the final campaign wave, in high awareness (88%) and message recall (68%), and positive attitudes and motivation. However, the campaign had mixed effects on self-efficacy and negative effects on risk perception (Wammes et al., 2007).

Mass-media campaigns adopt a variety of tactics to communicate their message, including emotional appeals, shock tactics and reassurance. The evidence on whether or not fear is an effective strategy is inconclusive. Early studies showed that people may attend to, comprehend and retain information when shocked, but may also become resistant or deny the relevance of the message (Montazeri et al., 1998). The use of fear appeals in social marketing has been criticized for its relative ineffectiveness and its unintended negative consequences (e.g. anxiety, complacency and increased social inequity; Hastings et al., 2004). However, a review of mass-media anti-smoking campaigns (Grey et al., 2000) concluded that 'threatening' and 'supportive' approaches could complement each other and contribute to overall effectiveness. What was important was an appeal to the emotions, coupled with supportive messages. It is also important to present a clear action which individuals feel confident they can take.

Extensive reviews of media campaigns now conclude that they may be successful if their goals are reasonable and there is no expectation of immediate results. Green et al. (2015) refer to the hierarchy of communication effects, which suggests that simple awareness or market penetration is relatively easy to achieve; to inform or reinforce attitudes is more difficult; and to have any effect on behaviour is even more difficult. They identify certain preconditions for success:

- favourable public opinion, which is most likely when there has been extensive market research at the design stage
- time available for the presentation of complex information
- support through interpersonal communication.

 Learning Activity 12.3 Evaluating mass-media campaigns

How would you evaluate a mass-media campaign to reduce drink-driving?

Evaluations of mass-media campaigns take many forms:
- coverage (the percentage of the target population who were exposed to the message)
- recall (the percentage of the population who could accurately recall the message)
- impact of the campaign on behaviour
- cost-effectiveness.

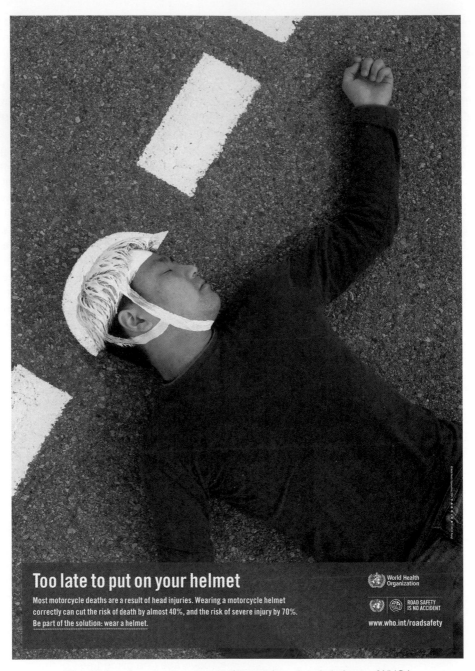

Too late to put on your helmet

Most motorcycle deaths are a result of head injuries. Wearing a motorcycle helmet correctly can cut the risk of death by almost 40%, and the risk of severe injury by 70%. Be part of the solution: wear a helmet.

World Health Organization

ROAD SAFETY IS NO ACCIDENT

www.who.int/roadsafety

Fig. 12.3 ● A poster to promote the wearing of cycle helmets. (WHO.)

Unpaid media coverage

The mass media have no responsibility to promote health, and so if they address such issues it is because the issues are inherently newsworthy or have been packaged by health promoters to become newsworthy. The tendency to sensationalize means that it is the emotional, the dramatic or the tragic that gets space. Stories tend to relate to individuals, and issues which concern population groups such as older people or the determinants of health tend to be ignored. The emphasis on behavioural journalism means that personalities or real-life case studies are also prominent.

The term 'unplanned' is used to describe media coverage that is not specifically paid for as part of a campaign. Health promotion has become increasingly concerned to generate news stories, and campaigns can extend their reach enormously through unpaid coverage. Chapman and Dominello (2001) found that newspaper coverage of tobacco and health issues could be significantly affected and increased through a strategy of proactive press reports. The key to increased media coverage was to use newsworthy aspects, for example, celebrities, moral panics or medical scares, to contextualize the story. Giving a local spin to general stories will also ensure coverage in regional media. Newsworthiness depends less on the importance of an issue than on its immediate impact, which is often heightened by being linked to celebrities in emotive ways. For example, the involvement of celebrity chef Jamie Oliver led to a dramatic increase in media coverage of children's diets and healthy school meals.

Although such tactics may increase coverage of the work of health promoters and put across health messages, the ability of the media to distort and sensationalize should always be remembered. An editorial in *The Observer* newspaper in 1994 commented: 'There is nothing quite so irresponsible as the media in hot pursuit of a health scare and nothing quite so gullible as the public presented with one.' The editorial was prompted by a concern about necrotizing fasciitis (a tissue-destroying disease caused by a strain of bacteria), which was neither new nor on the increase, but which had prompted headlines such as 'Killer bug eats my body' and 'Flesh-eater on the move'.

Media interest can be generated by surveys or research reports. However, such reports frequently result in health scares because of poor reporting and misunderstanding of statistics and the concept of risk. An example is the research study in 1998 led by Andrew Wakefield linking the measles, mumps and rubella (MMR) vaccine to the development of autism and Crohn's disease in young children, which led to a drop in MMR uptake immediately following the press reports.

 Case Study 12.2 Media coverage of swine flu

A/HINI, or swine flu, spread rapidly across the world and was classed as a global pandemic in June 2009. In contrast to other media reporting of major health issues, an analysis of the content and framing of the issue found that coverage was immense, but reflected scientific uncertainties about the cause of the pandemic. Risks were not exaggerated and coverage was measured (Hilton and Hunt, 2011).

Although the generation of unpaid publicity can be effective and have minimal cost, it is difficult to sustain a high level of coverage for more than a few days. Health promoters need persistence and creativity to keep issues prominent in the media. There is also a need for media training for health promoters in skills such as writing press releases, networking and design in order to access and use the media to their full potential.

Another way of gaining awareness is having health events. Most countries have a calendar of health awareness weeks or months designed to raise awareness of particular conditions, for example, Mental Health Awareness Week or Breast Cancer Awareness Month. Very few comprehensive evaluations of these events have been conducted. Public awareness of some events, which are supported by coloured ribbons, is high, for example, breast cancer and HIV/AIDS. The effect of such events on health behaviours is less clear, and unlikely to be significant if the desired health behaviour is not yet a social norm.

Media advocacy

Public policy is rarely a consequence of direct approaches to policymakers, and increasingly there is a recognition that public opinion can influence decisions. Media advocacy is a particular strategy of using the media to try to generate public concern about the ways in which the legislative, economic or environmental context affects public health. Examples include promoting the smoking ban in public places and the debate surrounding food-labelling regulations. Media advocacy is therefore a means of applying pressure for policy change to advance public health objectives (Wallack and Dorfman, 1996). Often there is major opposition from established economic interests to the proposed policy change. Media advocacy objectives are:

- to get an issue discussed
- to get an issue discussed differently
- to discredit opponents
- to bring in new voices
- to introduce new facts or perspectives
- to shift risk perceptions.

An example of successful media advocacy involving international cooperation was the Nestlé boycott of the 1970s and 1980s, which led to the World Health Organization's International Code of Marketing for Breast Milk Substitutes (McKee et al., 2005). Direct action can also be successful, as evidenced by Billboard Utilising Graffitists Against Unhealthy Promotions (BUGA-UP), an Australian group which targeted tobacco advertising (Fig. 12.4).

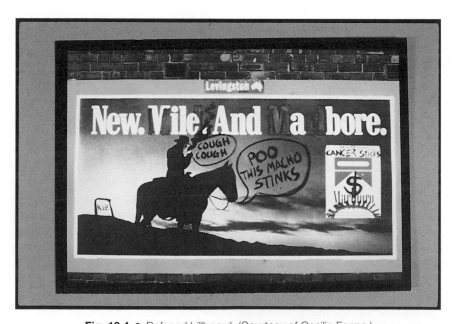

Fig. 12.4 ● Defaced billboard. (Courtesy of Cecilia Farren.)

'38 degrees' is a UK political activist movement that has gained 1.8 million members since 2009. It seeks to engage and mobilize the public on single-issue campaigns using email voting. One campaign, against the selling off of forests to private investors, got 500,000 people to vote and 100,000 to write to their Members of Parliament, while thousands paid for a national press advertising campaign. Within 8 months the plan was shelved.

Social marketing

Just as commercial companies are able to get the public to buy products (even those they may not really need), so health promoters should be able to get people to choose healthy behaviours. Some of the techniques of marketing are now being widely used in health promotion to influence the acceptability of healthy lifestyles so that they seem desirable and easy to adopt. One of the limitations of mass-media campaigns is that they are a one-way communication process and tend to adopt a uniform population message. Increasingly, health promoters are making use of social marketing techniques that allow specific groups to be targeted (Naidoo and Wills, 2010). The English public health white paper declared that 'Central government will sequence social marketing for public health throughout the life course… using emerging ideas from behavioural science, such as the use of social norms, changing defaults and providing incentives' (Department of Health 2010a, p. 44).

Marketing segments the population into different subgroups based on attitudes and behaviour as well as cruder socio-economic and demographic variables. Psychographic segmentation helps to reveal patterns or differences between groups of people who may be similar in age, gender or socio-economic status. Table 12.1 shows some ways in which segmentation has been used in recent studies of health behaviour.

Commercial marketing is based on the idea of 'exchange' – that the marketer tries to offer something the consumer wants at an acceptable price.

Health promoters are beginning to recognize the importance of formative research, which carefully identifies what people see as the benefits of particular health behaviours, so that these can be incorporated into the campaign message. In a sense this is merely an application of the health belief model (see Chapter 9), which suggests that for people to make a change in their health behaviour they need to see the benefits outweighing costs such as time and effort. For example, the marketing of condom use involves acknowledgement of the costs (money, embarrassment and loss of pleasure) and an emphasis on the benefits (protection against pregnancy and sexually transmitted infections, a sense of control and less anxiety).

 Learning Activity 12.4 Social marketing

How would you go about social marketing to raise awareness of a 'taboo' issue such as incontinence?

Marketing a commercial product is very different from trying to sell health. Advertising typically mobilizes existing predispositions, whereas health promotion typically tries to counter them. For example, advertising associates the product (beer, crisps) with something people desire, such as fun. All too often, health promotion messages are about not indulging, and therefore by implication not having fun (don't drink and drive, eat less fat). Advertising is selling things in the here and now, to be consumed and enjoyed immediately. By contrast, health promotion messages are often about forgoing present enjoyment for future benefits.

As we have seen, selling a product is a complex and carefully researched process. The needs of the market have to be identified, messages developed which will appeal to the market segment that is being targeted, and a comparison made of different media channels and their relative effectiveness in reaching the general and the targeted population. Together these aspects make up the marketing mix, which is said to comprise four Ps (Table 12.2).

Table 12.1 Psychographic segmentation and health behaviours

Segmentation type	Used by	Description	Sample segment
Geodemographic	Mosaic – UK profiling tool (Experian, 2004)	Classifications identify neighbourhood household types and person types based on demographic data (e.g. age, sex, socio-economic status, property characteristics, location) and financial measures indicating behaviour	*Bright Young Things:* well-educated young singles paying high rents to live in smart inner-city apartments
Psychographic	Sport England market segmentation (Sport England, 2009)	Used results from the Active People survey to identify 19 sporting segments and better understand the nation's attitudes to sports and motivations for action	*Sports Team Lads:* young blokes enjoying football, pints and pool
Life course	Healthy Foundations (Department of Health, 2010b)	Classification based on life stages which can encourage healthy or unhealthy behaviours; nine life stages were identified	*Young Settlers:* people aged 16–44 who have a partner, no children in the household, no caring responsibilities and are not retired
Pen portraits	Maximizing the appeal of weight management services (Department of Health, 2010c)	Based on interviews and focus groups, this study identified nine people segments based on motivations, barriers and ideal services	*Younger Women:* aspiring to 'body beautiful'; desire a youthful and glamorous service that is active and energizing

Wills et al. (2014).

Table 12.2 The marketing mix: The four Ps

Tool	Definition	Example
Product	The behavioural offer	Adoption of an idea or behaviour
Price	The value of the product and how important it is to the audience; the costs they may have to bear and the barriers they may have to overcome	Psychological, emotional, cultural, behavioural, practical, financial
Place	The channels by which the change is promoted and places in which change is encouraged	Media, personal communication, social media
Promotion	The means by which the change is promoted to the audience	Advertising, direct mail, publicity

The third national HIV testing week campaign took place in November 2014. Look at the poster below (Fig. 12.5).

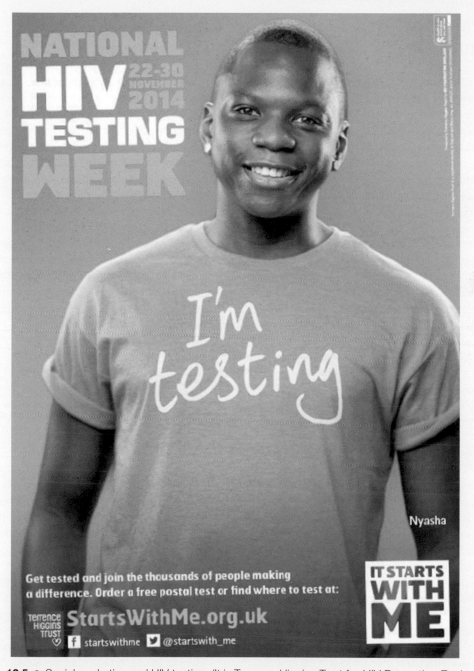

Fig. 12.5 ● Social marketing and HIV testing. (It is Terrence Higgins Trust for HIV Prevention England.)

What is the product?
What is the price?
What is the place?
What is the promotion?

What the mass media can and cannot do

Research and evaluation of the use of the mass media in health promotion have led to a reassessment of their potential and limitations (see particularly Green et al., 2015). It is now accepted that the mass media can:

- raise consciousness about health issues, for example, drink-driving
- contextualize an issue within a value framework, for example, childhood obesity as a result of parental negligence
- help place health on the public agenda, for example, nutritional content of fast food
- convey simple information and single messages, for example, put babies to sleep on their backs
- change behaviour if other enabling factors are present, for example, encourage smokers already committed to giving up.

Factors which enable behaviour change include existing motivation, supportive circumstances and advocating a simple one-off behaviour change (e.g. carry a donor card, install a smoke alarm).

Using the media is more effective if:

- they are part of an integrated campaign, including other elements such as one-to-one advice
- the information is new and presented in an emotional context
- the message resonates with popular values or is linked to celebrities
- the information is seen as being relevant for 'people like me'.

The mass media cannot:

- convey complex information, for example, the relative risks of different kinds of fat in the diet
- teach skills, for example, how to negotiate safer sex
- shift people's attitudes or beliefs – if messages are presented which challenge basic beliefs, it is more likely that the message will be ignored, dismissed or interpreted to mean something else
- change behaviour in the absence of other enabling factors.

Communication tools

A majority of patients actively seek information about how to cope with health problems, of whom three-quarters cite their doctor as the most important source of health information. About a third use the internet and a quarter look for information in leaflets and books (Coulter et al., 2006). Leaflets and pamphlets have been used to educate the public since the beginning of the twentieth century. When the Central Council for Health Education was established in 1927 it listed the provision of better and cheaper leaflets as its main aim. The greatest use of written material is to support one-to-one interactions with clients and patients. As only 50% of information can be recalled by patients 5 minutes after a consultation, this seems an effective use of leaflets. There is some evidence that written information can not only improve patients' understanding and recall, but also provide reassurance.

 Learning Activity 12.6 Health communication

What would be the key considerations for using written information as part of health communication?

Multimedia tools and other new technologies offer many new opportunities for the dissemination of information. The worldwide web offers the possibility of interactive dialogue and for the public to select the information they require at a time convenient for them. The Pew Internet Project in the USA (www.pewinternet.org and www.pewglobal.org) found that:

- 87% of US adults use the internet
- 90% of US adults own a cell (mobile) phone and 58% own a smartphone
- 95% of adults in China own a cellphone
- 59% of adults in Uganda own a cellphone and 12% own a smartphone
- 28% of people in Nigeria and 30% in Venezuela say they get information about health and medicines from the internet.

Case Study 12.3 Mobile midwife in Ghana

In Ghana the need to reduce infant and maternal mortality is acute. In 2008:

- the mortality rate for children under 5 years old was 79 per 1000
- the maternal mortality rate was 350 per 100,000
- the percentage of births attended by skilled staff was 57%, while the world average was 65% in 2009
- the adolescent (ages 15–19) fertility rate was 69 per 1000 births.

Mobile Technology for Community Health (Motech, see motechsuite.org) was launched in July 2010 in Ghana, funded by a grant from the Bill & Melinda Gates Foundation. The scheme involves pregnant women registering by providing their phone number, area in which they live, their estimated due date and language preference. They then receive information and advice via text and voice messages, including general information – such as the location of the closest health facility and treatments that they should receive – and messages tailored to antenatal history.

After each appointment, the nurse updates medical records electronically using a mobile phone. By reviewing a digitally generated monthly report, she can see who has had the correct vaccinations, for example. It also means that the health service can gather centralized data on maternal health. A desk-top nurse application has been developed to make it easier to enter large amounts of data, as well as an app for android smartphones.

Mobile technology is not a quick fix – many Ghanaians claim to have a mobile phone, but it is often shared with an entire family, drastically limiting access. Healthcare workers can regard automation such as this as extra work.

http://www.who.int/woman_child_accountability/ierg/reports/2012_08S_improving_access_to_maternal_child_health_service.pdf.

The rapid expansion of mobile phone ownership provides new opportunities for health communication.

Telemedicine, including the helpline NHS 111, offers a two-way dialogue allowing people who are unable to access primary care to ask questions and get feedback about their symptoms. These new technologies offer a simulation of human interaction – conversations, the café, support groups – all of which can be harnessed to link health information with the important element of sociability.

Research Example 12.3 Telehealth

Telehealth and telecare involve the use of technology to help people with a long-term condition to maintain independence and feel in control of their health, and to promote health and safety. Telehealth is equipment to monitor people's health in their own homes, for example a small device that can take readings such as blood pressure, oxygen levels, weight and temperature via a telephone line to a monitoring centre. Telecare includes a system of alarms, sensors and other equipment around the home that detects risks, for example, falls.

A study of the effects of telehealth on people with long-term conditions found that there was a small decrease in admissions to hospital compared to a control group. Other measures of hospital use (elective admissions, outpatient attendances and emergency department visits) were not significantly different between the groups, nor were the differences in notional hospital costs (Steventon et al., 2012). A review by the Centre for Reviews and Dissemination (2013, p. 11) concluded that:

although there is a large amount of evidence evaluating the effects of telehealth interventions, much of it is weak and/or contradictory. However, there is good evidence that telehealth monitoring can reduce mortality in patients with heart failure, particularly those recently discharged from hospital.

The proliferation of avenues of communication does not necessarily mean that people are better informed about health issues today. Quality control is often absent (e.g. in much of the worldwide web), and even when it exists, the criteria used are often not explicit. Commonly agreed criteria include being up to date, using reliable sources of information and information that is reliable, relevant, accurate and accessible (e.g. as assessed by readability tests).

Conclusion

Media are a significant partner and resource for health, but one that needs to be understood and used according to its own priorities. To expect a mass-media campaign to produce large shifts in behaviour and contribute directly to reduced morbidity and mortality is unrealistic. But the media can work for health by supporting individual and social change, and new technologies offer huge opportunities.

There are examples of mass-media campaigns impacting on behaviours, although effects are small and generally information seems to have more impact on knowledge and beliefs than on actual behaviour. Some messages that provoke changes in social norms have been effective but, as Robertson (2008) states, it is not clear exactly which messages do this and how.

On an individual level media can supplement, but not substitute for, one-to-one education and advice. Even with sophisticated marketing and audience research, media remain a fairly blunt instrument with little opportunity for feedback or clarification. However, the media can raise awareness, provide information and motivate people to change if their environment is supportive. The media can also be used to advocate for public health by shifting public opinion and encouraging the formation of healthy

public policies. The media can be used for social marketing, to promote attitudes, beliefs and behaviours that are conducive to health. Other forms of media, such as leaflets and posters, can provide a useful supplementary communication tool to inform, educate and advise people about health issues.

Questions for further discussion

In your practice how are media used to:
- raise awareness?
- provide information?

Summary

This chapter has looked at the ways in which the media, especially the mass media, are used to promote health. It has discussed different strategies, including information giving, advertising as part of a planned campaign, media advocacy and the marketing of health messages. There is now greater awareness of how to use the mass media more effectively, and the chapter looked at how media coverage can be generated and used to influence public opinion. It has reviewed evaluation studies that demonstrate how effective communication combines information with the key element of interaction.

 Feedback to learning activities

12.1 Studies of media representations show that alcohol consumption is presented as normal and unproblematic, with the portrayal of negative consequences being rare. The media may also influence behaviour by documenting nights out, when large amounts of alcohol are consumed (Atkinson et al., 2011).

12.2 It is likely that the greatest representation of health items, in both factual and entertainment programmes, will be about medicine. An Ebola outbreak raged across West Africa in 2014. Such diseases are often presented as uncontrollable, yet at the same time as posing little threat (Joffee and Haarhoff, 2002). Public health and health pro-

motion are unlikely to have received much media coverage.

12.3 Evaluation of a mass-media campaign to reduce drink-driving could take many forms, for example:
- coverage (the percentage of the target population who were exposed to the message)
- recall (the percentage of the population who could accurately recall the message)
- behaviour (changes in behaviour, such as statistics relating to the incidence of drink-driving)
- incidence of alcohol-related car accidents (this is the main cause for concern and is likely to be better monitored than drink-driving).
- cost-effectiveness of such a campaign.

12.4 Social marketing can seek to raise awareness or prompt a behaviour change. For an issue that is rarely discussed in public, the message must be made to seem relevant. It should identify a clear action the audience could take or some form of engagement, and make clear the benefits.

12.5 The product is an HIV test for which individuals take personal responsibility. The motivating declaration 'I'm testing' is intended to act as a social norm – people like themselves are taking the action. The benefits of an early diagnosis are also stressed.

The price includes barriers to testing such as stigma, lack of access, privacy and confidentiality, which are addressed.

The place includes social media, the press and outdoor advertising, for example, on London buses.

The promotion includes advertising, direct mailing and publicity, for example, stickers and t-shirts.

12.6 Any information should:
- be suitable for the target audience, for example, culturally sensitive and representative of the intended audience
- be available in different formats, for example, in different languages and in Braille
- be pitched at an appropriate literacy level
- have an effective design and structure
- have accurate and up-to-date content.

Further reading and resources

Corcoran, N. (Ed.), 2013. Communicating Health: Strategies for Health Promotion, second ed. Sage, London.

Chapter 4 examines the role of mass media in health promotion and engages with practical issues of how to design mass-media campaigns. Social marketing and media advocacy are also discussed.

French, J., Blair-Stevens, C., McVey, D., Merritt, R. (Eds.), 2009. Social Marketing and Public Health: Theory and Practice Oxford. Oxford University Press.

An analysis and case studies of social marketing applied to public health.

Naidoo, J., Wills, J., 2010. Public Health and Health Promotion: Developing Practice, third ed. Baillière Tindall, London.

Chapter 8, on information, education and communication, discusses how to target health messages so that they are effective, and how to use a social marketing approach.

References

Atkin, C.K., Rice, R.E., 2014. Theory and principles of media health campaigns. In: Rice, R.E., Atkin, C.K. (Eds.), Public Communication Campaigns, fourth ed. Sage, London.

Atkinson, A., Elliot, G., Bellis, M., Sumnall, H., 2011. Young People, Alcohol and the Media. Joseph Rowntree Foundation, York. Available online at: www.jrf.org.uk.

Bala, M., Strzeszynski, L., Cahill, K., 2008. Mass media interventions for smoking cessation in adults. Cochrane Database Systematic Reviews (1), CD004704. Available online at: http://onlinelibrary.wiley.com/doi/10.1002/14651858.CD004704.pub3/full (accessed 16.09.15).

Beattie, A., et al., 1993. The changing boundaries of health. In: Beattie, A., Gott, M., Jones, L. (Eds.), Health and Wellbeing: A Reader. Macmillan/Open University, Basingstoke.

Brinn, M., Carson, K., Esterman, A., 2010. Mass media interventions for preventing smoking in young people. Cochrane Database Systematic Reviews 11, CD001006.

Carter, M., 2014. How Twitter may have helped Nigeria contain Ebola. British Medical Journal 349, g6946.

Centre for Reviews and Dissemination, 2013. Telehealth for People with Long-term Conditions. CRD, York. Available online at: https://www.york.ac.uk/media/crd/Telehealth.pdf (accessed 16.09.15).

Chapman, S., Dominello, A., 2001. A strategy for increasing news media coverage of tobacco and health in Australia. Health Promotion International 16, 137–143. Available online at: http://m.heapro.oxfordjournals.org/content/16/2/137.full.pdf (accessed 16.09.15)

Coulter, A., Ellins, J., Swain, D., et al., 2006. Assessing the Quality of Information to Support People in Making Decisions about Their Health and Healthcare. Picker Institute, Oxford. Available online at: http://www.pickereurope.org/wp-content/uploads/2014/10/Assessing-the-quality-of-information-to-support-people-in-makin.pdf (accessed 16.09.15).

Craig, C.L., Bouman, A., Gauvin, L., Robertson, J., Murumets, K., 2009. ParticipACTION: a mass media campaign targeting parents of inactive children: knowledge, saliency, and trialing behaviours. International Journal of Behavioural Nutrition and Physical Activity 6, 88. Available online at: http://www.biomedcentral.com/content/pdf/1471-2458-12-404.pdf (accessed 16.09.15).

Croker, H., Lucas, R., Wardle, J., 2012. Cluster randomized trial to evaluate the "Change for Life" mass media/social marketing campaign in the UJK. BMC Public Health 12, 404. Available online at: http://www.biomedcentral.com/content/pdf/1471-2458-12-404.pdf (accessed 16.09.15).

Department of Health, 2010a. Healthy Lives, Healthy People: Our Strategy for Public Health in England. Department of Health, London. Available online at: https://www.gov.uk/government/uploads/system/uploads/attachment_data/file/216096/dh_127424.pdf (accessed 16.09.15).

Department of Health, 2010b. Ambitions for Health: A Strategic Framework for Maximizing the Potential of Social Marketing and Health Related Behaviour. Department of Health, London.

Department of Health, 2010c. Maximising the Appeal of Weight Management Services. Department of Health, London. Available online at: http://webarchive.nationalarchives.gov.uk/20130107105354/http://www.dh.gov.uk/prod_consum_dh/groups/dh_digitalassets/documents/digitalasset/dh_114723.pdf (accessed 16.09.15).

Dobkin, L., Kent, C., Klausner, J., et al., 2007. Is text messaging key to improving adolescent sexual health? Journal of Adolescent Health 40, S14.

Durkin, S., Brennan, E., Wakefield, M., 2012. Mass media campaigns to promote smoking cessation among adults: an integrative review. Tobacco Control 21, 127–138. Available online at: http://m.tobaccocontrol.bmj.com/content/21/2/127.full.pdf (accessed 16.09.15).

Experian, 2004. MOSAIC United Kingdom: The Consumer Classification for the UK Experian. Nottingham. Available online at: www.experian.co.uk/assets/business.

Franklin, V.L., Waller, A., Pagliari, C., et al., 2006. A randomized controlled trial of Sweet Talk, a text-messaging system to support young people with diabetes. Diabetic Medicine 23, 1332–1338. Available online at: http://onlinelibrary.wiley.com/doi/10.1111/j.1464-5491.2006.01989.x/epdf (accessed 16.09.15).

Gatherer, A., Parfit, J., Porter, E., et al., 1979. Is Health Education Effective? Health Education Council, London.

Green, J., Tones, K., Cross, R., Woodall, J., 2015. Health Promotion: Planning and Strategies, third ed. Sage, London.

Grey, A., Owen, L., Bolling, K., 2000. A Breath of Fresh Air: Tackling Smoking through the Media. National Institute of Health and Clinical Excellence, London. Available online at: https://www.nice.org.uk/proxy/?sourceUrl=http%3a%2f%2fwww.nice.org.uk%2fnicemedia%2fdocuments%2fsmokingmedia.pdf (accessed 18.09.15).

Hastings, G., Stead, M., Webb, J., 2004. Fear appeals in social marketing: strategic and ethical reasons for concern. Psychology and Marketing 21, 961–986.

Hicks, J., 2001. The strategy behind Florida's "truth" campaign. Tobacco Control 10, 3–5. Available online at: http://m.tobaccocontrol.bmj.com/content/10/1/3.full.pdf (accessed 18.09.15).

Hilton, S., Hunt, K., 2011. UK newspapers' representations of the 2009–2010 outbreak of swine flue: one health scare not overhyped by the media? Journal of Epidemiology and Community Health 65, 941–946. Available online at: http://m.jech.bmj.com/content/65/10/941.full.pdf (accessed 18.09.15).

Joffe, H., Haarhoff, G., 2002. Representations of far-flung illnesses: the case of Ebola in Britain. Social Science and Medicine 54, 955–969.

Katz, E., Lazarsfeld, P., 1955. Personal Influence: The Part Played by People in the Flow of Mass Communication. Free Press, Glencoe, Illinois.

Lasswell, H., 1948. The Structure and Function of Communication in Society. Institute for Religious and Social Studies, New York. Sourced in Fiske, J., 1990. Introduction to communication studies, second ed. Routledge, London.

Lupton, D., 2012. Medicine As Culture: Illness, Disease and the Body, third ed. Sage, London.

McKee, M., Gilmore, A.B., Schwalbe, N., 2005. International cooperation and health: part two: making a difference. Journal of Epidemiology and Community Health 59, 737–739. Available online at: http://m.jech.bmj.com/content/59/8/628.full.pdf (accessed 18.09.15).

McQuail, D., 2010. Mass Communication Theory, sixth ed. Sage Publications, London.

Montazeri, A., McGhee, S., McEwan, J., 1998. Fear inducing and positive image strategies in health education campaigns. International Journal of Health Promotion and Education 36, 68–75.

Naidoo, J., Wills, J., 2010. Public Health and Health Promotion: Developing Practice, third ed. Baillière Tindall, London.

Robertson, R., 2008. Using Information to Promote Healthy Behaviours. Kings Fund, London. Available online at: http://www.kingsfund.org.uk/sites/files/kf/field/field_document/information-promote-healthy-behaviours-kicking-bad-habits-supporting-paper-ruth-robertson.pdf (accessed 18.09.15).

Rogers, E.M., Scott, K.L., 1997. The Diffusion of Innovations Model and Outreach from the National Network of Libraries of Medicine to Native American Communities. Available online at: http://nnlm.gov/archive/pnr/eval/rogers.html (accessed 18.09.15).

Sport England, 2009. Market Segmentation. Available online at: http://segments.sportengland.org (accessed 19.03.15).

Steventon, A., Bardsley, M., Billings, J., Dixon, J., Doll, H., Hirani, S., et al., 2012. Effect of telehealth on use of secondary care and mortality: findings from the Whole System Demonstrator cluster randomised trial. BMJ 344, e3874. Available online at: http://www.bmj.com/content/344/bmj.e3874 (accessed 18.09.15).

Tones, K., 1993. Changing theory and practice: trends in methods, strategies and settings in health education. Health Education Journal 52, 126–139.

Wallack, L., Dorfman, L., 1996. Media advocacy: a strategy for advancing policy and promoting health. Health Education and Behaviour 23, 293–317.

Wammes, B., Oenema, A., Brug, J., 2007. The evaluation of a mass media campaign aimed at weight gain prevention among young Dutch adults. Obesity 15, 2780–2789. Available online at: http://onlinelibrary.wiley.com/doi/10.1038/oby.2007.330/epdf (accessed 18.09.15).

Wills, J., Crichton, N., Lorenc, A., Kelly, M., 2014. Using population segment to inform local obesity strategy in England. Health Promotion International. Available online at: http://dx.doi.org/10.1093/heapro/dau004.

Part Three
Settings for health promotion

This part of the book is concerned with the settings that can promote health. It is in settings that we live our lives – at school, at work, in neighbourhoods, in our contact with health services or in prisons. The Ottawa Charter (World Health Organization, 1986, p. 3) stated that 'health is created and lived by people within the settings of their everyday life: where they learn, work, play and love'. One of the five key action areas identified in the Ottawa Charter was creating supportive environments. As we have seen in this book, the focus of health promotion activity is moving away from identifying the diseases and conditions contributing to ill health and the groups at risk and towards identifying the complex interplay of factors which create health. It is in settings – at school, at work, in our neighbourhood, in hospital or in prison – that we live our lives, and it is these contexts or settings which need to be made more conducive to health.

Health promotion has been carried out in particular settings for many years. Workplaces and schools, for example, have provided established channels to reach defined populations. The concept of a settings approach to health promotion, however, is quite distinct and first emerged in the 1980s. The settings approach seeks to make systemic changes to the whole environment. This contrasts with using the setting as a convenient route to access individuals and provide traditional health education messages.

The settings approach builds a concern for health into the fabric of the system and makes sure that the routine activities of the system are committed to and take account of health. Adopting a healthy settings approach is fundamentally different to carrying out a one-off short-term health promotion project within a particular setting, and although the titles of the chapters in this part refer to health promotion *in* a setting, we are describing approaches to create 'health promoting settings'. Nutbeam (1998) describes a setting as

where people actively use and shape the environment and thus create, or solve problems relating to, health. Settings can normally be identified as having physical boundaries, a range of people with defined roles, and an organizational structure.

The settings approach is a long-term one. In most cases it is being implemented through defined projects which are designed to:

- introduce specific interventions to create healthy working and living environments

- develop health policies
- integrate health into quality, audit and evaluation procedures to build evidence of how health can make the system perform better.

The first and most well-known example of settings-based health promotion is the Healthy Cities project. Originally this was a small project initiated by the World Health Organization in 1986 to put the Ottawa Charter and Health for All (World Health Organization, 1985, 1986) principles into practice. It has subsequently expanded to become a worldwide movement incorporating over 1200 cities in more than 30 countries in the European region (www. euro.who.int/healthy-cities). Parallel initiatives have been developed and are coordinated by international networks in schools, hospitals, workplaces, prisons and universities. The UK health strategies have all referred to the importance of settings. *The Health of the Nation* (Department of Health, 1992) stated that settings 'offer between them the potential to involve most people in the country'. Schools, neighbourhoods, workplaces and prisons are also identified in *Choosing Health*: *Making Healthy Choices Easier* (Department of Health, 2004) as key settings through which inequalities in health should be tackled.

The settings approach is complex, and characterized by several unique factors (Dooris, 2005):

- an ecological model of health promotion that conceptualizes health as determined by a range of socio-economic, organizational, environmental and personal factors
- a focus on health and well-being rather than illness
- a focus on populations rather than individuals
- a holistic, salutogenic view of health rather than a mechanistic reductionist view that focuses on how health is created
- a systems perspective that sees settings as complex systems interacting dynamically with their environment and interconnected to other settings
- a whole-organization focus that seeks to change from within the organization.

As has been outlined in the rest of this book, health promotion draws upon ecological models of health that seek to explain the relationship and contributions of behaviour and the environment to the creation and maintenance of health and well-being, and points to the duality of structure and agency (Dooris et al., 2014). Implementing health promotion in settings requires the setting itself to change, and Poland et al. (2009) usefully set out a series of questions to guide practitioners in their understanding of the features of the setting. These include thinking about how the setting (e.g. hospitals) is different from (or similar to) other categories of settings (e.g. schools, workplaces), and how the setting interacts with other related settings and systems as well as the local environment to accomplish its goals. Poland et al. (2009) draw attention to not only the physical and built environment that may be causing ill health in this setting (ergonomics, noxious hazards, physical and social isolation or lack of opportunities for interaction, access to green space, etc.), but also the psychosocial environment that has a bearing on health and the possibilities for intervention in this setting, e.g. the workload and decision latitude, control over pace, status hierarchies and the quality of human relations (trust, reciprocity, local social capital and social cohesion, bullying). As we will see in the following chapters, it is important to consider the meaning of health from the different stakeholder perspectives in the setting and its salience to them.

The benefits of such an approach are hard to quantify, but appear to be significant. They include encouraging partnership working and collaboration, embedding health in organizational structures and systems, and taking account of broader determinants of health. Perhaps not surprisingly, given the complexity of this approach, evaluation and evidence for the effectiveness of the settings approach are rather scanty:

The settings approach has been legitimated more through an act of faith than through rigorous research and evaluation studies... much more attention needs to be given to building the evidence and learning from it

St Leger (1997), p. 100.

Part Three looks at health promotion in five key settings.

1. Workplaces.
2. Schools.
3. Neighbourhoods.
4. Hospitals.
5. Prisons.

Each setting is addressed in a separate chapter, but it is important to remember that the settings are not discrete but coexist as part of a wider independent system. Schools, workplaces and hospitals are all in neighbourhoods, and there is a constant flow of people within and between the settings. Prisons, although more separated from their neighbourhoods, are also sited in a specific locality and impact upon that locality in terms of employment and transport. And there are many other settings where health promotion interventions may be delivered, e.g. nightclubs, sports stadia and barbers' shops.

Each of the following chapters examines why the setting is appropriate for health promotion, identifying the factors of the settings which affect health and outlining some health promoting initiatives which have been developed in that setting.

References

Department of Health, 1992. The Health of the Nation. London, HMSO.

Department of Health, 2004. Choosing Health: Making Healthy Choices Easier. London, Stationery Office. Available online at: http://webarchive.nationalarchives.gov.uk/+/dh.gov.uk/en/publicationsandstatistics/publications/publicationspolicyandguidance/dh_4094550 (accessed 18.09.15).

Dooris, M., 2005. Healthy settings: challenges to generating evidence of effectiveness. Health Promotion International 21, 55–65. Available online at: http://heapro.oxfordjournals.org/content/21/1/55.full.pdf+html (accessed 18.09.15).

Dooris, M., Wills, J., Newton, J., 2014. Theorising healthy settings: a critical discussion with reference to healthy universities. Scandinavian Journal of Public Health 42(Suppl. 15), 7–16. Available online at: http://sjp.sagepub.com/content/42/15_suppl/7.long (accessed 18.09.15).

Nutbeam, D., 1998. Health Promotion Glossary. Geneva, WHO. Available online at: http://www.who.int/healthpromotion/about/HPR%20Glossary%201998.pdf?ua=1 (accessed 05.03.15).

Poland, B., Krupa, G., McCall, D., 2009. Settings for health promotion: an analytic framework to guide intervention design and implementation. Health Promotion Practice 10(4), 505–516. Available online at: http://hpp.sagepub.com/content/10/4/505.full.pdf (accessed 07.03.15).

St Leger, L., 1997. Health promoting settings: from Ottawa to Jakarta. Health Promotion International 12, 99–101. Available online at: http://heapro.oxfordjournals.org/content/12/2/99.full.pdf (accessed 18.09.15).

World Health Organization, 1985. Targets for Health for All. Copenhagen, WHO Regional Office for Europe.

World Health Organization, 1986. Ottawa Charter for Health Promotion. Geneva, WHO. Available online at: http://www.who.int/healthpromotion/conferences/previous/ottawa/en/ (accessed 05.03.15).

13

Health promoting schools

Learning Outcomes

By the end of this chapter you will be able to:
- understand how health promotion can be incorporated into the school setting
- understand how schools can enhance or inhibit health
- describe the elements of a health promoting school.

Key Concepts and Definitions

School-based health promotion Health promotion activities that take place within a school setting, for example sex education, traffic awareness education, physical activity sessions.

Health promoting school A health promoting school is one that constantly strengthens its capacity as a healthy setting for living, learning and working. A health promoting school seeks to provide a healthy environment that engages all parties (children, parents, teachers, communities).

Curriculum The lessons and academic content taught in a school or in a specific course or programme.

PSHE Personal, social, and health education was introduced as part of UK schools' national curriculum in 2000. In 2008 the subject was renamed as personal, social, health and economic education. PSHE promotes healthy living by providing young people with knowledge, understanding, attitudes and practical skills.

Importance of the Topic

The view that schools can promote the health and welfare of children and young people has a long history. The development of a school health service, the requirement for school boards to provide meals and, more recently, the inclusion of physical education in the national curriculum and the setting of nutritional standards for school meals are examples of how the school was, and is, seen as a key setting in which a captive audience could be encouraged to adopt lifestyles conducive to good health.

The World Health Organization (WHO) defines a health promoting school as 'one that fosters health and learning, strives to provide a healthy environment; implements policies and practices that respect well-being and dignity' (www.who.int/school_youth_health/gshi/hps/en). The school is seen as a total environment in which many aspects affect the health of its pupils and staff, including its organization, ethos, culture and layout, in addition to any teaching about health issues and the provision of medical and nursing services. Schools also act as referral agencies, signposting children and parents to other health, welfare and voluntary services when appropriate. This chapter looks at the physical, mental and social well-being of children and young people, and how schools can be powerful agents in the promotion of good health through the curriculum and everyday practices.

Why the school is a key setting for health promotion

Education is a resource for health. This is recognized by the WHO, and the United Nations included 'achieving universal primary education' as one of its eight Millennium Development Goals. Equally, health is a prerequisite for education: 'Children who face violence, hunger, substance abuse, and despair cannot possibly focus on academic excellence. There is no curriculum brilliant enough to compensate for a hungry stomach or distracted mind' (National Action Plan for Comprehensive School Health Education, 1992).

School is seen as an important context for health promotion, principally because it reaches a large proportion of the population for many years. The emphasis on schools is also a recognition that the learning of health-related knowledge, attitudes and behaviour begins at an early age.

 Learning Activity 13.1 The aims of health promotion in schools

Consider each of the following statements about the aims for health promotion for young people, and indicate how important you would rate each.

Health promotion should:	Very important	Important	Not very important	Not important at all
1. Provide information about how the body works				
2. Foster positive personal and social relationships				
3. Teach young people to keep fit and feel good				
4. Equip young people with the skills to make informed and responsible decisions				
5. Inform young people about local services and how to get help				
6. Teach young people about the dangers of certain behaviours, such as taking drugs				
7. Help young people to express their feelings and emotions				
8. Teach young people how to say 'no'				
9. Show young people the wonders of the human body so they do not damage it				
10. Put young people off unhealthy behaviour by emphasizing the risks to their health				
11. Prepare young people for parenthood				
12. Provide information about human sexuality, puberty and contraception				
13. Teach young people how to reduce their risk from drug taking or sexual activity (safer sex and safer drug taking)				
14. Prepare young people to be active citizens				
15. Show young people how to cope with stress				
16. Equip young people with the skills to negotiate and be assertive in relationships				
17. Help to build young people's self-esteem				

Research Example 13.1 The Health Behaviour of School-Aged Children (HBSC) study

The WHO study on health behaviour in school-aged children (HBSC) looks at patterns of health in 43 countries in Europe and North America. The HBSC findings show that those who perceive their school as supportive are more likely to engage in positive health behaviours and have better health outcomes, including lower smoking prevalence.

www.euro.who.int/_data/assets/pdf_file/0003/163857/social-determinants-of-health-and-well-being-among-young-people.pdf.

Childhood and adolescence are times of great change, when young people often acquire lifetime habits and attitudes. One function of a healthy school environment is to enable children to develop healthy behaviours. While adolescence is characterized by powerful peer-group attachments, the school setting provides an opportunity to communicate with young people and gives learning opportunities and a safe environment to practise new skills.

Learning Activity 13.2 The relationship between health and learning

In what ways might a child's educational potential and achievement be influenced by his or her health?

Health promotion in schools

The development of health education and promotion in schools has reflected many approaches to health promotion. Health education has tended to reflect the medical view of health, and in many countries is almost exclusively concerned with hygiene, nutrition and fitness. Education in the 1960s saw a swing to being child-centred, and educational methods sought to develop autonomy and responsibility through discovery learning. Health education emerged as a complex theme of well-being and fulfilment of maximum potential. Health promotion in schools is now closely linked to personal and social development, and delivered in the curriculum as personal, social health and economic education (PSHE). The aim is for young people to be in charge of their own lives, and the role of the school is to develop self-esteem and self-awareness. Emphasis is placed on the *process* of education, and finding teaching and learning strategies which encourage reflection and personal awareness. The direction and organization of the health promotion programme also aim to reflect the needs of the children and young people. The provision of PSHE in schools remains patchy, and often focuses on knowledge rather than skills and attitudes. There are many reasons for this, including the lack of training for teachers in this subject and mixed messages from government as to the importance of PSHE within the curriculum (PSHE is not mandatory but is strongly encouraged).

Alongside these attempts to promote autonomy and decision-making skills are more traditional information-giving approaches. Behind such an approach is the simple assumption that people are rational decision-makers whose behaviour will change once they have information about how to live more healthily. Much health promotion in schools therefore entails the provision of information about the health-damaging effects of certain behaviours, such as smoking and taking drugs.

The provision of sex education in schools reflects these views of health promotion. Sex education is now commonly referred to as 'sex and relationships education' (SRE), in recognition of the need to move away from a focus on biology to a focus on emotional health, values and life skills. SRE is a contentious area. The Department for Education's popular questions website provides the following information on the current position relating to SRE in schools (updated 9 October 2014).

- SRE is compulsory from age 11 onwards. It involves teaching children about reproduction, sexuality and sexual health. It does not promote early sexual activity or any particular sexual orientation.
- Some parts of SRE are compulsory – these are part of the national curriculum for science. Parents can withdraw their children from all other parts of SRE if they want.
- All schools must have a written policy on sex education, which they must make available to parents for free.

Table 13.1 Health education in school versus the health promoting school

Traditional health education	The health promoting school
• Health education is delivered in the classroom only	• The life of the school is considered health promoting
• Emphasizes physical health and hygiene	• Sees health as interaction of physical, mental, social and emotional dimensions
• Uses didactic and instructional methods	• Uses participatory methods that seek to empower students
• Tends to respond to perceived problems or crises, for example drug use or violence on a one-off basis	• Recognizes that skills and processes are common to all health issues and should be incorporated into the curriculum
• Takes little account of psychosocial aspects of health	• Developing positive self-image and self-efficacy is important
• Does not involve parents	• Considers parent support as central
• Views school health services only in relation to disease prevention and screening	• Helps to integrate services within the curriculum and to enable students to be consumers of health services

In delivering sex education, schools are currently required to have regard to the *Sex and Relationship Education Guidance*, published in 2000 (https://www.gov.uk/government/uploads/system/uploads/attachment_data/file/283599/sex_and_relationship_education_guidance.pdf).

The distinction between schools that offer health education and those that are health promoting was made by Young and Williams (1989), and is shown in Table 13.1.

The health promoting school

The health promoting school (HPS) is an international approach to addressing the health of pupils and teachers in a comprehensive and strategic manner. If education for the health of young people is to focus on more than individual behaviour and be health *promoting*, it needs to acknowledge the influence of the school itself as a health promoting environment and as part of a wider community.

The whole-school context, as illustrated in Figure 13.1, includes its:
- ethos
- organization
- management structures
- relationships
- physical environment
- taught curriculum.

In the HPS all these aspects will reinforce and support each other, leading to a synergistic effect.

In reality, different aspects of the school may give conflicting messages. Many aspects of a school can be health promoting or health inhibiting. Educationalists have long talked of a 'hidden curriculum', and the way in which messages can be transmitted through children and young people's daily experience of their surroundings and relationships at school. For example, the state of many school toilets might suggest that hygiene is not valued or the pupils do not require (or deserve) cleanliness or care. Knowing that someone (e.g. personal tutor, school nurse) is always available to talk to about any personal concerns or incidents at school such as bullying or teasing is important for mental health and well-being.

The International Union of Health Promotion and Education guidelines for HPSs (www.iuhpe.org/images/PUBLICATIONS/THEMATIC/HPS/HPSGuidelines_ENG.pdf) include the following principles:
- promote the health and well-being of students
- uphold social justice and equity concepts
- involve student participation and empowerment
- provide a safe and supportive environment
- link health and education issues and systems
- address the health and well-being issues of staff
- collaborate with the local community
- integrate into the school's ongoing activities
- set realistic goals
- engage parents and families in health promotion.

In common with other settings, effective health promotion in schools happens when it is coordinated

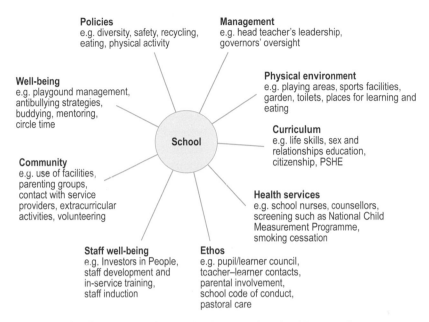

Policies
e.g. diversity, safety, recycling, eating, physical activity

Management
e.g. head teacher's leadership, governors' oversight

Well-being
e.g. playgound management, antibullying strategies, buddying, mentoring, circle time

Physical environment
e.g. playing areas, sports facilities, garden, toilets, places for learning and eating

School

Curriculum
e.g. life skills, sex and relationships education, citizenship, PSHE

Community
e.g. use of facilities, parenting groups, contact with service providers, extracurricular activities, volunteering

Health services
e.g. school nurses, counsellors, screening such as National Child Measurement Programme, smoking cessation

Staff well-being
e.g. Investors in People, staff development and in-service training, staff induction

Ethos
e.g. pupil/learner council, teacher–learner contacts, parental involvement, school code of conduct, pastoral care

Fig. 13.1 ● The whole-school approach to health promotion.

and takes place within structured frameworks. Many countries have HPS networks. In England the Healthy Schools Standard award scheme, which, as with other award schemes for hospitals and workplaces, encourages institutions to work towards specific targets, was discontinued in 2011, although local awards continue.

Case Study 13.1 A health promoting nursery school

A tool to assess the health promoting aspects of a nursery school has been produced by the education authority in Fife, Scotland (www.fife-education.org.uk/fhps/). Health promoting aspects include:

- lunch service
- fruit being available
- free access to fresh water
- playing fields
- safe drop off/collection area
- clinical protocols on the administration of medicines
- an Epi or Ana pen
- nut allergy policy
- a strategy for communication and engagement.

Policies and practices

The policies that a school develops represent its values. Schools may have policies on equal opportunities, discipline and rewards, health and safety, bullying, healthy food and various curriculum issues, including sex education. Policies may be merely 'paper exercises' unless they have been influenced by wide consultation within the school and community, have been clearly written and disseminated and are consistently applied. The practices of a school can be evidenced in its daily life and the ways in which decisions are taken. Democratic participation by pupils is a key element in an HPS.

Learning Activity 13.3 Student participation in schools

The Ottawa Charter describes health promotion as a process of 'enabling people to take more control over and improve their health' (WHO, 1986). How can pupils in schools be enabled to make decisions about their education and their health?

Social environment

The quality of social interactions among pupils, between staff and pupils and between the staff contributes to the ethos or climate in a school. Increasingly, schools are recognizing that healthy schools which value positive relationships, prioritize learning and build self-esteem also drive up educational standards.

Curriculum

The formal curriculum includes knowledge and understanding of health-related topics (e.g. biology and nutrition) at a level appropriate for pupils' ages and social and cognitive development. The informal curriculum refers to areas not formally taught or examined, including pastoral care and extracurricular activities in areas such as sports and arts. In England and many other countries there is no statutory provision for health promotion, and its integration into the curriculum is patchy.

Physical environment

The physical environment and layout of a school may be stimulating or depressing. Schools should provide a clean and safe environment with no litter or graffiti, clean toilets and a welcoming but secure entrance. There should be areas for play, for social interaction and for quiet study or reading. In many countries the provision of basic amenities such as sanitation, water and air cleanliness may be priorities.

Learning Activity 13.4 Health promoting playgrounds

Think back to your primary school and try to picture the playground area. Was it a health promoting environment? What would constitute a health promoting playground?

Links with the community

How well the school communicates and connects with its local community, where its pupils and their families live, is an important criterion for the HPS. Partnerships with parents may vary from information about school events, fundraising requests and consultation about uniform or meals' provision to the active involvement of all parents in decision-making about the curriculum, pastoral care and resource issues. Parents may also become involved in school life through reading schemes, practical parenting classes and breakfast clubs. Schools are part of a wider community and should be open to that community. Many agencies and services can provide support to schools. For example, the police and emergency services often provide educational sessions concerning accident prevention.

Learning Activity 13.5 School healthy-eating policies

In the broad areas of policy, curriculum, social and physical environment and community links, what would demonstrate that the school was health promoting in its approach to healthy eating?

Effective interventions

Health promotion interventions in schools differ substantially in their nature, ranging from programmes providing physiological information and life skills to abstinence-oriented programmes, in addition to the comprehensive whole-school approaches outlined above. Many curriculum programmes aim to have outcomes relevant to risk reduction, such as increased knowledge or changes in behaviour. Programmes may thus be specific to a particular health issue (e.g. smoking education) or more generic life-skills programmes aiming to develop self-esteem and social and communication skills. They may target pupils only, or extend their reach to include teachers, parents and the wider community.

Schools are dynamic communities, and there are many varied influences on young people both within and outside the school setting, so demonstrating the particular effect of health promotion is extremely difficult. The majority of interventions aim to develop health-enhancing behaviours. These health outcomes will not be apparent until later in life. For example, the Australian 'no hat – no play' policy will not demonstrate an effect on skin cancer rates until well into adulthood. Evidence shows that increasing children's knowledge is feasible, but changing their attitudes and behaviour, even in the short term, is far more difficult (Lister-Sharp et al., 1999).

A Cochrane review of HPSs (Langford et al., 2014) found that the settings approach was effective for certain outcomes related to fruit and vegetable intake, tobacco use, physical activity and bullying. An earlier review (Stewart-Brown, 2006) found that mental health promotion programmes were among the most effective. Factors associated with increased effectiveness included long duration, high intensity, involvement of the whole school, a focus on the school environment, multifactoral interventions and peer-led health promotion (Stewart-Brown, 2006). There is evidence that integrated, holistic and strategic programmes are more effective than classroom education programmes (St Leger, 2005).

Conclusion

Schools are widely seen as having a key role in health promotion. Young people are seen as a key target group for the provision of information and encouragement of responsible and health promoting attitudes and behaviour. The habits acquired in childhood and adolescence may prove influential for the rest of one's lifespan. Adolescence is also a time of development and risk taking, and a fine balance needs to be struck between encouraging the development of autonomy alongside responsible and health promoting attitudes and behaviour. However, PSHE has always been marginalized within the formal curriculum. Currently PSHE is not a mandatory subject, although its inclusion is encouraged. Research suggests that narrow information-based programmes are less effective than broader programmes addressing the school as a whole. This is the direction taken by the HPS initiative, which seeks to promote a whole-school approach, encompassing not just the formal curriculum but also the informal curriculum, the school's physical and social environment, and its links with its community.

The evolving evidence base suggests that the HPS approach is effective and contributes to children and young people's health, education and welfare.

Questions for further discussion

- You are a newly appointed teacher in a failing secondary school in an inner-city area with an ethnically and culturally diverse intake of students. You are asked to produce a strategy to make your school an HPS. How would you go about this task? What areas would you prioritize, and why? How would you integrate the following health promotion principles within school structures:
  - equity?
  - empowerment?
  - collaboration?
  - participation?

Summary

This chapter has examined the reasons why schools are a key setting for health promotion. Health and education have a reciprocal relationship, so that enhancing either one will impact favourably on the other. The holistic HPS approach has been identified as providing the most promising strategy. There is an accumulating evidence base to support the whole-school integrated approach.

Further reading and resources

Noble, C., Toft, M., 2012. How effective are schools as settings for health promotion? In: Scriven, A., Hodgins, M. (Eds.), Health Promoting Settings: Principles and Practice. Sage, London.

Whitman, C., Aldinger, C., 2009. Case Studies in Global School Health Promotion. Springer, USA. *A review of case examples from over 20 developing and developed countries.*

The International Union for Health Promotion and Education publishes guides on HPSs: www.iuhpe.org/index.php/en/iuhpe-thematic-resources/298-on-school-health.

The Schools for Health in Europe network supports the development of school health promotion: www.schools-for-health.eu/she-network.

Many countries have networks to provide information and good practice examples.

Australia: www.ahpsa.org.au.

New Zealand: hps.tki.org.nz/.

Canada: www.phecanada.ca/programs/health promoting-schools.

Wales: wales.gov.uk/topics/health/improvement/schools/?lang=en.

Scotland: www.educationscotland.gov.uk/resources/b/genericresource_tcm4242182.asp.

 ## Feedback to learning activities

13.1 Children spend a large proportion of their waking lives in school, so it is an important setting for them. Schools can create a healthy environment, for example by providing healthy lunches and snacks and encouraging children to walk to school. The school curriculum can also foster health, for example by teaching children about healthy lifestyles. The school ethos is important in fostering self-respect and helping children to be happy and healthy.

13.2 There is a relationship between health and education and the ability to learn. Young people's experiences in school influence the development of their self-esteem, self-perception and health behaviours. Pupils with low school performance and educational aspirations and high levels of absence from school are more likely to engage in earlier risk-taking behaviour such as drug use. School attendance is particularly important, and provision of food at school, for example through breakfast clubs, can improve attendance rates. Equally, health can impact on educational performance. There is evidence that providing good nutrition in school can improve attention, concentration and overall cognitive development (Powney et al., 2000).

13.3 Participation is recognized as a desirable feature in school inspections. Participation can range from supporting children to express their views to enabling them to share decision-making through school councils.

13.4 Health promoting playgrounds seek to encourage children to be active. Strategies include playground markings for games; child 'buddies' to discourage bullying; areas for reflection; and protection from the sun (e.g. Australia has a 'no hat – no play' policy).

13.5 Indicators of a school healthy-eating policy might include:

- a whole-school food policy
- a welcoming eating environment
- consultation with children about food choices
- a breakfast club
- water fountains to promote hydration and reduce plastic waste
- healthy school lunches with fruit and vegetables and low levels of salt, sugar and fat.

References

Department for Education, 2000. Sex and Relationship Education Guidance. HMSO, London. https://www.gov.uk/government/.../sex-and-relationship-education.

Langford, R., Bonell, C.P., Jones, H.E., Pouliou, T., Murphy, S.M., Waters, E., Komro, K.A., Gibbs, L.F., Magnus, D., Campbell, R., 2014. The WHO Health Promoting School Framework for Improving the Health and Wellbeing of Students and Their Academic Achievement (Review). Cochrane Collaboration. Wiley.

Lister-Sharp, D., Chapman, S., Stewart-Brown, S., Sowden, A., 1999. Health promoting schools and health promotion in schools: two systematic reviews. Health Technology Assessment 3(22). Available online at: http://www.journalslibrary.nihr.ac.uk/__data/assets/pdf_file/0010/64657/FullReport-hta3220.pdf (accessed 18.09.15).

National Action Plan for Comprehensive School Health Education, 1993. Working together for the future: 1992 comprehensive school health education workshop. Journal of School Health 63, 46–66.

Powney, J., Malcolm, H., Lowden, K., 2000. Health and Attainment: A Brief Review of Recent Literature. Scottish Council for Research in Education, Edinburgh. Available online at: https://dspace.gla.ac.uk/bitstream/1905/222/1/101.pdf (accessed 18.09.15).

Stewart-Brown, S., 2006. What Is the Evidence on School Health Promotion in Improving Health or Preventing Disease and, Specifically, What Is the Effectiveness of the Health Promoting School Approach. WHO, Copenhagen.

St Leger, L., 2005. Protocols and guidelines for health promoting schools. Promotion and Education 12 (3–4), 145–146.

World Health Organization, 1986. Ottawa Charter for Health Promotion. WHO, Geneva. Available online at: http://www.who.int/healthpromotion/conferences/previous/ottawa/en/.

Young, I., Williams, T., 1989. The Healthy School. Scottish Health Education Group, Edinburgh.

Chapter Fourteen

Health promoting workplaces

Learning Outcomes

By the end of this chapter you will be able to:
- describe the relationship between work and health
- understand how the workplace can enhance or inhibit health
- describe the elements of a health promoting workplace.

Key Concepts and Definitions

Work A job or paid employment. It may include unpaid or voluntary work, education and training, and caring.

Workplace The physical environment where work takes place.

Employer A person or business that employs one or more people and in return gives that person or people wages or a salary.

Worker A person employed to carry out specific functions, usually in return for a wage or salary.

Importance of the Topic

A comprehensive review of how health is influenced by work identified that work is good for health (Black, 2008). A key recommendation of the review was to encourage people to remain in work and those off sick to return to work. The workplace is significant both in affecting people's health and as a context in which to promote health. UK statistics for the first quarter of 2014 show that 72.9 percent of people aged 16 to 64, or 30.54 million people, were in work (www.ons.gov. uk/ons/dcp171778_363998.pdf). Promoting health in the workplace will therefore reach a large percentage of the adult population, and will have an impact on a setting where many adults spend a considerable amount of their time.

In common with the other settings in this part of the book, this chapter looks at the workplace as a social system and ways in which it can contribute to ill health and health. It goes on to look at ways in which health promotion has been implemented in the workplace. Most health promotion interventions have tended to focus on individual lifestyle risk factors and employers' legal responsibilities to provide a safe working environment. Interventions that address the workplace organization and culture as a whole are less common, but evaluation shows they are more effective. The different partners and stakeholders involved in workplace health promotion are identified, and their contribution to interventions discussed.

Why is the workplace a key setting for health promotion?

A global survey of workplace health promotion strategies (www.ncbi.nlm.nih.gov/pubmed/18173386) found that improving productivity and reducing staff absence rates were the main priorities. There are five main reasons for prioritizing the workplace.

1. The workplace gives access to a target group – healthy adults, especially men – who are often difficult to reach in other ways. Employees in the workplace are a captive audience for health promotion. It is easy to follow up interventions and encourage participation in health programmes because there are established modes of communication. The cohesion of the working community also provides peer pressure and support.
2. Promoting health in the workplace ensures that people are protected from the harm to their health that certain jobs may cause.
3. There are economic benefits associated with healthy workplaces (Wanless, 2004). American research studies provide evidence that workplace health promotion programmes are associated with lower medical and insurance costs, decreased absenteeism and enhanced performance, productivity and morale (www.uclan. ac.uk/facs/health/hsdu/settings/workplace/htm). The Health and Safety Executive (HSE) identifies the costs of work-related ill health, which include sick pay, damage from injuries, compensation and insurance costs, and recruitment costs. Research has shown that employees who have three or more risk factors (e.g. smoking, overweight, excessive alcohol intake, physical inactivity) are likely to have 50 percent more sickness absence from work than employees with no risk factors (Shain and Kramer, 2004). Investing in health and preventing ill health increase productivity and staff retention. Adopting a healthy

workplaces approach therefore makes sound business sense.

4. The workplace provides a resource for health that is relevant to a large percentage of the adult population. Creating a healthy environment at work will benefit employees' health and have positive spin-offs for their families and communities. The traditional focus on the workplace has centred on hazards and illnesses, but a health promoting approach to the workplace has great potential.
5. Enabling people to work and stay in work and safeguarding their health at work are beneficial to them. Presenteeism (when people are at work but not productive) due to poor mental health is an invisible but substantial cost.

 Case Study 14.1 Work-related ill health

HSE statistics for the UK for 2013 to 2014 showed that:
- 133 workers were killed at work (a 19 percent decrease on the previous five years)
- 148,000 employees suffered serious injuries at work
- 1.2 million people were suffering from an illness they believed was caused or made worse by their work; of these, 535,000 were new cases in the last 12 months
- 80 percent of work-related conditions were musculoskeletal disorders (MSDs) or stress, depression or anxiety
- 31 million days were lost due to sickness absence in 2013, an average of 4.4 days per worker
- There are on average 10.7 working days lost per year per staff member in the National Health Service (NHS).

 Research Example 14.1 Economic benefits of workplace health promotion programmes

Many evaluation studies of workplace health promotion programmes have reported positive results, including the following.
- Prudential Insurance Company reports that its major medical costs dropped from $574 to $312 for each participant in its wellness programme.
- A two-year study by the DuPont Corporation reports that blue-collar employees involved in

its comprehensive health promotion programme showed a 14 percent decline in sick leave, compared to a 5.8 percent decline for controls.

- The Canadian Life Assurance Company demonstrated a 4 percent increase in productivity for workplaces with employee fitness programmes compared to controls. Nearly half (47 percent) of participants in the programme reported benefits, including enjoying work more, better rapport with co-workers and feeling more alert (www.uclan.ac.uk/facs/health/hsdu/settings/workplace/htm).

The relationship between work and health

The relationship between work and health is complex. In general, attention has focused on the effects of work on health, although it is also acknowledged that poor health will have negative effects on the capacity for paid employment. There is evidence that paid work is good for your health and unemployment can be linked to ill health (Waddell and Burton, 2006). Work is beneficial for health because it provides an income, a sense of self-worth and social networks of colleagues and friends. However, work may also harm health, and most research has concentrated on this aspect of the relationship.

 Learning Activity 14.1 The impact of work on health

Think of a recent work experience.

In what ways do you think work contributed to your health?

In what ways do you think work had a negative impact on your health?

The workplace can affect health in many different ways. Figure 14.1 provides a means of classifying these different kinds of relationship.

Hazards tend to be what people think of first when health in the workplace is mentioned. Most legislation is directed towards the containment of hazards,

and safety legislation has been enshrined in numerous Factory Acts in the UK since the mid-nineteenth century. Work that involves handling hazardous or toxic materials may have a direct negative effect on health (e.g. cancers caused by asbestos or occupational asthma). Work which provides easy access to hazardous substances is also linked to associated ill health. For example, doctors and pharmacists have high rates of suicide caused by drug overdose. There is a downward trend in fatal and non-fatal injuries at work, probably due to automation and fewer physical jobs that present hazards. Almost one-third of deaths occur in the construction sector, with agriculture, waste and recycling industries also implicated.

The workplace is characterized by fragmented information that is collected by different bodies (including the HSE and occupational health services). This poses obvious difficulties when trying to plan and implement a health promotion intervention. Health is often affected through risky behaviour or changed routines. Risky behaviour is the preferred explanation for most official accounts of accidents and injuries sustained in the workplace. There are extensive regulations to cover manual handling (Manual Handling Operations Regulations, amended in 2002), which require employers to provide training and equipment. Nevertheless, employees are expected to 'take reasonable care for the health and safety of themselves and any others who may be affected by their acts and omissions'. This approach extends to the workplace the victim-blaming ideology of some brands of health promotion. Behaviour which carries health risks may be an integral part of the job or part of the work culture. For example, bartenders have high rates of alcohol-related ill health because drinking heavily is associated with work (Wilhelm et al., 2004).

The general work environment and its effects on health are the most neglected aspects of the work–health relationship. This is due in part to ideological or political reasons, and in part to the fact that such a generalized relationship is hard to research or prove. Because the relationship between work and health is to a large extent indirect, it is often difficult to trace ill health to what happens in the workplace. This in turn leads to the true impact of work on health being underestimated. Focusing on the work environment instead

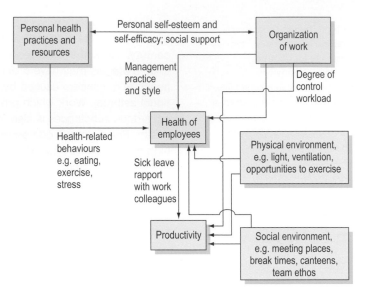

Fig. 14.1 ● The relationship between health and productivity in the workplace. (Adapted from Shain, M., Kramer, D.M., 2004. Health promotion in the workplace: Framing the concept; reviewing the evidence. Occupational and Environmental Medicine 61, 643–648.)

of individual workers' behaviour shifts responsibility on to the employer and has resource implications.

Although the relationship is difficult to quantify, strong evidence implicating the importance to health of the general work environment is becoming available (Marmot, 2010). There is a body of research demonstrating that certain factors associated with some types of work, such as repetitive tasks, lack of autonomy and pressures to meet deadlines, have harmful effects on health. In particular, low control by workers over what they do and how they do it is associated with increased risk of ill health (Marmot and Wilkinson 2006). The concept of well-being at work is also receiving attention. Key components of well-being relate to being valued, having opportunities to engage in decision-making and being able to work productively and creatively (Foresight, 2008). Working environments may also pose risks for mental well-being. For example, an imbalance between the effort required at work and the rewards received can lead to stress. Long-term exposure to stress results in poor health and may also lead to less healthy lifestyle choices, such as smoking. There is a growing acknowledgement of the impact of workplace stress on health:

● work-related stress accounts for over a third of all new incidents of ill health

● 11.3 million working days were lost due to stress, depression and anxiety in 2013 to 2014.

The occupations reporting the highest rates of work-related stress were health professionals (especially nurses), teaching and education professionals, and social care professonals (www.hse.gov.uk/statistics/causdis/stress/stress.pdf).

There are two main ways in which workplace stress is being addressed. The traditional approach has been to see the individual as unable to cope with the demands and pressures, and therefore in need of support. Many large workplaces offer stress management courses, counselling services and employee assistance programmes to help people adjust to new skills. Organizational approaches to stress are still rare despite a growing literature linking stress with organizational factors, such as lack of control or lack of consultation over changes. These approaches start from the view that illness and stressed behaviour are responses to factors in the workplace of which individuals may not even be aware. As the Department of Health (2004, Chapter 7, para. 16) points out:

A focus on individual stress can be counter-productive, leading to a failure to tackle the underlying causes of problems in the workplace.

Evidence has shown that poor working arrangements, such as lack of job control or discretion, consistently high work demands and low social support, can lead to increased risks of CHD [coronary heart disease], musculoskeletal disorders, mental illness and sickness absence. The real task is to improve the quality of jobs by reducing monotony, increasing job control, and applying appropriate HR [human resources] practices and policies – organisations need to ensure they adopt approaches that support the overall health and well being of their employees.

The HSE (Health and Safety Executive, 2012) identifies seven stressor areas that contribute to stress in the workplace.

1. Demands – workloads, work patterns.
2. Control – how much of a say employees have over things that affect them.
3. Support – encouragement, appreciation, sponsorship, resources.
4. Relationships at work – managing conflict or unacceptable behaviour.
5. Role – understanding of role and no conflicting roles.
6. Change – how it is managed and communicated.
7. Culture – management commitment, and open and fair procedures.

 Learning Activity 14.2 Stress at work

What could your organization do to reduce stress at work?

 Research Example 14.2 Unemployment and health

Figure 14.2 charts unemployment rates by previous occupation and shows that unemployment is unevenly distributed across society, with those in lower socio-economic positions more likely to be without work. Unemployed people have higher rates of long-term illness, mental illness and cardiovascular disease. Unemployment has also been linked to increased suicide rates, although research shows that countries with strong systems of social protection including active

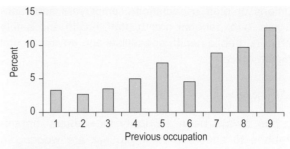

1. Management and senior officials
2. Professional
3. Associate professional and technical
4. Administrative and secretarial
5. Skilled trades
6. Personal service
7. Sales and customer service
8. Process, plan and machine operatives
9. Elementary

Fig. 14.2 ● Unemployment and Health. (Office for National Statistics licensed under the Open Government Licence v.3.0.)

labour market programmes were able to maintain long-term declines in suicide rates despite rapid increases in unemployment (Stuckler et al., 2009). Unemployment affects mortality and morbidity rates in three main ways.

1. Increased financial problems, which lower living standards and may reduce social integration.
2. Unemployment can be a trigger for distress, anxiety and depression.
3. Unemployment can lead to other unhealthy behaviours, such as smoking and drinking alcohol.

A summary of this evidence can be found in the Marmot Review (2010), Section 2.6.3.

Responsibility for workplace health

The relationship between work and health may appear substantial, but it is viewed in different ways by different groups of people. One of the defining characteristics of the workplace setting is that it brings together a variety of groups who have different agendas with regard to work and health. The key parties are workers or employees and their trade unions or staff associations, employers and managers, occupational health staff, health and safety officers, public health specialists and environmental health officers.

Workers

It has always been a priority for workers' organizations to ensure that employees are working in safe and healthy conditions. Membership of trade unions has, however, declined since the mid-1970s, when membership was just under two-fifths, to just over a quarter of the working population in 2013 (www.gov.uk/government/publications/trade-union-membership-statistics-2012-to-2013-user-survey). Changing patterns of employment also mean that part-time (mainly female) workers make up a significant percentage of the working population. So, although consultation with unions is an important means of reaching workers, it does not reach everyone. As the key target group, workers need to be fully involved as partners in decision-making processes. This is recognized by the European Network for Workplace Health Promotion (ENWHP), which states that effective workplace health promotion involves employees in decision-making processes and develops a working culture based on partnership (www.enwhp.org).

Employers and managers

Employers and managers have as their first priority the viability of the organization. Health is relevant in so far as it can be shown to be linked to organizational goals. Examples of 'hard' benefits are improvements in productivity due to lower rates of sickness, absenteeism and staff turnover, and improved recruitment and retention of trained staff. 'Soft' benefits, such as enhanced corporate image, are also influential.

Employers are responsible for the health, safety and welfare of all their employees under the Health and Safety at Work Act (1974). There is evidence of a shift in attitudes to and awareness of health and safety issues in the workplace. The Investors in People standard is an example of the government's strategy to use awards to provide incentives for employers, and has been widely adopted. The Improving Working Lives standard is another example that sets a model of good human resources practice against which employers can be measured. The Workplace Charter (http://wellbeingcharter.org.uk/index.php [accessed 20.09.15]) sets a series of standards for workplaces. Leadership and commitment at senior management level have been shown to be vital for effective health promotion initiatives and the creation of healthy workplaces. An organizational audit of NHS trusts in 2014 found that trusts with high levels of patient mortality had high rates of staff absence due to ill health, 24 percent of trusts do not monitor the mental well-being of staff and 28 percent do not have an obesity plan for staff (www.rcplondon.ac.uk/sites/default/files/implementing_nice_web_0.pdf).

 Learning Activity 14.3 Employers and healthy workplaces

What might be employer responsibilities to encourage a healthier workplace?

Occupational health staff

In many European countries occupational health is a statutory part of healthcare. In the UK there is no requirement for employers to provide an occupational health service, other than first aid. Occupational health nurses (OHNs), who are specialist nurses with post-qualification training, form an important element of the occupational health staff. OHNs are responsible for the health and well-being of employees in the workplace.

The main functions of an occupational health service are:

- surveillance of the work environment, e.g. the effects of new technologies
- initiatives and advice on the control of hazards
- surveillance of the health of employees, e.g. assessment of fitness to work, analysis of sickness absence
- organization of first aid and emergency response
- adaptation of work and the environment to the worker.

The workplace has experienced considerable change and uncertainty in the last 20 years. There has been a rapid growth in the service sector, a fragmentation of large organizations and a huge increase in information technology. The provision for health in companies thus needs to be seen alongside policies on employment, the work environment and overall company policy.

Health and safety officers and environmental health officers

Health and safety officers and environmental health officers are responsible for ensuring that workplaces conform with safety legislation. They have powers to force workplaces to comply with health and safety regulations, and to impose penalties in the case of non-compliance. Responsibility for workplaces is divided between the HSE and environmental health officers employed by local authorities. There is now a developed body of European Union (EU) occupational health and safety legislation.

 Case Study 14.2 European agency for safety and health at work campaigns

The European Healthy Workplaces campaigns raise awareness of issues related to occupational safety and health. Recent campaigns include 'Lighten the Load' to promote an integrated approach to tackling MSDs, which are the most common form of work-related illness in Europe. In the EU 25 percent of workers suffer from backache and 23 percent from muscular pains. In 2012 to 2013 the campaign focused on risk prevention through measures such as linking insurance premiums to safety performance. In 2014 to 2015 the campaign focused on stress at work, including work overload, uncertainty and low levels of job control (https://osha.europa.eu/en/campaigns/index_htm/).

Worker participation is an important part of managing health and safety, and safety representatives prevent many injuries and work-related illnesses annually. Yet safety representatives are not universal. Only 46 percent of workplaces (92 percent of public sector and 39 percent of private sector) and 68 percent of employees (98 percent of public sector and 59 percent of private sector) are covered by employee representation.

Health promotion in the workplace

There are two approaches to health promotion in the workplace. The most common is to target individual lifestyles and behaviour within a workplace setting. This approach sees the workplace primarily as a site through which programmes can be delivered. The more challenging, but potentially more effective, approach is to target the workplace and its organization and culture. Health promotion in the workplace falls into the following categories:

- first aid and medical treatment
- screening, e.g. bone-density scanning
- protection from accidents
- control of hazards and infections
- education and advice about healthy lifestyles and practices
- policies and regulations to provide a healthier environment, e.g. catering choices
- provision of services, e.g. exercise facilities, screening, counselling, smoking cessation.

 Case Study 14.3 Examples of healthy workplace initiatives

- Provision of an online personalized health advice and information service.
- Provision of an 'MoT' clinic at a railway station during rush hours, to encourage women and especially men to attend for health check-ups.
- Initiating physical activities in the workplace during lunch breaks, e.g. speed walks.
- Encouraging healthy lifestyles through, for example, the provision of cycle racks, shower rooms, stair prompts to encourage staff to take the stairs rather than the lift and healthy options in staff canteens and vending machines.
- Changing the physical environment of the workplace to encourage exercise, e.g. situating key locations at an appreciable distance from one another.

Dooris and Hunter (2007).

There is evidence that health promotion targeting the whole organization is more effective than targeting individual lifestyles (Noblet and LaMontagne, 2006). Changing organizational culture and practice, through more flexible working hours and break times, for example, has a more significant impact than programmes that assume individuals can make the necessary changes themselves, e.g. offering relaxation classes after working hours.

Workplace health promotion elements include:

- health education, e.g. tobacco use, alcohol/drug use, physical activity, overweight/obesity, primarily addressed through risk assessments and information
- supportive social and physical environments addressed through healthy catering, shower facilities and staff rooms
- screening programmes
- safety, including wellness champions.

The whole-organization approach has been recognized and endorsed at the highest level and by international bodies. For example, the ENWHP adopted the Luxembourg Declaration on Workplace Health Promotion in 1997. The declaration states that successful initiatives should follow these guidelines:

- participation – all staff should be involved
- integration – embedding health in all organizational areas, policies and decisions
- project management – programmes to follow a problem-solving cycle of needs analysis, planning, implementation and evaluation
- comprehensiveness – embraces individually focused and environmentally focused initiatives.

To maximize the impact of workplace health promotion, the approach needs to shift from an exclusively individually focused lifestyle approach to a more comprehensive approach that includes whole-organization activities as well.

The evidence for effective health promotion interventions in the workplace is building, although it remains rather scanty. The usual rationale for workplace health programmes is that they improve employees' health and increase productivity. A meta-analysis of 56 studies (Chapman, 2005) found that workplace health programmes can lead to:

- a 27 percent reduction in sick leave
- a 32 percent reduction in compensation and disability cost claims
- a 6:1 return on investment.

Various systematic reviews have pulled together evidence related to nutrition interventions in the workplace, and found only limited or moderate evidence of effectiveness of interventions such as health education and changing the physical workplace environment (through provision of healthier options in cafeterias and vending machines) (Maes et al. 2011; Ni Mhurchu et al., 2010). There is likewise some evidence that workplace physical activity interventions such as pedometers and initatives to encourage active travel to work can lead to individual physical activity choices which can then contribute to increased overall fitness, improved physical activity behaviour, reduced body measurements, improved work attendance and reduction in job stress (Dugdill et al., 2008).

Conclusion

The workplace is recognized as a key setting in which to promote health, due to both its reach (three-quarters of the working-age population are employed) and its importance in contributing directly and indirectly to people's health. Traditionally the focus has been on individually targeted programmes centred on hazards and the prevention of ill health. The challenge today is to broaden the focus to include the whole organizational setting, and to move from ill health to positive health and well-being. There is a developing evidence base demonstrating that such a comprehensive and multicomponent approach is effective. The proven benefits include not just better employee health but also increased productivity and economic benefits to industry and society as a whole. Many different groups have a role to play in promoting health in the workplace, including workers, managers, employers, occupational health staff, health and safety officers and environmental health officers.

Questions for further discussion

- Think of a workplace with which you are familiar. What areas would you prioritize to promote health, and why? Are there different workforces or work patterns (e.g. shift work) that you would target? Who would you involve, and how?

Summary

This chapter has looked at the potential benefits to be gained from implementing health promotion within the workplace setting. The tension between interventions that focus on individual lifestyles and those that address the whole organization has been discussed. Evaluation studies have demonstrated that the whole-organization approach is more effective. The role of different partners in workplace health promotion has been identified and discussed.

Further reading and resources

European Network for Health Promotion website www.enwph.org. *This website is a useful resource for up-to-date information.*

National Institute for Health and Care Excellence (NICE), www. nice.org.uk. *NICE has produced various documents synthesizing research evidence of effective health promotion practice in the workplace. Topics covered include smoking in the workplace, physical activity and mental health.*

Black, C., 2008. Working for a Healthier Tomorrow London, TSO and Department for Work and Pensions (2013) Improving Health and Work: Changing Lives the Government's Response. Department of Work and Pensions, London. *These two reviews identify the impact of work on health, and the reforms on sickness, unemployment and early interventions.*

Boorman, S., 2009. NHS Health and Wellbeing Review. Department of Health. London. Available online at: http://www.nhshealthandwellbeing.org/FinalReport.html (accessed 07.03.15).

Scriven, A., Hodgins, M. (Eds.), 2012. Health Promotion Settings: Principles and Practice. Sage, London. *Part Three of this book is devoted to the workplace setting.*

 ## Feedback to learning activities

14.1 The benefits of work include pay, the contribution of work to an individual's identity and social status, and the opportunities work provides to meet people. However, work can also be detrimental to an individual's health, due to work-related hazards, job insecurity and long working hours.

14.2 Task and work reorganization is the most successful form of intervention. It describes various system solutions to improve communication, the creation of autonomous work groups and whole-organization interventions to restructure relations between management and unions. These interventions do not obviate the need for individual support, but follow an earlier stage of raising staff awareness of stress and its causes.

14.3 Employer responsibilities might be:
- making healthy choices easy for staff
- creating flexible working arrangements that are compatible with employees' home lives
- ensuring a smoke-free work environment
- ensuring that any catering offered on-site has healthy options
  - mental health awareness for managers
  - an active travel plan to encourage physical activity
  - a 24-hour canteen for shift workers. The wellbeing charter standards (http://wellbeing charter.org.uk/Whats-Involved.php) focus on three areas of leadership, culture and communication.

References

Black, C., 2008. Working for a Healthier Tomorrow. TSO, London. Available online at: https://www.gov.uk/government/uploads/system/uploads/attachment_data/file/209782/hwwb-working-for-a-healthier-tomorrow.pdf (accessed 07.03.15).

Chapman, L.S., 2005. Meta-evaluation of worksite health promotion economic return studies: 2005 update. American Journal of Health Promotion 19 (6), 1–11.

Department of Health, 2004. Choosing Health: Making Healthy Choices Easier. TSO, London. Available online at: http://webarchive.nationalarchives.gov.uk/+/dh.gov.uk/en/publicationsandstatistics/publications/publicationspolicy andguidance/dh_4094550 (accessed 07.03.15).

Dugdill, L., Brettle, A., Hulme, C., McCluskey, S., Long, A.F., 2008. Workplace physical activity interventions: a systematic review. International Journal of Workplace Health Management 1 (1), 20–40. Available online at: http://eprints.whiterose.ac.uk/3578/ (accessed 07.03.15).

Dooris, M., Hunter, D.J., 2007. Organisations and settings for promoting public health. In: Lloyd, C.E., Handsley, S., Douglas, J., et al. (Eds.), Policy and Practice in Promoting Public Health. Sage and the Open University, London (Chapter 4).

European Network for Workplace Health Promotion, 1997. The Luxembourg Declaration on Workplace Health Promotion in the European Union. European Network for Workplace Health Promotion, Luxembourg. Available online at: http://www.enwhp.org/fileadmin/downloads/free/Luxembourg_Declaration_June2005_final.pdf (accessed 21.09.15).

Foresight, 2008. Mental Capital and Wellbeing: Making the Most of Ourselves in the 21st Century. Government Office for Science, London. Available online at: https://www.gov.uk/government/publications/mental-capital-and-wellbeing-making-the-most-of-ourselves-in-the-21st-century (accessed 07.03.15), Sudbury, HSE books.

Health and Safety Executive, 2012. The Causes of Stress. Available online at: http://www.hse.gov.uk/stress/furtheradvice/causesofstress.htm (accessed 20.01.16).

Maes, L., Van Cauwenberghe, E., Van Lippevelde, W., Spittaels, H., De Pauw, E., Oppert, J-M., Van Lenthe, F.J., Brug, J., De Bourdeaudhuij, I., 2011. Effectiveness of workplace interventions in Europe promoting healthy eating: a systematic review. European Journal of Public Health 1–6. Available online at: http://eurpub.oxfordjournals.org/content/eurpub/early/2011/07/22/eurpub.ckr098.full.pdf (accessed 07.03.15).

Marmot, M., 2010. Fair Society, Healthy Lives. Institute of Health Equity, London. Available online at: http://www.instituteofhealthequity.org/projects/fair-society-healthy-lives-the-marmot-review (accessed 07.03.15).

Marmot, M., Wilkinson, R., 2006. The social determinants of health, second ed. World Health Organisation, Geneva. Available online at: http://www.euro.who.int/__data/assets/pdf_file/0005/98438/e81384.pdf (accessed 20.01.16).

Ni Mhurchu, C., Aston, L., Jebb, S., 2010. Effects of worksite health promotion interventions on employee diets: a systematic review. BMC Public Health 10, 62. Available online at: http://www.biomedcentral.com/1471-2458/10/62 (accessed 07.03.15).

Noblet, A., LaMontagne, A.D., 2006. The role of workplace health promotion in addressing job stress. Health Promotion International 21, 346–353. Available online at: http://heapro.oxfordjournals.org/content/21/4/346.full.pdf+html (accessed 21.09.15).

Office for National Statistics, 2009. Economic and Labour Market Review: Further Labour Market Statistics, Unemployment Rates by Previous Occupation. (Cited in Marmot 2010, page 68.)

Shain, M., Kramer, D.M., 2004. Health promotion in the workplace: framing the concept; reviewing the evidence. Occupational and Environmental Medicine 61, 643–648. Available online at: http://oem.bmj.com/content/61/7/643.full.pdf+html (accessed 21.09.15).

Stuckler, D., Basu, S., Suhrcke, M., et al., 2009. The public health effect of economic crises and alternative policy responses in Europe: an empirical analysis. Lancet 374, 315–323.

Waddell, S., Burton, A.K., 2006. Is work good for your health and well being? Occupational Health Review 24, 30–31. Available online at: https://www.gov.uk/government/uploads/system/uploads/attachment_data/file/214326/hwwb-is-work-good-for-you.pdf (accessed 21.09.15).

Wanless, D., 2004. Securing Good Health for the Whole Population. Stationery Office, London. Available online at: http://webarchive.nationalarchives.gov.uk/+/http:/www.hm-treasury.gov.uk/media/D/3/Wanless04_summary.pdf (accessed 07.03.15).

Wilhelm, K., Koves, V., et al., 2004. Work and mental health. Social Psychiatry and Epidemiology 39 (11), 866–873.

Health promoting neighbourhoods

Learning Outcomes

By the end of this chapter you will be able to:
- define what is meant by a neighbourhood
- discuss neighbourhoods as settings for health promotion
- distinguish between interventions in a neighbourhood and a settings approach
- understand what is meant by a place-based approach.

Key Concepts and Definitions

Neighbourhood is a geographically defined community within a larger area (city, town, suburb or rural area). There is often a high level of social interaction and networking between people in a neighbourhood.

Community is a group of people living in the same place or sharing a common characteristic (e.g. the gay community).

Social capital The social networks linking people, characterized by shared values and behaviour and mutually advantageous cooperation.

Place-based approach is an approach that brings together different stakeholders, including the local community, to address the issues of a specific location (usually a disadvantaged and deprived area).

Importance of the Topic

As we have seen in other chapters in this part of the book, healthy settings are physical and social settings which serve as supportive environments for health and health promotion activities. This chapter examines the concept of neighbourhood and how different factors – physical, social and economic – contribute to the concept. The linked concept of social capital to describe neighbourly relationships and networks is explored. The popularity of neighbourhoods in different policy and practice arenas in recent years and the usefulness of the neighbourhood as a setting for health promotion are discussed. Neighbourhoods include different levels or structures, such as the neighbourhood environment, services and people, which may all be used as a springboard for health promotion. Various initiatives which focus on the neighbourhood setting are described as examples of good practice. Evaluating such a multidimensional strategy poses many challenges, and issues regarding the evaluation and evidence base for neighbourhood health promotion are discussed.

Healthy Cities is arguably the best-known and largest of the settings approaches. The programme is a long-term international development initiative that aims to place health high on the agendas of decision-makers and to promote comprehensive local strategies for health improvement and sustainable development. The Healthy Villages programme in rural areas addresses similar issues as the Healthy Cities programme. Health is again defined by the area's residents; however, the generally accepted definition of a healthy village includes a community with low rates of infectious diseases, access to basic healthcare services and a stable, peaceful social environment (see http://www.who.int/healthy_settings/types/en/index.html). In addition, the holistic and multifaceted linking of activities that characterizes the settings approach is used in schools, workplaces, hospitals (discussed in other chapters in Part Three), universities, markets, islands and homes. The neighbourhood provides a link between these and the other settings explored in this part. Neighbourhoods have been identified as important settings for health promotion in a number of English policy documents.

> *The environment we live in, our social networks, our sense of security, socio-economic circumstances, families and resources in our local neighbourhood can affect individual health.*
>
> Department of Health (2004), p. 77

 Learning Activity 15.1 Neighbourhood or community?

The terms neighbourhood and community are frequently used. Are they the same thing?

Defining neighbourhoods

Neighbourhoods are defined as small localities with a distinct identity forged by a community of people who know each other, and the provision of essential services such as post offices, shops and health centres. Lay networks and support systems are important elements. Neighbourhoods will often be bounded by geographical features such as major roads, railways or green areas, and may be urban or rural. The key factor is that residents define their local neighbourhood themselves and feel they have an investment in its future, the services provided and its appearance. In the modern world where transactions are increasingly fragmented and anonymous, and where the overarching symbols of community, such as religion and nationhood, are less cohesive and meaningful, the role of the neighbourhood in promoting identity and self-esteem is more important. Neighbourhoods provide the immediate environment where people live, work and play, and for many more vulnerable groups, such as older people and those on low income, most of their lives are lived in one neighbourhood.

Neighbourhood identity is established at an early stage in each neighbourhood's history, and is resilient to change (Robertson et al., 2008). Neighbourhood identity is largely based on residents' socio-economic status, which in turn is often based on employment patterns, as well as physical characteristics such as housing. Neighbourhoods are often internally differentiated, and the sense of community is based on everyday social interactions and networks of friends, families and neighbours. Neighbourhoods therefore combine objective and subjective components.

There are many ways to get to know neighbourhoods, ranging from the objective gathering of statistics to the subjective collection of people's thoughts, feelings and memories. Local statistics on topics such as housing and crime are collected (see www.ons.gov.uk) and can be used to compare different neighbourhoods. The website https://neighbourhood.statistics.gov.uk provides detailed information about postcode areas in England. Community profiles or observation walks, where notes are taken of local facilities, the physical environment, transport routes and social networking opportunities, provide a more holistic picture of neighbourhoods.

Why neighbourhoods are a key setting for health promotion

 Learning Activity 15.2 Can neighbourhoods be used as a setting to address inequalities?

The Marmot Review on inequalities (2010) had a policy objective to create and develop healthy and sustainable places and communities. Why might neighbourhoods be identified as a key route through which to tackle health inequalities?

Neighbourhoods are a key setting for health promotion because they provide the infrastructure for health. Neighbourhoods are where the physical and social environments interact with service provision to provide an overall environment which has enormous potential to support people's health. Neighbourhoods have several aspects.

- *The physical environment*, for example the degree of air and noise pollution, quality of housing including its energy efficiency, amount of traffic and the availability of green space.
- *The social environment* – the amount of social interaction between residents, the number of community or voluntary groups or organizations operating in the area and the extent of mutual self-help activities. The concept of social capital, which refers to relationships of trust and regard between people and organizations they have contact with, is relevant to both the social environment and services provided.
- *Services* provided in neighbourhoods include places such as shops, post offices, health services, places of worship, sports facilities and community halls. They also cover transport systems and outreach workers from statutory agencies, for example housing and welfare officers' weekly sessions held in the community hall.

Identifying what exactly it is about neighbourhoods that has an impact on well-being is difficult. Research suggests that people value neighbourhoods for their effect on quality of life, reflected through aspects such as friendliness, safety and quiet (Bowling et al., 2006; Office for National Statistics, 2007). In addition to providing the context for health, neighbourhoods are a popular setting because they are seen as a means to engage people in addressing their own health needs. A neighbourhood focus therefore fosters empowerment and independence, which are themselves health promoting.

 Case Study 15.1 Belfast Healthy City

In contrast to other settings such as schools or hospitals, a healthy city has not achieved a particular status. A healthy city is defined by a process – putting health high on the political and social agenda. Belfast Healthy City was established in 1988 and joined the World Health Organization European Healthy Cities Network, which now includes 99 cities. One of Belfast's programmes is 'life course and empowering people', which focuses on developing an age-friendly environment. This includes:
- involving older people in the design of the city
- having dropped kerbs and tactile paving that is well maintained
- providing public seating
- a review of pedestrian crossings and crossing times.

www.belfasthealthycities.com

The physical environment

Many aspects of the physical environment, such as buildings and land use, affect health. Transport patterns and car usage are linked to health. Cars contribute to climate change and have a negative impact on individuals' health. For example, in one rapidly developing area of China, those who bought a car gained on average 1.8 kg in weight (Rice and Grant, 2007). Tackling issues such as dependence on private cars can seem a daunting proposition. UK car users, although a smaller percentage of the population than in other European countries, use their cars more frequently. However, the importance of weaning ourselves away from overdependence on cars is being recognized. Goals include ensuring the provision of high-quality routes for walkers and cyclists, and making public spaces and the countryside seem more attractive. Local authorities in England are required to produce local transport plans; increasingly, these focus on sustainable transport and active travel.

 Case Study 15.2 Walking for Health

Walking for Health was launched by the British Heart Foundation and the Countryside Agency to encourage people to take part in locally designed walks. Healthcare professionals are encouraged to 'prescribe' pedometers to act as an incentive. The benefits of this programme include:

- promotes active lifestyles and physical exercise
- improves self-image and social relationships
- promotes neighbourliness and social interaction – helping to turn places into communities
- tackles social isolation
- discourages antisocial behaviour through more people being out and about
- is a reason to conserve wildlife and enhance the character of local places.

www.walkingforhealth.org.uk

The impact of housing on health has been known since the nineteenth century, and the role of housing as a key determinant of health is discussed in our companion volume (Naidoo and Wills, 2010) and in Chapter 2. Poor-quality housing is often sited in deprived neighbourhoods with few local amenities. Graffiti, litter, boarded-up premises and dog mess are all signs of a neglected environment which, in turn, affects people's perception of the safety of their neighbourhood and hence their willingness to be active participants within it. These issues often rank high on community agendas. Part of the health disadvantage in relation to housing relates to the quantity of affordable housing. As rents increase, the amount of social housing declines. Cold housing is also a health risk. Cold is the main explanation for the excess winter deaths that occur each year in England and Wales. Being able to afford a warm house is clearly a factor. Half of single pensioners and two-thirds of households with no-one in work were in fuel poverty in 2007 to 2008, spending more than 10% of their income on fuel (Marmot, 2010).

The social environment

The quality of life in a community is a powerful determinant of health. By studying several healthy communities, Wilkinson (1996) identified a number of factors which contribute to quality of life.

 Case Study 15.3 Quality of life in communities

The small town of Roseto, Pennsylvania, USA (1600 inhabitants) is cited as an example of a community with markedly lower death rates from heart attacks than neighbouring areas. The population of Roseto is made up of Italian-Americans descended from migrants from the town of Roseto in southern Italy. It differed from other towns because it was 'remarkably close knit... with a sense of common purpose... [with] a camaraderie which precluded ostentation... [and] a concern for neighbours ensuring no one was ever abandoned... the family as the hub and bulwark of life provided a security and insurance against any catastrophe'. Roseto's considerable health advantage only seems explicable in relation to these social characteristics. As the younger people moved away, community and family ties broke down and people became more concerned with material values and conspicuous consumption (Bruhn and Wolf, 1979, cited in Wilkinson (1996, p. 116)).

Social capital refers to social cohesion and the cumulative experience of relationships, with both those known to us and those who are strangers, that are characterized by mutual trust, acceptance, approval and respect. People are social beings, and the quality of social interaction is vital to both personal and communal well-being. Social capital provides the foundation for collective action in the public sphere for the public good. Although definitions of social capital vary, the main indicators are:

- social relationships and social support
- formal and informal networks
- community and civic engagement, including voluntary associations
- trust and neighbourliness
- a sense of belonging for all communities

- the diversity of people's backgrounds and circumstances is appreciated and valued
- those from different backgrounds have similar life opportunities
- strong and positive relationships are developed between people from different backgrounds.

Community networks may be built around activities associated with school, leisure or living in a particular locality. Parents, especially mothers, have been identified as particularly active in forging neighbourhood links (Robertson et al., 2008). In addition to their primary purpose, buildings such as schools and leisure facilities are often used to house additional community events and networks. The closure of services such as schools and post offices therefore has a negative impact on neighbourliness, and this might help to explain the strength of feeling voiced whenever communities are threatened with the closure of such amenities.

There is evidence that building social capital is only possible above a certain threshold of income. If people are preoccupied with survival in its crudest meaning (i.e. ensuring they are fed, warm, sheltered and safe), they will be unable to focus beyond, on broader communal issues. The fact that social capital is not always benign also has to be acknowledged. Drug dealing and criminality on many housing estates rely on strong, closely integrated networks. Neighbourhoods with less social capital differ from stronger communities in many ways. There is likely to be less volunteering, the neighbourhood is perceived to be less safe and there will be less socializing and trust in others.

Research Example 15.1 Social capital and health

As the Marmot Review, 'Fair Society Healthy Lives' (2010), points out, 'we live, grow, learn, work and age in a range of environments, and our lives are affected by residential communities, neighbourhoods and relational communities and social structures'. (p. 126). Section E2.3 summarizes the evidence linking social capital with health. It cites Wilkinson and Pickett (2009), stating that the most powerful sources of stress are low status and lack of social networks. Low levels of integration and

loneliness increase mortality. Social capital can provide a source of resilience and social support, and connections act as a buffer against particular risks of poor health and other difficulties. Several studies show that social networks act as a protective factor against dementia and cognitive decline. Living longer with more complex health needs means older people will be more reliant on such social support systems and networks. People's participation in their communities gives added control over their lives, which contributes to their psychosocial well-being and, as a result, to other health outcomes.

Both crime and the fear of crime are health hazards associated with negative effects, including depression and mental ill health. It has been suggested that negative effects are both direct, for example stress and depression, and indirect, for example mental ill health linked to social isolation and feelings of vulnerability. Excessive noise or petty disputes with neighbours, although less severe than violence or the threat of violence, can have a large impact on quality of life. Tackling what came to be called 'antisocial behaviour' became problematized and part of an ideological position by the New Labour government in the early twenty-first century (Squires, 2006). The Scottish government framework 'Promoting Positive Outcomes' aims to address the causes of antisocial behaviour, which it identifies as drink, drugs and deprivation (www.scotland.gov.uk/Topics/archive/law-order/asb).

Services

An adequate service infrastructure is essential to the health and life of a neighbourhood. If essential services such as shops and post offices are not available locally, people are forced to travel outside the area, leading to a loss of social contacts as well as incurring additional costs (time and travel). This has been recognized by many communities fighting to retain local schools or shops. However, many planning decisions appear not to recognize this fact. In particular, the increase in out-of-town supermarkets has had a severe impact on both small local shopping outlets and traffic rates. Proximity to fast-food outlets is greater in deprived neighbourhoods. For example, a study of the location of McDonalds' outlets in England found provision was four times higher in the most deprived areas (Cummins et al., 2005).

Evaluating neighbourhood work

Numerous activities take place *in* neighbourhoods to improve them such as housing regeneration or community facilities. There is great potential in building health into community activities, such as adult education and leisure and cultural activities.

It could be argued that any neighbourhood development work has the potential to promote health by increasing social contacts and trust, or social capital.

Case Study 15.4 Community gardens

Community gardens exist in many nations and in both urban and rural areas. They may fulfil a number of functions, including leisure gardens, child and school gardens, healing and therapy gardens, demonstration gardens and those concerned with ecological restoration. They are actively supported by specific communities, reflecting some form of mutual aid and communal reciprocity, they probably have had a fair degree of altruism in getting them started and, very often, they are supported by charitable or municipal grant aid. They may also be grassroots initiatives aimed at revitalizing low- to moderate-income neighbourhoods in urban settings. Community gardens have been shown to improve health by increasing participants' access to fruit and vegetables, providing the opportunity for regular exercise and communal interaction, and enabling economic self-reliance through using the gardens for training and recreation purposes and selling surplus produce (McGlone et al., 1999; Ferris et al., 2001; Dickinson et al., 2003).

Place-based approaches or approaches that see the neighbourhood as a setting, attempt to address the social and physical environment and targets an entire community. The aim is to make the neighbourhood more engaged, connected and resilient.

Learning Activity 15.3 Evaluation of neighbourhood work

What might be some of the challenges in the evaluation of neighbourhood development programmes?

Additional spin-offs in terms of direct support for healthy lifestyles are common, as the following example shows.

In any consideration of the effect of neighbourhood on health it is very difficult to separate the effects of compositional factors (those relating to the kinds of individuals being studied, including their socio-economic status and lifestyles) from the effects of contextual factors (those relating to the environment) (Kawachi and Berkman, 2003). Compositional explanations for health disadvantage state that it is the demographic profile of an area that determines the health outcomes of its residents. There is a clear bias in research towards considering the impact of compositional factors. The complexity of relationships between individuals and environments, plus the long timescale in which effects become apparent, militates against research investigating whether differences in health outcomes result from characteristics of the place. There are some attempts to carry out research into contextual factors, including multilevel analysis, but it remains very difficult to attribute cause and effect in neighbourhood work.

However, even given these caveats, the evidence base for targeted responses to spatial concentrates of inequality, termed neighbourhood renewal or place-based approaches, having a positive impact on health is rather thin (Macintyre and Ellaway, 2003; Blackman, 2006).

Conclusion

The relationship between people, place and health has long been recognized in the effects of poor physical environments and social exclusion. The recognition that this health inequity stems from location, geography and place is more recent. The neighbourhood is not just a physical environment but also a psychosocial environment, as is a workplace or school. The neighbourhood provides a valuable setting for accessing many vulnerable groups, including older people and people on low incomes. Neighbourhoods are real-life settings with the potential for priorities to be defined by residents rather than professionals. Addressing health on a neighbourhood basis means addressing core determinants of health, such as the social fabric and quality of people's lives. It is important that in a focus on neighbourhood settings the opportunity to address people's self-defined needs is taken. It would be easy to use neighbourhoods merely as a means of professional outreach work, but this would be to neglect one of the great strengths of this setting.

 Learning Activity 15.4 The role of community healthcare professionals

Many members of the primary care team (especially health visitors and general practitioners) regard themselves as working with neighbourhood communities. How might their role change if they were to focus on community capacity building and building social capital?

While there are many advantages to working within a neighbourhood setting, it is not a universal panacea. Many factors which affect people's lives are determined at national level, for example level of benefit entitlement or availability of employment. However, the neighbourhood setting does offer opportunities for creative and imaginative ways of working which support the core principles of health promotion – participation, equity, empowerment and collaboration.

Question for further discussion

- Think of your neighbourhood. What are its health promotion resources and assets?

Summary

This chapter has identified neighbourhoods as a key setting for health promotion and discussed reasons for its popularity. Examples of innovative practice centred on neighbourhood work have been given, and the problems of evaluating such work discussed.

Further reading and resources

Biddle, S., Seymour, M., 2012. Healthy neighbourhoods and communities: policy and practice. In: Scriven, A., Hodgins, M. (Eds.), Health Promotion Settings: Principles and Practice. Sage, London, pp. 92–110. *A useful chapter that outlines the role of local government in England in place-based approaches.*

Gowman, N., 1999. Healthy Neighbourhoods. Kings Fund, London. Available online at: http://www.kingsfund.org.uk/sites/files/kf/field/field_publication_file/healthy-neighbourhoods-natasha-gowman-kings-fund-1-february-1999.PDF (accessed 07.03.15). *Although dated, this is a useful summary of the arguments for neighbourhoods as a healthy setting.*

Macintyre, S., Ellaway, A., 2003. Neighbourhoods and health: an overview. In: Kawachi, I., Berkman, L.F. (Eds.), Neighbourhoods and Health. Oxford University Press, Oxford, pp. 20–43. *A useful summary of the evidence for neighbourhoods impacting on health, covering both theoretical and methodological issues.*

Stewart, M., 2007. Neighbourhood renewal and regeneration. In: Orme, J., Powell, J., Taylor, P., et al. (Eds.), Public Health in the 21st Century: New Perspectives on Policy, Participation and Practice, second ed. McGraw Hill/Open University Press, Berkshire, pp. 170–184. *An account of the development of neighbourhood intitiatives, exploring their role in tackling inequalities and building social capital and partnership working.*

Wilkinson, R., Pickett, K., 2009. The Spirit Level: Why Equality Is Better for Everyone. Penguin, London. *This book argues that greater equality in society is directly linked to better health outcomes for everyone.*

Government departments have neighbourhood strategies, for example, Department for Social Development, Northern Ireland at www.dsdni.gov.uk/index/urcdg-urban_regeneration/neighbourhood_renewal.htm.

Useful websites include the following:

Joseph Rowntree Foundation, www.jrf.org.uk/, which conducts research into neighbourhoods and communities.

London Healthy Urban Development Unit, www.healthyurbandevelopment.nhs.uk, which works to create healthy sustainable communities through the use of planning regulations and processes.

 Feedback to learning activities

15.1 Neighbourhood and community are often used interchangeably. Neighbourhood refers to a geographical area and the people living within that area. Community refers to people who share a common characteristic, which may be the geographical area they live in but may be another shared characteristic, such as religion or ethnicity (as in the Christian or Black communities). The

Continued

phrase 'place-based approaches' is also used to describe strategies that address complex determinants of health within a specific location.

15.2 The Marmot Review (2010) identified the following aspects of a neighbourhood as having a significant impact on health: pollution, green and open space, transport, food, housing and community participation. People living in the poorest neighbourhoods will, on average, die seven years earlier than people living in the richest neighbourhoods (Marmot, 2010). Tackling inequalities through neighbourhood interventions can be a cost-effective strategy, reaching a large number of people who might otherwise be hard to reach.

15.3 Evaluation of neighbourhood and community work is extremely difficult for several reasons. Firstly, neighbourhood work involves long-term processes to promote social cohesion and regeneration. Funding long-term evaluation projects and maintaining continuity of focus and resources are difficult. Many projects are set up under time-limited funding initiatives which then compromise their sustainability (e.g. Healthy Living Centres were funded through lottery money). Projects may find they are diverted from their core business into fundraising in order to keep going. Funding streams may also specify certain activities or outcomes, leading to the neglect of long-term activities to build community capacity and networks.

15.4 Chapter 10 on community development describes how empowerment can help to achieve healthier neighbourhoods. It shows how involving people in decisions about health provision increases wellbeing. However, many health professionals would argue this role should be undertaken by dedicated community development workers rather than community health workers, as such a role does not require medical knowledge and expertise.

References

Blackman, T., 2006. Placing Health: Neighbourhood Renewal, Health Improvement and Complexity. Policy Press, Bristol.

Bowling, A., Barber, J., Morris, R., et al., 2006. Do perceptions of neighbourhood environment influence health. Journal of Epidemiology and Community Health 60, 476–483.

Bruhn, J.G., Wolf, S., 1979. The Roseto Story. University of Oklahoma Press, Norman, OK.

Cummins, S., McKay, L., Macintyre, S., 2005. McDonalds restaurants and neighbourhood deprivation in Scotland and England. American Journal of Preventive Medicine 4, 308–310.

Department of Health (DoH), 2004. Choosing Health: Making Healthy Choices Easier. DoH, London. Available online at: http://webarchive.nationalarchives.gov.uk/+/dh.gov.uk/en/publicationsandstatistics/publications/publicationspolicyandguidance/dh_4094550 (accessed 07.03.15).

Dickinson, J., Duma, S., Paulsen, H., Rilveria, L., Twiss, J., Weinman, T., 2003. Community gardens: lessons learned from California's healthy cities and communities. American Journal of Public Health 93, 1435–1438.

Ferris, J., Norman, C., Sempik, J., 2001. People, land and sustainability: community gardens and the social dimensions of sustainable development. Social Policy and Administration 35, 559–568.

Kawachi, I., Berkman, L.F. (Eds.), 2003. Neighbourhoods and Health. Oxford University Press, Oxford.

Macintyre, S., Ellaway, A., 2003. Neighbourhoods and health: an overview. In: Kawachi, I., Berkman, L.F. (Eds.), Neighbourhoods and Health. Oxford University Press, Oxford, pp. 20–43.

McGlone, P., Dobson, B., Dowler, E., et al., 1999. Food Projects and How They Work. Joseph Rowntree Foundation, York.

Marmot, M., 2010. Fair Society, Healthy Lives. London Institute of Health Equity. Available online at: http://www.instituteofhealthequity.org/projects/fair-society-healthy-lives-the-marmot-review (accessed 07.03.15).

Naidoo, J., Wills, J., 2010. Public Health and Health Promotion: Developing Practice, third ed. Baillière Tindall, London.

Office of National Statistics, 2007. West of Scotland Twenty-07 Study NOS, London. See details at: http://www.sphsu.mrc.ac.uk/research-programmes/ss/sineq/20-07.html (accessed 07.03.15).

Rice, C., Grant, M., 2007. The Potential of Car-free Developments: Practicalities and Health Impacts. WHO Collaborating Centre for Healthy Cities and Urban Policy, Bristol.

Robertson, D., Smyth, J., McIntosh, I., 2008. Neighbourhood Identity: People, Time and Place. Joseph Rowntree Foundation. Available online at: http://www.jrf.org.uk/system/files/2154-neighbourhood-identity-regeneration.pdf (accessed 07.03.15).

Squires, P., 2006. New Labour and the politics of antisocial behavior. Critical Social Policy 26 (1), 144–168.

Wilkinson, R.G., 1996. Unhealthy Societies: The Afflictions of Inequality. Routledge, London.

Wilkinson, R., Pickett, K., 2009. The Spirit Level: Why Equality Is Better for Everyone. Penguin, London.

Chapter Sixteen

Health promoting health services

Learning Outcomes

By the end of this chapter you will be able to:
- understand the concept of a health promoting health service
- discuss the potential of health services to promote health.

Key Concepts and Definitions

Health promoting hospital A hospital which provides high-quality medical care and seeks to develop its health promoting capacity, including its organizational structure and identity, active participation from its staff and patients, its physical environment and its role within the community.

Healthy pharmacy A pharmacy which provides high-quality pharmaceutical services, including proactive health advice and interventions within the community it serves.

Importance of the Topic

In this part of the book we look at schools, prisons, neighbourhoods and workplaces, all settings where health and health promotion are not part of the core business or primary goals. Hospitals are concerned with health, yet to change a large and complex organization such as a hospital from being a place of treatment to one where health gain is valued and seen as part of its purpose is a major reorientation and a challenging process (see also Chapter 8). Instead of being a place for curing disease which values patient compliance, a health promoting hospital would be a place for promoting health, empowering patients and concerned with the whole community of patients, relatives, friends and staff. Health promoting hospitals (HPHs) incorporate a variety of different projects, but with the same overall aims.

- To make the hospital a healthier working and living environment for its large workforce and for patients.
- To expand self-management, recuperation and rehabilitation programmes.
- To encourage participation by staff and patients.
- To provide information and advice on health issues.
- To act as a community resource and an agent of social cohesion.
- To act in a socially responsible manner, especially in relation to environmental impact.

A hospital, like a school or a workplace, is a social system with its own procedures, culture and values. The process of developing an HPH will thus involve the adaptation of management structures, top-level political commitment and the facilitation of greater participation by staff and patients.

Defining a health promoting hospital

Settings can normally be identified as having physical boundaries (including geographical), a range of people with defined roles and an organizational structure. As we have seen earlier in this part of the book, a settings approach is not about doing a health promotion project such as a display for World AIDS Day, nor is it about delegating health promotion to specific departmental or staff 'champions' (Johnson and Baum, 2001), although both activities may be used as part of wider development. The settings approach to health promotion focuses on bringing about holistic organizational and practice changes to create a more health promoting environment. The challenge lies in convincing hospital authorities that health promotion does not constitute an additional burden but is very much part of its core business and approach.

The World Health Organization (WHO) definition of an HPH (Nutbeam, 1998) provides a useful starting point for understanding what is required:

> A health promoting hospital does not only provide high quality comprehensive medical and nursing services, but also develops a corporate identity that embraces the aims of health promotion, develops a health promoting organizational structure and culture, including active, participatory roles for patients and all members of staff, develops itself into a health promoting physical environment, and actively cooperates with its community.

The hospital as a setting for health was validated by the launch of the Health Promoting Hospitals initiative in 1990 by the WHO Regional Office for Europe. This network now includes 669 institutions in 39 countries. While hospitals represent the greatest challenge to become health promoting, primary care services and pharmacies can also promote health. In this chapter the potential of health services to promote health is examined, and examples of good practice are given to illustrate what can be achieved.

Why hospitals are a key setting for health promotion

Many health practitioners assume that health promotion has always been a core task of medicine in general and hospitals in particular. Yet health promotion can be at odds with the hospital context, which is based on a medical model of care with an orientation towards cure and treatment.

- The expectation of the patient role has generally been one of passivity.
- Staff competencies, job remits and time are mainly dedicated to clinical work and care.
- Patients' contact with the hospital staff is generally based on brief 'consultations' related to their particular diseases.
- Patients in hospital are at a late stage in their diseases, and highlighting prevention may make them feel responsible and blameworthy.
- Hospitals are not in themselves healthy environments.

Yet hospitals are also a natural focus for health promotion.

- Twenty per cent of the population will visit a local hospital as a patient within a single year, and a further percentage will visit the hospital as family and friends (NHS Confederation, 2014).
- Hospitals are often the biggest employer in their community: 8% of all jobs in Europe are in the healthcare sector (European Commission, 2012).
- Contact with patients is at a time of heightened awareness about health and illness, when they may be motivated to make major lifestyle changes.
- Staff are respected and credible.

There has been a shift in recent years away from an emphasis on the compliant patient to one which is more patient-centred and acknowledges patients' concerns and expertise (see Chapter 9 for an outline of the Expert Patient programme). Considerable evidence exists to show that patient outcomes are much improved when patients are involved in their own care and have adequate explanations and time to discuss their concerns (Coulter and Ellins, 2007; Coulter et al., 2008; www.nationalvoices.org.uk). A major proportion of hospital admissions are related to patients suffering from one or more chronic diseases. These patients require support to cope with their diseases and achieve some changes in lifestyle, adherence to possibly complicated drug and nutrition regimens and management of their condition. There is evidence that patients are more receptive to information and advice in situations of acute ill health. Although hospitals may appear to be 'downstream', the hospital thus provides a 'window of opportunity' for patients to understand the potential benefits of behaviour change.

 Learning Activity 16.1 Emergency care and health promotion

The role of an emergency department (ED) or accident and emergency (A&E) unit is to provide prompt treatment and care for the acutely ill and injured at any time. How could an ED or A&E promote health?

An HPH will also have benefits for its staff and community. Staff sickness/absence rates are likely to be lower, and staff retention is likely to be better. Local communities will benefit from having a large, responsible and responsive employer in their area. HPHs will bring income into local communities (through workforce wages), demonstrate how large organizations can be environmentally aware (through, e.g. recycling and local sourcing of food) and provide an accessible and local source of expertise regarding health matters.

 Learning Activity 16.2 Indicators of a health promoting hospital

Existing performance management measures for hospitals relate to productivity, for example number of emergency admissions, unnecessary procedures and inpatient bed stays. What might be indicators of a health promoting hospital?

The WHO Health Promoting Hospital Network was launched in recognition of the impact that a hospital can have, and focuses on four areas (WHO, 2007).

1. Promoting the health of patients.
2. Promoting the health of staff.
3. Changing the organization to a health promoting setting.
4. Promoting the health of the community in the catchment area of the hospital.

Promoting the health of patients

The main focus of most health promotion in hospitals is disease management and prevention for patients. But even in cases of severe diseases, patients are always partly healthy (whether emotionally, socially or spiritually) when they enter the hospital, and these aspects (e.g. self-care, psychological well-being or social contact) can be maintained.

In many healthcare settings, including hospitals, health promotion strategies are often referred to as opportunistic when a chance has arisen to offer health education or other preventive advice during a clinical visit, such as the Making Every Contact Count (MECC) initiative. There are other opportunities for more coordinated intervention strategies, such as risk assessment for alcohol-related problems or the offer of chlamydia screening.

 Case Study 16.1 Making every contact count

MECC is a national initiative intended to extend radically the delivery of public health advice to the public by training all NHS and local authority staff in the basic skills of giving simple and timely advice to patients and service users. A short intervention, from 30 seconds to 3 minutes, is delivered opportunistically to raise awareness of, and assess a person's willingness to discuss, lifestyle issues. It is claimed that across NHS Midlands and East, for example, there are
- 288,000 staff who collectively have millions of contacts with the public every year. If each staff member

Continued

delivers MECC just 10 times each year, there will be 2.88 million new opportunities to change lifestyle behaviour every year.
- If one in 20 of these people goes on to make a positive change to his/her behaviour, a total of 144,000 people would be improving their health and well-being.

www.makingeverycontactcount.com.

Professionals play a minor role in promoting the health of their patients, however; the major contributors to patients' health are themselves, their relatives and friends. Empowering patients to get involved as partners and (co-)producers of their health in decision-making and diagnostic and therapeutic processes, through the provision of information and education, is therefore an important health promotion strategy.

Actions such as co-designing pre-admission information with patients, offering computer-based decision aids for treatment options, and patient involvement in infection control illustrate how health promotion principles of being equitable, empowering and participatory can become the basis of hospital practice. Maintaining patients' positive health with greater consideration of their quality of life and psychosocial functioning includes:

- securing personal privacy (e.g. data protection, curtains around beds)
- relationship-centred caring
- providing animal therapy
- providing offers and options to encourage psychosocial activities of patients (e.g. cultural activities, religious services, patient libraries, discussions, patient internet café)
- bringing humour into the hospital, for example by clown doctors
- using art therapy
- providing adequate visiting hours for family members, friends, peers and lay carers
- providing facilities for caring relatives or friends to stay in the hospital (especially for very vulnerable groups of patients, for example children and the terminally ill)

- organizing visiting and lay support services for unattended patients
- providing psychological and social assistance to cope with stress or anxieties related to the hospital stay or the patient's specific disease (e.g. cancer, terminal illness) or general life situation (e.g. loss of work due to disease) by specialized personnel (e.g. clinical psychologists, social workers, pastoral carers) (www.hph-hc.cc; Hancock, 2012).

Case Study 16.2 Hospital food

One of the poorer aspects of hospital care that is frequently cited by patients is the quality of food. Intake of nutritious food is crucial for patients recovering after surgery or medical interventions. The campaign for better hospital food (http://www.sustainweb.org/hospitalfood/) claims that the NHS spends about £250 million a year on food alone, or £500 million on food, contract and catering staff costs. It serves about 300 million patient meals a year in about 1200 hospitals, as well as several million meals to staff and visitors. Poor-quality food that is overcooked or lukewarm by the time it reaches patients often ends up in the bin. Uneaten meals cost about £18 million a year. If food preparation waste and labour are included, the price of uneaten food rises to over £144 million a year. Over the past few years there has been considerable concern about patient malnutrition, poor-quality food and poor hygiene standards among hospital food suppliers. The Council of Europe passed Resolution ResAP (2003) on food and nutritional care in hospitals, and clinical standards are now established for food, fluid and nutritional care. However, food quality is not included. Scotland has recently introduced a statutory requirement to report on food quality, and there are calls to have this monitored in England by the Care Quality Commission.

Although the NHS is the only health system in the industrialized world where wealth does not determine access to care, accessing healthcare is still a concern for patients. Six percent of people in the UK (compared to 33% in the USA and 5% in Holland) do not see a doctor when sick or fail to get a prescription because of the cost (www.commonweathfund.org); and 1.4 million people miss, turn down or do not seek hospital appointments because of problems with transport. With the concentration of acute facilities into fewer and larger units, such problems are likely to increase. Others may not access care because of barriers of language or fears of discrimination. A low service uptake may be due to a service not meeting needs. The articulated needs of minority groups, including gypsies and travellers, people with learning disabilities and new migrants, who all experience difficulties accessing healthcare, focus on communication, information and account to be taken of religion, dietary preferences and obtaining consent (Bhopal, 2007).

Stating that every second person in Europe has limited health literacy, the WHO has called for action in transforming healthcare into health-literacy-friendly settings, and acknowledged that the health sector must remove barriers to information, services and care (WHO, 2013). Brach et al. (2012) identified the attributes of a health-literate healthcare organization as one that:

- Recognizes that people may have difficulty without stigmatization, and so offers everyone help with health literacy tasks.
- Uses communication strategies such as the *teach-back technique*, for example ensuring patients' understanding by asking them to repeat back the information provided in a non-shaming manner; and *Ask me 3*, a tool encouraging patients to ask three main questions that enable them to understand and manage their care better (What is my problem? What do I have to do? Why is it important for me to do that?).
- Provides easy access to health information and services and navigation assistance, for example using electronic patient portals.
- Designs print, audio-visual and social media content that is easy to understand and act upon.
- Recognizes high-risk situations for people with low literacy, for example care transitions, invasive procedures and communications about medicines.

Promoting the health of staff

The hospital as a physical and social setting has an impact on the health of staff. Hospitals are potentially dangerous workplaces, encompassing physical risks (e.g. exposure to biological, chemical and nuclear agents), mental risks (e.g. stress, night shifts) and social risks (e.g. night shifts have a negative effect on social life, bullying and violence against staff).

 Learning Activity 16.3 Obese staff in the NHS

The chief executive of the NHS claimed in 2014 that a third of the NHS workforce are obese. If this is true, does it matter?

Other aspects of the environment that affect the health of staff are less addressed. For example, patients, staff, visitors and the local community are affected by the physical environment of the hospital setting, including its functionality and aesthetic design. In 1859 Florence Nightingale commented:

People say the effect is on the mind. It is no such thing. The effect is on the body, too. Little as we know about the way in which we are affected by form, colour, by light, we do know this, that they have a physical effect. Variety of form and brilliancy of colour in the objects presented to patients is the actual means of recovery.

For many of today's patients, visitors and staff, however, the hospital environment remains soulless, drab and depressing. One report (Commission on Architecture and the Built Environment, 2004) highlighted the following as key factors in the poor working environment:
- fluorescent lighting
- noise
- lack of independent control over ventilation
- no facility for exercise.

Research Example 16.1 Hospitals as health promoting environments

A review of numerous studies found that the physical design of hospitals can influence a variety of patient outcomes, including cross-infection rates, sleep, length of stay, privacy, communication and social support. The studies conclude that:

- single rooms lower the rate of acquired infections, improve patient confidentiality and facilitate social support
- noise levels can be reduced by sound-absorbing ceilings, noiseless paging and single rooms
- views of natural landscapes reduce stress
- improved ventilation and lighting improve patient outcomes

Ulrich et al. (2004).

The Boorman Report (2009), which was an inquiry into the health of NHS staff, found high levels of sickness absence and a clear relationship between workers' self-reported well-being, patient satisfaction, and NHS trust performance.

Learning Activity 16.4 Violence in hospitals

Violence against health staff is increasingly common, and may include verbal abuse, threats and physical assaults. Those working in A&E and psychiatry are most likely to suffer abuse. What could a hospital do to protect the health of its staff?

Research Example 16.2 Creating a health promoting hospital

The NHS is a round-the-clock service with caring staff who do work which is often physically and psychologically demanding and can involve risks. A needs assessment of staff at one London hospital found:

- a low percentage use a car to get to work
- low levels of physical activity, and no access to facilities to encourage physical activity at work
- low levels of consumption of fruit and vegetables, which were thought to be overpriced in work canteens; and over 50% of staff do not take a lunch break

- 10% staff are smokers.
  The report includes the following recommendations:
- improve the psychosocial environment, with a culture of concern, reward for work and rest breaks
- better management of bullying and harassment at work
- promote a cycle-to-work scheme and cycling between sites
- reduce the availability of unhealthy food in the canteen and vending machines
- have health champions to lead on public health issues
- focus occupational health and human resources services towards the prevention of ill health.

Institute of Health Equity/Barts and the London Trust (2011).

The hospital and the community

The hospital has an impact on the health of people living and working in the surrounding neighbourhood. In recent years the largest capital development programme in the history of the NHS has led to large car parks, energy-intensive air conditioning, heating and lighting and huge quantities of waste. Sustainability is central to the development of an HPH.

Hospitals can further promote health in their community by:

- systematically contributing to health reporting (e.g. frequency and causes of accidents on roads help to create a data linkage with transport and planning)
- organizing specific action programmes (e.g. information, counselling, training) in cooperation with schools, other healthcare providers and local community groups, for example dump campaigns (getting rid of unused medicines), promoting baby carseats, asthma management
- being a responsible, health promoting and ethical employer.

Organizational health promotion

The hospital is not just a site for health promotion activities, but a social entity that creates health. An

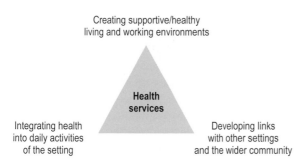

Creating supportive/healthy living and working environments

Health services

Integrating health into daily activities of the setting

Developing links with other settings and the wider community

Fig. 16.1 ● Health promoting health services.

HPH must therefore incorporate the vision, concepts, values and basic strategies of health promotion (equity, empowerment, participation and collaboration as well as sustainability) into the structures and culture of the hospital, and thus health becomes its outcome (as shown in Figure 16.1).

An ecological social systems approach to developing a healthy setting requires change from both the top, in relation to organizational development and political commitment, and from the bottom, in high-visibility innovative projects, the active engagement of all users and embedding the values of HPH into the hospital's institutional agenda and core business. HPH can be embedded into the structure and philosophy of hospitals through being linked and combined with other strategies of hospital development (e.g. health education, patients' rights, self-help movements, health at work, hospital hygiene, the ecological and sustainable development movement, strategies for personal and organizational development, and quality management) (Dooris, 2006).

 Learning Activity 16.5 The arguments for becoming a health promoting hospital

Give three reasons why a hospital should become an HPH, and then three reasons why an HPH is not a good idea.

The HPH movement

The HPH network, launched by the WHO Regional Office in Europe in 1990, now operates in 39 countries on all continents. This initiative seeks to promote good practice by developing concepts and strategies, developing and disseminating model projects and networking via conferences and newsletters (www.healthpromotinghospital.org). The HPH focuses on the health of staff, patients and its local community.

Hospitals accepted into the HPH network have to meet certain conditions (WHO, 2004):

- develop a written policy for health promotion, and develop and evaluate an HPH action plan to support the introduction of health promotion into the culture of the hospital/health service during the four-year period of designation
- identify a hospital/health service coordinator for the coordination of HPH development and activity, and pay an annual contribution fee for the coordination of the international HPH network
- share information and experience on national and international levels, i.e. HPH development, models of good practice (projects) and the implementation of standards/indicators.

The complex organizational structures of many hospitals and the fact that most health professionals in the hospital setting do not readily associate health promotion as being part of their roles make the HPH a challenging setting. Whitehead (2004) argues that the hospital is the least visible of all the Ottawa Charter settings, and 'there is little empirical evidence of a measurable health impact' of policies focused on creating healthy environments as part of an HPH (Dooris, 2006, citing McKee, 2000). A review of health promoting health services found few studies on the benefits and effects (McHugh et al., 2010). To realize its full potential, the HPH strategy needs not only to be implemented within limited projects but also embedded as an integral aspect of hospital service (quality) management systems (WHO, 2004).

 Case Study 16.3 A health promoting hospital in Africa

A district hospital in rural South Africa has become a model HPH, demonstrating that the concept can be applied in different contexts. The South African HPH's activities include educational workshops on occupational safety and infection control, health education delivered via a closed-circuit network on HIV/AIDS and healthy eating, and weekly health walks for staff (Delobelle et al., 2010).

Table 16.1 Pharmacy services and health promotion

Primary prevention	Health education	Health promotion
• Advice on immunizations and vaccinations • Chlamydia screening • Access to emergency contraception • Provision of statins for people who would benefit	• Maintaining medications • Advice on managing long-term conditions, e.g. asthma • Skills training, e.g. use of inhalers for asthma • Symptom management • Participation in media campaigns • Local knowledge of statutory and non-statutory services	• Tobacco cessation programmes that use nicotine replacement • Monitoring the use of antibiotic prescriptions • Pregnancy testing • Ensuring the pharmacy is user-friendly, e.g. appropriate location, opening times, atmosphere

Health promoting pharmacies

Pharmacies are known as places where medicines and prescriptions are collected. A UK pharmacy white paper (DH, 2008) proposes that pharmacies should move from dispensing medicines to promoting health, well-being and self-care. Pharmacies will be the first port of call for minor illnesses and ailments, and will support patients with long-term conditions. Community pharmacies are well placed to do this for the following reasons:

- an estimated 1.2 million people visit a pharmacy each day
- many pharmacists have established good relationships with their regular customers, who include people with long-term conditions and those with physical and mental disabilities
- pharmacists are acknowledged as experts on medicine by the public and health workers, putting them in an influential position to promote health and prevent ill health.

Learning Activity 16.6 Health promoting pharmacies

How might a pharmacy promote health?

There is clearly potential for a pharmacy to promote health, as shown in Table 16.1, but there are also obstacles to the development of health promoting pharmacies. Obstacles include:

- the lack of a confidential space for discussion
- the lack of training for pharmacists on health promotion and behaviour change
- the pharmacy's priority function as a commercial business.

Case Study 16.4 The Healthy Living Pharmacy initiative

The Healthy Living Pharmacy (HLP) initiative started in 2010 in Portsmouth. The criteria for a healthy living pharmacy include staff trained as health champions; suitable facilities, for example a private consultation area; and high-quality NHS services, such as emergency contraception, stopping-smoking programmes, weight management and NHSD health checks, in addition to the core services of medicine supply and self-care advice. Evaluation of the HLP initiative is promising, with HLP customers twice as likely to set a quit-smoking date as customers in traditional pharmacies. In just one month, pharmacies in Portsmouth made more than 3600 alcohol interventions and directly referred 29 individuals to a specialist alcohol service (http://www.hantslpc.org.uk/uploads/Portsmouth%20 HLP%20interim%20outcomes.pdf).

Research Example 16.3 The role of the community pharmacist

A scoping study identified a wide range of roles that community pharmacists were providing in public health, with the dominant themes being in the areas of smoking-cessation services, healthy eating and lifestyle advice, provision of emergency hormonal contraception, infection control and prevention, promoting cardiovascular health and blood-pressure control and prevention, and management of drug abuse, misuse and addiction. There was no evidence of pharmacies involved in preventing falls in the elderly, emergency preparedness for and response to bioterrorism, climate change and potential pandemics, immunization and vaccination services of prevention and risk assessment of osteoporosis.

Agomo (2012).

Conclusion

Although core activities of health services remain focused on medical diagnosis and treatment, the HPH concept has taken root and there are many examples of hospitals, and more recently pharmacies, embracing health promotion principles. Health promoting initiatives occur at all levels, from individual practitioners using checklists to include health promotion systematically in client contacts to hospital-wide initiatives to increase service user participation and reduce environmental impact. In between lie a range of activities at ward or departmental level, including the use of arts therapies and the provision of healthy locally sourced food. All initiatives are guided by core health promotion principles: a holistic concept of health, empowerment, participation, intersectoral collaboration, equity and sustainability.

The HPH needs to be supported by an organizational structure: support from management, a budget, specific aims and targets, and action plans for implementing health promotion into everyday business. All hospital staff need to make health promotion their business. This can be a challenge, particularly for staff in acute settings who are trained in other (diagnosis and treatment) priorities. Treating health promotion as one specific quality aspect to be monitored can aid its incorporation into core processes. Integrating health impact assessments into all decision-making within the hospital will also help to advance the HPH.

Questions for further discussion

- Think of a health facility you use or work in. Can you identify activities that promote equity, collaboration, participation, engagement and empowerment?
  What factors might impede the development of the service becoming health promoting? How could these factors be addressed?

Summary

This chapter has looked at the reasons for prioritizing hospital settings for health promotion. Recent national and international policy developments which affect the delivery of health promotion in health service settings, and the range of professionals involved, have been identified. Ways in which health promotion principles may be applied in health service settings have been discussed, and illustrated with examples.

Further reading and resources

Gröene, O., Garcia-Barbero, M. (Eds.), 2005. Evidence and Quality Management. WHO, Copenhagen. Available at: http://www.euro.who.int/__data/assets/pdf_file/0008/99827/E86220.pdf (accessed 08.03.15). *Summarizes evidence on HPHs and knowledge on implementation of the concept implementation.*

Hancock, T., 2012. The healthy hospital: a contradiction in terms? In: Scriven, A., Hodgins, M. (Eds.), Health Promotion Settings: Principles and Practice. Sage, London, pp. 126–140. *An interesting discussion of the potential of the hospital as a health promotion setting.*

McHugh, C., Robinson, A., Chesters, J., 2010. Health promoting health services: a review. Health Promotion International 25, 230–237. *A useful summary of the evidence on the benefits of health promoting services. Available online at: http://heapro.oxfordjournals.org/content/25/2/230.full.pdf+html (accessed 21.09.15)*

World Health Organization, 2004. Standards for Health Promotion in Hospitals. WHO Office for Europe, Copenhagen. Available online at: http://www.euro.who.int/__data/assets/pdf_file/0006/99762/e82490.pdf (accessed 08.03.15).

World Health Organization, 2006. Putting HPH Policy into Action: Working Paper. WHO Collaborating Centre on Health Promotion in Hospitals and Health Care, Vienna. Available at: http://www.hph-hc.cc/fileadmin/user_upload/HPH_BasicDocuments/Working-Paper-HPH-Strategies.pdf (accessed 08.03.15). *Theory-driven background paper on 18 HPH core strategies, including examples and selected evidence.*

World Health Organization, 2007. Integrating Health Promotion into Hospitals and Health Services. Concept, Framework and Organization. WHO Office for Europe, Copenhagen.

Available at: http://www.euro.who.int/__data/assets/pdf_file/0009/99801/E90777.pdf (accessed 08.03.15). Health Promotion Hospital website: www.hph-hc.cc.

 ## Feedback to learning activities

16.1 The ED can be a suitable setting for health promotion because it is an established entry point to the health system and it tends to have good links with the community. Bensburg and Kennedy (2002) offer numerous examples of health promotion strategies, from risk assessment (young people and alcohol) to health information (triage nurses providing information to carers who are high users of emergency paediatric services, including a follow-up appointment after discharge) and health education (asthma management training and follow-up telephone calls, and using the waiting room to promote reading and literacy to children).

16.2 An HPH would adhere to the following core principles, outlined in the Vienna Recommendations (WHO, 1997):
- acknowledges differences in the needs, values and cultures of different population groups
- promotes dignity and empowerment
- forms as close links as possible with other levels of the healthcare system and the community.

16.3 The NHS workforce is similar to the rest of the population, which also has a high level of obesity. The Health and Social Care Information Centre (2013) estimated that one-quarter of the adult population are obese. If the NHS chief executive's claims are true, NHS staff have an above-average rate of obesity. This could be due to some aspects of the NHS work environment, for example shift work and lack of access to healthy food in work canteens. Being obese compromises health and impacts on certain aspects of care, for example manual handling and a lack of willingness to deliver health promotion messages about diet and healthy eating. High levels of obesity among NHS staff are therefore a matter of concern.

16.4 The most common response is one of zero tolerance, a message which is promoted through publicity campaigns and education programmes for staff, who are encouraged to report violent incidents with formal protocols for documentation of violent episodes. Although such programmes are seen to be protecting the health of staff, they are not tackling the systemic issues that give rise to these events. Early studies of nursing, for example, focused on the profession's lack of power. The explanation for this was said to lie in nursing's predominantly female workforce, its function as the alleged handmaiden to medicine and because it had absorbed the values of its own activities, which assumed a level of passivity and compliance.

16.5 Reasons why an HPH is a good idea include:
- it accords with the vision of the hospital as committed to staff and patient well-being
- it can help to improve patient outcomes
- it could help with staff retention
- it reduces carbon waste.

16.6 Pharmacies are known as places where medicines and prescriptions are collected. However, pharmacies provide many more services, including stopping smoking, sexual health and alcohol support services. The benefits of pharmacies as health promoting settings include their availability (no appointments are required) and their anonymity. Pharmacists are professionals with expertise in medicines and health promotion. Some pharmacies provide additional services, such as minor ailments schemes and healthy heart clinics.

References

Agomo, C.O., 2012. The role of community pharmacists in public health: a scoping review of the literature. Journal of Pharmaceutical Health Services Research 3 (1), 25–33.

Bensberg, M., Kennedy, M., 2002. A framework for health promoting emergency departments. Health Promotion International 17, 179–188. Available online at: http://heapro.oxfordjournals.org/content/17/2/179.full.pdf+html (accessed 21.09.15).

Bhopal, R., 2007. Ethnicity, Race and Health in Multicultural Societies. Oxford University Press, Oxford.

Boorman, S., 2009. NHS Health and Wellbeing. Department of Health, London. Available at: www.nhshealthandwellbeing.org/pdfs/staff%20H&WB%20case%20studies%20vFinal%2023-11-09.pdf (accessed 06.02.15).

Brach, C., Dreyer, B., Schyve, P., Herrnandez, L.M., Baur, C., Lemerise, A.J., Parker, R., 2012. Attributes of a Health Literate Organization. Institute of Medicine. Available online at: https://www.iom.edu/~/media/Files/Perspectives-Files/2012/Discussion-Papers/BPH_HLit_Attributes.pdf (accessed 07.03.15).

Commission on Architecture and the Built Environment, 2004. The Role of Hospital Design in the Recruitment, Retention and Performance of NHS Nurses in England. Available online at: www.cabe.org.uk.

Coulter, A., Ellins, J., 2007. Effectiveness of strategies for informing educating, and involving patients. Patent Medical Journal 335, 24–27.

Coulter, A., Parsons, S., Astra, J., 2008. Where Are the Patients in Decision Making about Their Own Care? WHO, Copenhagen. Available online at: http://www.who.int/management/general/decisionmaking/WhereArePatientsinDecisionMaking.pdf (accessed 06.02.15).

Delobelle, P., Onya, H., Langa, C., Mashamba, J., Depoorter, A., 2010. Advances in health promotion in Africa; Promoting health through hospitals. Global Health Promotion 17, 33–36.

Department of Health, HM Government, 2008. Pharmacy in England: building on strengths-delivering the future. Cm 7341, Stationary Office, London. Available online at: https://www.gov.uk/government/uploads/system/uploads/attachment_data/file/228858/7341.pdf (accessed 21.09.15).

Dooris, M., 2006. Healthy settings: challenges to generating evidence of effectiveness. Health Promotion International 21, 55–65. Available online at: http://heapro.oxfordjournals.org/content/21/1/55.full.pdf+html (accessed 21.09.15).

European Commission, 2012. Action Plan for the EU Health Workforce. Available online at: http://ec.europa.eu/dgs/health_consumer/docs/swd_ap_eu_healthcare_workforce_en.pdf (accessed 06.02.15).

Hancock, T., 2012. The healthy hospital: a contradiction in terms? In: Scriven, A., Hodgins, M. (Eds.), Health Promotion Settings: Principles and Practice. Sage, London, pp. 126–140.

Health and Social Care Information Centre (HSCIC), 2013. Statistics on Obesity, Physical Activity and Diet – England, 2013. Published online February 20, 2013. Available at: http://www.hscic.gov.uk/catalogue/PUB10364.

Institute of Health Equity/Barts and the London, 2011. Strategy for Health promoting Hospitals. Available online at: http://www.instituteofhealthequity.org/projects/barts-and-the-london-nhs-trust--health promoting-hospitals-strategy (accessed 06.02.15).

Johnson, A., Baum, F., 2001. Health promoting hospitals: a typology of different organizational approaches to health promotion. Health Promotion International 16, 281–287.

McHugh, C., Robinson, A., Chesters, J., 2010. Health promoting health services: a review of the evidence. Health Promotion International. Available online at: http://heapro.oxfordjournals.org/content/early/2010/02/23/heapro.daq010.full.pdf+html (accessed 07.03.15).

McKee, M., 2000. Settings 3 – health promotion in the health care sector. In: International Union for Health Promotion and Education. The Evidence of Health Promotion Effectiveness. Shaping Public Health in a New Europe. Part Two: Evidence Book. ECSC-EC-EAEC, Brussels.

NHS Confederation, 2014. Key Statistics on the NHS. Available online at: http://www.nhsconfed.org/resources/key-statistics-on-the-nhs.

Nightingale, F., 1859. Notes on Nursing. What It Is and What It Is Not 84. Lippincott, Williams and Wilkins, Philadelphia.

Nutbeam, D., 1998. Health Promotion Glossary. WHO, Geneva. Available online at: http://www.who.int/healthpromotion/about/HPR%20Glossary%201998.pdf?ua=1 (accessed 06.02.15).

Ulrich, R., Simring, C., Joseph, A., Choudhary, R., 2004. The Role of the Physical Environment in the Hospital of the 21st Century: A once in a Lifetime Opportunity. Available online at: https://www.healthdesign.org/chd/research/role-physical-environment-hospital-21st-century (accessed 06.02.15).

Whitehead, D., 2004. The European health promoting hospitals (HPH) project: how far on? Health Promotion International 19, 259–267. Available online at: http://heapro.oxfordjournals.org/content/19/2/259.full.pdf+html (accessed 21.09.15).

World Health Organization, 1997. Vienna Recommendations on Health Promoting Hospitals. WHO, Vienna.

World Health Organization, 2004. Standards for Health Promotion in Hospitals. WHO, Copenhagen.

World Health Organization, 2007. Integrating Health Promotion into Hospitals and Health Services: Concept, Framework and Organization. WHO, Copenhagen. Available online at: http://www.euro.who.int/_data/assets/pdf_file/0009/99801/E90777.pdf.

World Health Organization, 2013. Health Literacy: The Solid Facts. WHO, Copenhagen. Available online at: http://www.euro.who.int/__data/assets/pdf_ file/0009/99801/E90777.pdf (accessed 08.03.15).

Health promoting prisons

Learning Outcomes

By the end of this chapter you will be able to:
* understand the concept of a health promoting prison
* discuss the challenges of implementing a health promotion approach in prisons
* identify the factors that can enhance or inhibit the health of prisoners.

Key Concepts and Definitions

Healthy prison is where the staff, ethos and regime of the prison environment builds up and reinforces the health and well-being of prisoners.

Prisoner A person held in custody while on trial or serving a custodial sentence for criminal offences.

Importance of the Topic

Prisons have been identified as a health promotion setting in a variety of policy documents over the last 25 years. Over 30 European countries are now members of the World Health Organization (WHO) Health in Prisons Project (HIPP) network. Prisons have been identified as a key setting for health promotion for several reasons. Prisoners are one of the most socially excluded groups in society, so addressing their health is a means of addressing health inequalities. However, there are also challenges to promoting health within prisons, and there are many features of prison life that would seem to militate against a healthy lifestyle. There is a range of possible interventions, and a growing body of evidence for their effectiveness. As with all settings, the evidence suggests an integrated whole-systems approach works best within the prison setting to promote the health of prisoners, staff and the wider community.

Why prisons have been identified as a setting for health promotion

While it may seem that health promotion runs counter to the setting of a prison, which curtails freedom and choice, there are several reasons why prisons have been identified as a suitable setting for health promotion:

- prisoners are a socially excluded group with demonstrable health inequalities
- the prison population is a 'captive audience'
- prisoners typically comprise the 'harder-to-reach' segments of the population
- prisoners often service multiple and short-term sentences, so improving their health will also impact on their families and communities.

 Case Study 17.1 Prisoners as a socially excluded group

The following statistics clearly demonstrate that many prisoners have experienced a lifetime of social exclusion:

- prisoners are 13 times more likely than the general population to have been in care as a child and to be unemployed
- 20% to 30% of all offenders have learning disabilities or difficulties that interfere with their ability to cope
- one-third of prisoners were not in permanent accommodation prior to their imprisonment
- 49% of female and 23% of male prisoners suffer from anxiety and depression
- half of women prisoners have suffered domestic violence and one-third have suffered sexual abuse
- half of male prisoners have no qualifications
- nearly half of all prisoners' reading age is at or below the level expected of an 11-year-old
- prisoners are more likely than the general population to engage in high-risk behaviours such as smoking, hazardous drinking and unprotected sex.

Prison Reform Trust (2013) and Condon et al. (2006).

The rate of ill health in the prison population is higher than in the wider community. Mental health problems and drug and alcohol issues are commonplace. Imprisonment tends to exacerbate social exclusion and mental ill health, and increase the risk of behaviours such as shared use of needles for drug injections. Overcrowding is an ongoing problem within prisons. The Howard League estimate suggests that in the UK 12,000 prisoners (out of a total prisoner population of around 75,000) are being held two to a cell in cells designed for one (www.howardleague.org). Overcrowding leads to unsafe and degrading conditions, increases the risk of transmission of infectious diseases, and impedes prisoners' access to purposeful training opportunities, exercise and fresh air. From a health inequalities perspective, prisoners are thus a key target group.

 Learning Activity 17.1 Health promoting prisons: an oxymoron?

Is there a contradiction between using prisons as a penal system to remove people's liberty and using prisons as a health promoting setting?

Barriers to prisons as health promoting settings

Prisons are by their nature closed communities. For some this may mean the use of prisons as a health promoting setting is a contradiction in terms, as key principles of health promotion such as free choice and empowerment are severely restricted (De Viggiani, 2006a). The prison regime allows prisoners little opportunity to make decisions, exert their autonomy or become empowered. The monotony and boredom of prison life may predispose some prisoners towards risk-taking behaviour (such as smoking or drug use). Prison culture is known for its bullying, victimization and violence – all factors that contradict health promotion principles. As Woodall et al. (2014, p. 480) put it: 'The paradox is that prisons are by their nature disempowering yet are tasked with creating more empowered individuals capable of taking control of their lives on release'.

Other commentators, however, see the nature of the prison setting as offering potential to promote health, as it guarantees access to prisoners and a long-term stable environment where any changes will impact directly on inmates (Ramaswamy and Freudenberg, 2007). Prisoners have very high rates of physical and mental ill health and risky behaviours. For example, smoking rates among prisoners (estimated at over 80%) are much higher than for the general population (RCP, 2013). The UK is moving towards smoke-free prisons, which have been implemented in most US prisons and in Canada and New Zealand (ASH, 2014). Targeting prisoners also potentially enables health promotion programmes to reach out beyond the prison to prisoners' families and deprived communities. There are an estimated 1 million relatives affected by imprisonment each year (Williams, 2006). The imprisonment of a family member often leads to emotional, psychological and financial stress for the rest of the family. The availability of support in prison may prompt offenders to seek help when they are released.

Finally, targeting the prison as a setting enables interventions to reach prison staff as well. Prison staff are an important, if neglected, target group in their own right. The positive health and well-being of staff can also be expected to impact favourably on the prisoners in their charge.

Health promoting prisons

A focus on the health of prisoners and the prison setting is a relatively new phenomenon. The first-ever seminar on prison health, organized by the Council of Europe and the Ministry of Justice in Finland, was held in 1991. A European initiative, HIPP, was launched by the WHO in 1995. This early programme identified three key priority areas: communicable diseases, mental health and drugs. HIPP also stated some of its underlying principles, for example 'All prisoners have the right to health care, including preventive measures, without discrimination and equivalent to what is available in the community' (World Health Organization/UNAIDS, 1998).

Case Study 17.2 Health in Prisons Project strategies

- To integrate public health and prison health systems in order to reduce health inequalities and promote overall public health.
- To encourage prisons to operate their services within recognized international and national codes of human rights and medical ethics.
- To use prison health services to contribute towards prisoners' rehabilitation and resettlement, especially with regard to drug addiction and mental health problems, and thereby reduce reoffending.
- To reduce prisoners' exposure to communicable diseases.
- To ensure that the standard of all prison health services, including health promotion services, is equivalent to those in the wider community.

WHO (2004).

The HIPP (WHO, 1998) is an international strategy that has been endorsed in England and Wales (DH, 2002). The WHO strategy has three priorities: health promoting policies, environments supportive of health and access to preventive healthcare. Prison health was identified in the UK as a key public health target in the public health white paper in 2004 (DH, 2004), although it was conceptualized rather narrowly as access to health services. In the UK the health of prisoners remains a responsibility of the National Health Service (NHS) after the transfer of public health functions to local government.

The challenge is to use the prison setting to tackle long-term inequalities in health, and to go 'upstream' to address the social and systemic determinants of health (De Viggiani, 2006b). While integrating the prison health system within the NHS might ensure comparability of service provision, it does not facilitate this movement upstream towards the determinants of health. The wider determinants of health – for example low educational attainment, poor literacy and little work experience – need to be tackled by a whole-prison approach. It has been argued that a relatively narrow medical perspective still prevails in prisons, with an emphasis on disease control, screening and testing (Woodall and South, 2012).

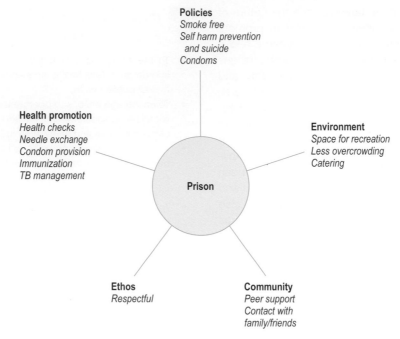

Policies
Smoke free
Self harm prevention
and suicide
Condoms

Health promotion
Health checks
Needle exchange
Condom provision
Immunization
TB management

Environment
Space for recreation
Less overcrowding
Catering

Prison

Ethos
Respectful

Community
Peer support
Contact with
family/friends

Fig. 17.1 ● A health promoting prison

Learning Activity 17.2 Decency and health promotion

The concept of decency has been identified as an important foundation for promoting health. What do you understand by this concept?

The settings approach is based on an ecological model of health that sees health as created in the interaction of personal, organizational and environmental factors (Dooris, 2009). A health promoting prison, just like a health promoting school, will therefore focus on all aspects of life, from individual health needs to the social community it represents for prisoners and as a workplace for staff, as shown in Figure 17.1.

Examples of effective interventions

The novelty of the prison as a health promoting setting means that the evidence base for effective interventions is rather scarce. However, in common with the settings approach as applied to other settings, theory suggests that a whole-systems approach, involving the prison's social and physical environment as well as individual behaviours, is likely to prove most effective. Developing a whole-prison approach involves three components:

- policies that promote health, for example no smoking, prevention of communicable diseases
- an environment that is supportive of health, for example the opportunity to undertake meaningful work
- prevention and health education programmes, for example avoiding sexually transmitted infections, anger management, immunization against TB and hepatitis B.

What evidence there is suggests prisons can be an effective setting for health promotion. For example, a review of evidence of the effectiveness of needle-exchange programmes in prisons concluded that they were effective in reducing reported needle sharing and did not undermine institutional safety or security (Lines et al., 2005). These programmes remain controversial, and the first trial of such a scheme only started in Australia in 2012. There is also evidence that substitution therapy is beneficial, and that together these measures can reduce the spread of HIV and help support the health of drug-addicted prisoners (Gatherer et al., 2005). Smoking-cessation services targeted at prisoners have achieved quit rates equal to, or better than, rates for other groups in the community, with average quit rates of 41% in prisons in north-west England (MacAstrill and Hayton, 2007). Other projects provide a variety of opportunities for offenders to participate in gardening and cooking activities that increase physical activity and improve mental well-being (www.groundwork.org.uk).

A coordinated approach is necessary to address the multiple determinants – individual, social and environmental – that affect prisoners' health. This in turn requires an infrastructure, including supportive policies, senior support and leadership, coordination of efforts and engaging with both staff and prisoners.

Conclusion

The prison setting poses many challenges for health promotion, yet it also presents an opportunity to tackle health inequalities and address a socially marginalized and excluded group in conditions of relative security and predictability. Over the last 25 years the prison has been identified as a health promoting setting by the WHO, the European Community and the UK government in a number of policy and strategic documents. Various projects tackling health behaviours have been launched, but evaluation suggests the most effective programmes are those that address the whole prison system, including the prison culture and its physical and social environment. Funding prison health promotion programmes is likely to be a sound economic investment, as it will help prevent reoffending as well as improving health.

Summary

This chapter has examined the reasons why the prison has been identified as a health promoting setting and outlined some of the most important policies and strategies. The barriers to promoting health in prisons have been identified and discussed. Some examples of successful projects have been given to illustrate the potential for the prison as a healthy setting.

Questions for further discussion

'Health promotion in prisons is a contradiction in terms'. Construct an argument either for or against this proposition.

Further reading and resources

World Health Organization, 2014. Prisons and Health Copenhagen, WHO. Available online at: http://www.euro.who.int/_ data/assets/pdf_file/0005/249188/Prisons-and-Health.pdf?ua=1 (accessed 08.03.15).

De Viggiani, N., 2006. A new approach to prison public health? Challenging and advancing the agenda for prison health. Critical Public Health 16 (4), 307–316. *A persuasive proposal to advance prison health through moving 'upstream' to address the determinants of health.*

Woodall, J., South, J., 2012. Health promoting prisons: dilemmas and challenges. In: Scriven, A., Hodgins, M. (Eds.), Health Promotion Settings: Principles and Practice London. Sage, pp. 170–185. *A useful summary of some of the challenges faced by health promotion in the prison setting.*

Feedback to learning activities

17.1 The key elements of a health promoting setting are choice and empowerment. Many would argue that health promotion is impossible in a setting which curtails freedom and choice (De Viggiani, 2006a).

17.2 It has been argued that decency underpins all aspects of prison life (Wheatley, 2001). Decency includes clean facilities, attending promptly to prisoners' concerns, protecting prisoners from harm and fair and consistent treatment by staff.

References

Action on Smoking and Health, 2014. Smokefree Prisons. Fact sheet Available online at: www.ash.org.uk/files/documents/ASH_740.pdf.

Condon, L., Hek, G., Harris, F., 2006. Public health, health promotion and the health of people in prison. Community Practitioner 79 (1), 19–22.

Department of Health, 2002. Health promoting prisons: a shared approach. Department of Health, London. Available online at: http://webarchive.nationalarchives.gov.uk/20130107105354/http://www.dh.gov.uk/prod_consum_dh/groups/dh_digitalassets/@dh/@en/documents/digitalasset/dh_4034265.pdf (accessed 21.09.15).

Department of Health, 2004. Choosing Health: Making Healthier Choices Easier. Cm 6374. Stationery Office, London. Available online at: http://webarchive.nationalarchives.gov.uk/+/dh.gov.uk/en/publicationsandstatistics/publications/publicationspolicyandguidance/dh_4094550 (accessed 21.09.15).

De Viggiani, N., 2006a. Surviving prison: exploring prison social life as a determinant of health. International Journal of Prisoner Health 2 (2), 71–89.

De Viggiani, N., 2006b. A new approach to prison public health? Challenging and advancing the agenda for prison health. Critical Public Health 16 (4), 307–316.

Dooris, M., 2009. Holistic and sustainable health improvement: the contribution of the settings approach to health promotion. Perspectives in Public Health 129, 29–36.

Gatherer, A., Moller, L., Hayton, P., 2005. The World Health Organisation European Health in Prisons Project after 10 years: persistent barriers and achievements. American Journal of Public Health 95 (10), 1696–1700.

Lines, R., Jurgens, R., Betteridge, G., Stover, H., 2005. Taking action to reduce injecting drug-related harms in prisons: the evidence of effectiveness of prison needle exchange in six countries. International Journal of Prisoner Health 1 (1), 49–64.

MacAstrill, S., Hayton, P., 2007. Stop Smoking Support in HM Prisons: The Impact of Nicotine Replacement Therapy. University of Stirling.

Prison Reform Trust, 2013. Prison Fact File. Available online at: www.prisonreformtrust.org.uk/Publications/Factfile.

Ramaswamy, M., Freudenberg, N., 2007. Health promotion in jails and prisons: an alternative paradigm for correctional health services. In: Greifinger, R.B., Bick, J., Goldenson, J. (Eds.), Public Health behind Bars. From Prisons to Communities. Springer, New York, pp. 229–248.

Royal College of Physicians and Royal College of Psychiatrists, 2013. Smoking and Mental Health. RCP, London. Available online at: https://www.rcplondon.ac.uk/sites/default/files/smoking_and_mental_health_-_full_report_web.pdf (accessed 21.09.15).

Williams, M., 2006. Improving the Health and Social Outcomes of People Recently Released from Prisons in the UK. The Sainsbury Centre for Mental Health, London.

Wheatley, P., 2001. Prison Service Conference Speech. HM Prison Service Internal Communications Unit.

Woodall, J., South, J., 2012. Health promoting prisons: dilemmas and challenges. In: Scriven, A., Hodgins, M. (Eds.), Health Promotion Settings: Principles and Practice. Sage, London.

Woodall, J., Dixey, R., South, J., 2014. Control and choice in English prisons: developing health promoting prisons. Health Promotion International 29 (3), 474–482. Available online at: http://heapro.oxfordjournals.org/content/29/3/474.full.pdf+html (accessed 21.09.15).

World Health Organization, 1998. Promoting Health in Prisons – a Good Practice Guide. WHO, Geneva.

World Health Organization Regional Office for Europe, 2004. Strategic Objectives for the WHO Health in Prisons Project: 2004-2010. WHO, Copenhagen.

World Health Organization/UNAIDS, 1998. HIV/AIDS, Sexually Transmitted Diseases and Tuberculosis in Prisons; Joint Consensus Statement. WHO, Geneva.

Part Four

Implementing health promotion

The final part of this book is concerned with the practical task of how to implement health promotion. Good practice depends on the coexistence of many factors: adherence to core health promoting principles, personal skills and training, and the use of suitable models and frameworks to guide action. Health promotion programmes and activities should be guided by the following principles.

- Empowering, to enable individuals and communities to take control over the factors affecting their health.
- Participatory, involving all concerned in all stages of the process of development and evaluation.
- Equitable, and guided by a concern for social justice.
- Intersectoral, involving the collaboration of many sectors and agencies.
- Sustainable, such that any change can be continued once initial funding has ended.
- Multistrategy, combining policy development, legislation and regulation, organizational change, community development, advocacy,

communication and education (Rootman et al., 2001).

Good practice also depends on a systematic and structured approach to interventions, which is the focus of this part of the book. There are several stages in programme planning.

1. **Defining the problem to be addressed.** What is the problem? What are its causes and the contributory factors? What are people's needs and what is the nature of the context and communities in which people live?
2. **Solution generation.** How might the problem be solved or addressed? What is known about what works? What do practitioners believe might work? What resources are available?
3. **Intervention testing.** Did the intervention work? How do we know?
4. **Intervention dissemination.** Can the intervention or programme be repeated or should it be refined? Is it feasible to implement given the resources available? Can it be sustained?

Nutbeam (1998) shows the stages of planning in six steps with associated questions in Figure 1.

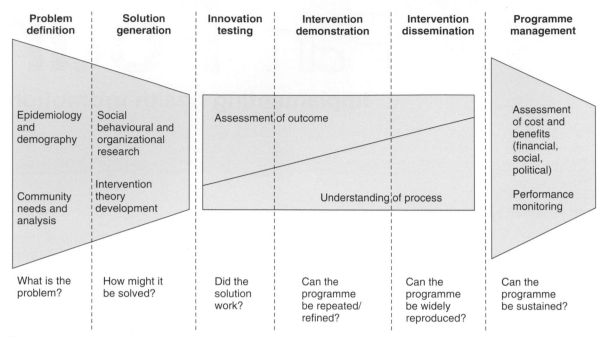

Fig 1. ● The stages of programme planning and evaluation. (Nutbeam, D., 1998. Evaluating health promotion progress, problems and Solutions. Health Promotion International 13 (1), 27–44. Available online at: http://heapro.oxfordjournals.org/content/13/1/27.full.pdf+html [accessed 09.03.15].)

As seen in the figure, there are three major stages in carrying out interventions: needs assessment, planning and evaluation. In Part Four we consider each of these stages in turn, devoting a chapter to each. Chapter 18 explores how needs – whether identified by communities, practitioners or researchers – underpin the actions we take. The process of assessing needs includes soliciting subjective perceptions from clients as well as accessing objective factual indicators such as mortality, morbidity or service-use statistics. Needs assessment methods should be health promoting in themselves, including a variety of participatory methods to support empowerment and capacity building, and a focus on equity of inputs and outputs. Resource and organizational constraints tend to prioritize disease-reduction targets, but understanding the determinants of health will help orient health promotion activities towards 'upstream' interventions.

A systematic approach to planning will help the health promoter to analyse clearly the problem or area of need, set appropriate aims and objectives, and identify an appropriate plan of action. Chapter 19 discusses the factors that need to be taken into account when planning a health promotion intervention at any level (individual intervention, project or strategy). Planning is an important tool for the practitioner, enabling a structured and rational approach to one's workload. It enables transparency and accountability, allowing all stakeholders to assess the proposed plan and monitor its progress. Planning also contributes towards reflective practice, enabling practitioners to develop their expertise and build their capacity to promote health.

Evaluation has long been recognized as fundamental to good practice, but is often neglected. From the point of view of practitioners, reviewing progress and making changes to ensure a project or intervention proceeds as envisaged is all part of sound planning and professional practice. For other stakeholders, evaluation is a means to have their voices heard and their values and priorities recognized. Evaluation helps to build an evidence base, identifying interventions that are not only effective and cost-effective but also acceptable and sustainable. Such evidence should inform decision-making, but is often missing in the field of health promotion. Evaluation is therefore a vital stage in developing professional health promotion practice. Chapter 20 discusses the importance of identifying appropriate outcomes and indicators of success, and how practitioners may evaluate their health promotion activities.

Together these three chapters provide a reflective and critical account of the practice of health promotion, combining 'how-to' information with a critique of underlying assumptions and values. The intention is to help practitioners develop effective and reflective practice that operationalizes core health promotion principles, produces the desired results and helps build a solid evidence base for health promotion.

References

Nutbeam, D., 1998. Evaluating health promotion progress, problems and Solutions. Health Promotion International 13(1), 27–44. Available online at: http://heapro.oxfordjournals.org/content/13/1/27.full.pdf+html (accessed 09.03.15).

Rootman, I., Goodstadt, M., Hyndman, B., et al., 2001. Evaluation in Health Promotion. Principles and Perspectives. Copenhagen, WHO Europe. Available online at: http://files.eric.ed.gov/fulltext/ED460081.pdf (accessed 22.09.15).

Chapter Eighteen

18

Assessing health needs

Learning Outcomes

By the end of this chapter you will be able to:
- understand the concept of need
- evaluate critically different approaches to identifying needs
- discuss the ways in which policy and practice respond to, and develop, programmes that reflect needs.

Key Concepts and Definitions

Need is something which is required or essential rather than merely desired or wanted.

Needs assessment A systematic process to identify needs or the gap between existing and desired conditions.

Want A lack or deficiency of something.

Supply Provide or make available something which is wanted or essential.

Community profile A representation (written or graphical) of information regarding the characteristics of a place or community.

Quality-adjusted life year (QALY) The quality-adjusted life year combines both the quality and the quantity of life lived and is used as a measure of the impact of disease, and in assessing the value of medical interventions.

Importance of the Topic

The first phase in health promotion planning is an assessment of what a client, community or population group needs to enable them to become healthier. Healthcare usually takes the individual as its starting point. Public health concerns the health and welfare of groups of people. Practitioners do not assess individuals in isolation from the communities in which they live. As we have seen in previous chapters, the health experiences of individuals are affected by where they reside. The knowledge of practitioners about the range of local services, facilities and networks is an important part of needs assessment. Within a neighbourhood there will be people in settings such as schools and workplaces, and population groups with specific health needs. Practitioners need to know how to assess individuals, how to manage their care and how to encourage healthier lifestyles. They also require an understanding of people's ways of life and the health problems and opportunities they experience, and they need to know how to use this understanding to assess the needs of people in groups systematically.

The term 'needs assessment' describes the process of gathering information. It has been defined as a 'systematic method of reviewing the health needs and issues facing a given population leading to agreed priorities and resource allocation that will improve health and reduce inequalities' (Cavanagh and Chadwick, 2005, p. 3). The purpose of health needs assessment at national, regional or local level is twofold.

1. To identify which actions to improve health should have greatest priority.
2. To choose which particular groups or communities should have priority, and so help in targeting interventions and commissioning services.

National Health Service (NHS) and local government reforms have emphasized the participation of local people in setting priorities, signalling a philosophical shift from a paternalistic medical model to a participatory consumer-led model. Recognition of the right to participate in defining health needs and healthcare was also acknowledged in the 1978 World Health Organization Alma Ata Declaration, and one of the underlying principles of Health For All is community participation (World Health Organization, 1985).

This chapter considers the ways in which local health needs are assessed and applied in planning for health promotion. It should be read in conjunction with Chapter 3, which outlines the principal sources of information about health status.

Defining health needs

The concept of need is widely used but often not well understood. People may believe they 'need' a new coat because someone observed that their old one is worn out, or because it looks old compared to other people's coats, or simply because they would like one. A need may thus be something people want or something that is lacking in comparison to others.

Learning Activity 18.1 Defining health needs

How would you define need?

Economists tend to avoid the use of the term 'needs' altogether, arguing that it is overlaid with emotion, and what is really meant by a health need is actually a matter of people's wants and demands, and these are limitless (Cohen, 2015). Identifying health needs therefore becomes a question of identifying priorities.

An alternative view is that there are universal needs. Maslow's (1954) hierarchy of needs suggests that all human needs, whether they are related to safety or self-esteem, are in fact health needs (Figure 18.1).

Learning Activity 18.2 Human needs

- Make a list of 10 important human needs.
- Are some more fundamental than others?
- Are these needs relative to a particular country, or are they universal?

For a person to be self-actualizing, physical, social and emotional needs must be met. Doyal and Gough (1992) similarly argued that the ultimate goal of human beings is to participate fully in society, and to do this the basic needs for physical health and autonomy must be met. These needs are not relative to a particular country or period of time, but are fundamental rights and include the prerequisites for health – peace, shelter, education, food, income, a stable ecosystem, sustainable resources, social justice and equity (World Health Organization, 1986) – and social security, social relations, the employment of women, respect for human rights and the alleviation of poverty (World Health Organization 1997). The United Nations Declaration of the Rights of the Child (1959, Article 6) declares that 'the child, for the full and harmonious development of his personality, needs love and understanding'. But these needs are not undisputed. How healthy do people have to be before we can say that their needs have been met?

Bradshaw (1972), in a widely used taxonomy, distinguished four types of health and social need.

1. Normative needs, as defined by experts or professional groups, e.g. a patient needs an operation.
2. Felt needs, as defined by clients, patients, relatives or service users, e.g. a person feels he or she needs pain relief.

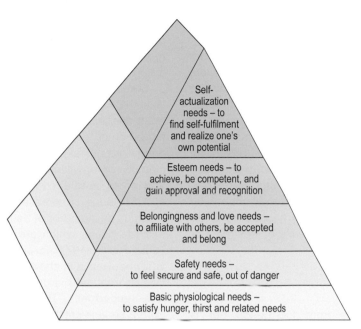

Fig. 18.1 ● Maslow's hierarchy of needs

3. Expressed needs, when felt needs become a demand, e.g. a person who expects and seeks a service.
4. Comparative needs, identified when people, groups or areas fall short of an established standard, e.g. a service should be provided as it is available elsewhere.

Normative needs

Normative needs are objective needs as defined by professionals, who also identify the ways in which these needs can be met. A normative need reflects a professional judgement that a person or persons deviate from a required standard. This may be against some external criteria such as occupational or legal requirements – thus the manager of a restaurant is in need of training because she has not completed a course in food hygiene. Or it may be that a person deviates from what is defined by medical staff as the range of 'clinically normal' physiological indicators.

Normative needs are not absolute or objective 'facts' – they reflect the judgement of professionals, which may be different from that of their clients. Healthcare workers will judge a need relative to what they are able to provide. The ability to judge normative needs also contributes to the notion of professionalism and the authority and status of professionals.

 Case Study 18.1 Normative needs and child development

Growth charts are based on data collected in different populations and time periods. The WHO growth charts published in 2006 (www.rcpch.ac.uk/research/uk-WHO-Growth-Charts) are meant to act as a normative standard, as they are based on children who fulfil specific criteria – being breastfed, born at gestational age and weight, living in adequate socio-economic conditions and born to non-smoking mothers. The data on growth were gathered from infants in the USA, Norway, Oman, Brazil, India and Ghana, and there was a similar linear growth pattern for all the infants. However, a professional may plot a child's growth differently, e.g. by not taking account of gestational prematurity or not assessing neonatal weight loss.

Felt needs

Felt needs are what people really *want*. They are needs identified by clients themselves and may relate to services, information or support, which can be termed service needs. Moves towards bottom-up approaches in health and social care have meant a greater acceptance of service users' views. Chapter 6 in our companion volume (Naidoo and Wills, 2010) discusses some of the policy drivers for patient and public involvement. Needs may be limited by the perceptions of an individual. Individuals may not believe themselves to be in need simply because they do not know what is available in terms of treatment or services.

Expressed need

Expressed need arises from felt needs but is expressed in words or action – it has become a *demand*. Thus clients or groups are expressing a need when they ask for help or information, or when they make use of a service. Expressed need is often used to measure the adequacy of service provision, even though it is not a comprehensive or complete measure. There are also objective needs which exist

but are not expressed. Only a proportion of patients make contact with health services and they are merely the tip of an iceberg of potential need, as illustrated in Figure 18.2.

Sometimes people will use a service because it is all that is available, even if it does not adequately meet needs. The best example of expressed need (and unmet demand) is the waiting list. Some needs are not expressed, perhaps because of an inability or unwillingness to articulate the need. This could be due to language difficulties or a lack of knowledge. Expressed needs should not be taken as an indicator of demand because they also exclude needs which are felt but not expressed. Tudor Hart's (1971) inverse-care law has been of vital importance in showing that just because a service or treatment is used less does not mean that it is needed less. Those who could most benefit from a service are often those least likely to use it. People may express different needs, and there is a tendency to listen to those with loud and powerful voices, such as views which come from an established group or which appear to express a popular need. Responding to expressed needs may also therefore have the effect of increasing inequalities in service provision.

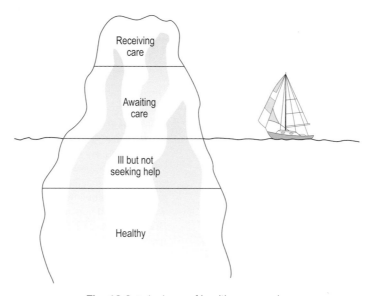

Fig. 18.2 ● Iceberg of healthcare needs.

Comparative needs

Individuals or groups are said to be in need if their situation, when compared with that of a similar group or individual, is found wanting or lacking with regard to services or resources. For example, if a person with dementia in area A is living in sheltered accommodation and receiving day care, but in area B this was not available, we would say that people with dementia in area B were in need. In the NHS, although people may be assessed to be in absolute need (normatively), in practice comparative needs assessment will often dictate whether their needs will be met. Areas may be compared on the basis of provision of services or length of waiting lists to see if the health needs of their populations are being met. In a sense, then, comparative need is about equity, or equal provision for equal need. As stated by Nutbeam (1998, p. 7): 'Equity is about fairness. Equity in health means that people's needs guide the distribution of opportunities for wellbeing.' This kind of analysis of need does, of course, also assume that those in receipt of a service are receiving adequate provision and that their needs are being met. Yet health services are provided in a market environment and are more likely to be led by demand rather than need.

The NHS uses the term 'health gain' in association with health needs to signal that the meeting of needs is related to a person's ability to benefit. Health gain is defined as:

- adding years to life by reducing premature mortality
- adding life to years by enhancing the quality of life and improving well-being.

The concept of health gain is rooted in a medical model which defines health quite narrowly as the absence of disease. Consequently, health needs tend to be defined as problems which may be successfully met by services or treatment, and the gain is measured by concepts such as quality adjusted life years (QALYs) or disability adjusted life years (DALYs) (these are discussed in Chapter 3). Because need is seen as infinite and resources as limited, health authorities confine themselves to what is known to be effective care. Yet community surveys often show that the public define ill health far more broadly than simply problems requiring treatment by health services. Many priorities for health go beyond the narrow outcomes encompassed by adding 'years to life' and require health authorities to take account of the structural influences on health, such as housing, community safety and transport links. The meeting of needs is also related to what can be offered (what the state can supply). Health economists thus distinguish need from supply. As we have seen, need is influenced by contemporary culture; demand is influenced by the abilities of a person or group to express needs and by the media; supply may be influenced by political pressure. These differing interpretations are illustrated in Figure 18.3.

Bradshaw's (1994) work is useful in showing that different groups in society, whether the public, professionals or commissioning or providing organizations, all hold different definitions of need. We can see that needs are not objective and observable entities to which we must just match our interventions. The concept of need is a relative one, and is influenced both by values and attitudes and by other agendas.

 Learning Activity 18.3 Needs and health service interventions

Consider these interventions available to women in childbirth. Has medicine created these needs or are they needed improvements in technology?
- Prostaglandin to induce labour.
- Epidural to reduce pain.
- Electronic fetal monitoring.
- Belt monitoring of contractions.
- Elective caesarean section.

What is clear from this discussion is that definitions of need vary depending on whose interpretation and values are used. People's health needs are not the same as those of 20 years ago – the nature and prevalence of diseases may change, as do the expectations of the population and the capacity of health services to meet them.

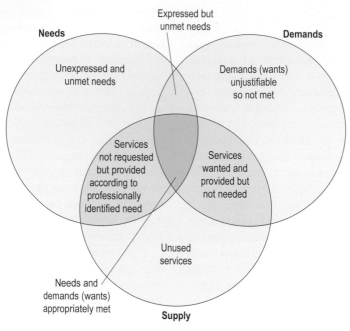

Fig. 18.3 ● Needs, wants, supply and demand.

The purpose of assessing health needs

The process of assessing needs is nothing new. As we shall see in Chapter 19, understanding needs is integral to a basic process approach to planning. Needs assessment including the collection of data is the first step, from which subsequent aims will be derived. Assessing the health and social needs of local populations is a means of obtaining accurate and appropriate information on which to base priorities, and ensures that decisions are based on solid information and evidence. This overall purpose can be broken down into different elements, as follows.

Help in directing interventions appropriately

Within clinical practice assessing needs is routine and accepted. Assessment takes place to determine what care is required through the gathering of data about:

- the individual, e.g. age

- health history, e.g. medical, surgical, activities of daily living
- current health, e.g. self-reported symptoms
- current health measurement, e.g. blood pressure, pain assessment, oxygen saturation.

An integrated care pathway gives a single record of assessment for all the many professionals and agencies who may be involved with a patient, and also provides a map of care for all patients with a similar set of symptoms or diagnosis. It is intended to reduce variations in interpretations of need and treatment offered. The 'common assessment framework' is an assessment tool shared across all children's services and areas in England. Its aim is to identify a child's additional needs which may not be met by the services he or she is receiving.

For those practitioners who work with individual clients, there is increasing recognition of the importance of client participation in the assessment of needs. Nursing practice, for example, has frequently been criticized for being too inflexible and routine – doing things *to* people rather than *with* them. Prescription has now given way to negotiation, alongside the move from sick nursing to health nursing. Understanding the thoughts, feelings and experiences of individuals has become an important part of the therapeutic and nursing process.

Learning Activity 18.4 Expressed needs

For what reasons might clients find it difficult to express their needs in a clinical situation?

The needs of patients may not accord with the needs identified by professionals, who may be confined by what they feel they can provide. There are many examples where needs are expressed very differently. For example, the main goal of sanitation programmes in low-income countries is to improve health and reduce diarrhoeal diseases, but according to the summary of the evidence by Mara et al. (2010), householders rarely adopt and use toilets for health-related reasons. Instead, needs in relation to sanitation include the desire for privacy and convenience, to avoid embarrassment, wanting to be modern, to avoid the discomforts or dangers of the bush (e.g., snakes, pests, rain and risk of rape or attack for women) and wanting social acceptance or status.

Learning Activity 18.5 Meeting patient needs

A male patient who is young and fit has a heart attack. The nurse on the ward offers the patient advice on cardiac rehabilitation and information on healthy eating, exercise and safe drinking.
- Is the nurse meeting the patient's needs?
- Is health education information an appropriate intervention?

Identifying population needs and reducing inequalities

To meet community health needs it is essential to have a clear understanding of what the needs are, what capacity communities have for addressing these needs and whether particular groups face specific challenges in meeting their needs. A health equity audit is a requirement of planning in which local strategic partnerships and other organizations systematically review the role of inequities in the causes of ill health and the access to services for defined population groups (NICE, 2003). Health equity audits show whether different groups of people (categorized by socio-economic status, geographical area, age, sex, disability or minority ethnic group) are having their needs met in an equal manner and whether the most appropriate services are being provided. The process entails systematically reviewing inequities in the causes of ill health, and access to effective services and their outcomes, for a defined population (see for example a health equity audit of the NHS health check programme in the London Borough of Lewisham www.healthcheck.nhs.uk/document.php?o=4430 [accessed 22.09.15]).

Case Study 18.2 Health profiles

Local Health (www.localhealth.org.uk) is produced by Public Health England. It provides health information at small-area and local authority levels. It includes:
- the total resident population and the numbers of people in different age groups
- the percentage of the population who cannot speak English well or at all
- the percentage of the population living in income-deprived households
- the crude rate of births per 1,000 females of child-bearing age
- the percentage of children aged 0 to 15 living in income-deprived households.

Identifying and responding to the specific needs of minority groups and socially excluded groups

There are recognizable social, demographic or identity-based groups who have traditionally avoided, or been excluded from, service needs assessments.

Such harder-to-reach groups may think that services do not care about them, do not listen or are irrelevant. For example, studies of the health of gypsies and travellers have shown that:

> *There are widespread communication difficulties between health workers and gypsy travellers, with defensive expectation of racism and prejudice. Barriers to health care access were experienced with several contributory causes, including reluctance of GPs to register travellers or visit sites.*

Parry et al. (2004), p. 8

While early intervention in relation to maternal and child health might be acknowledged as important, there remain some gypsy and traveller families who have complex and ongoing needs that are not addressed. Many parents face barriers to support, including:

* a lack of services
* poor signposting
* fear of stigmatization
* low level of literacy.

 Research Example 18.1 Health literacy

One in 33 people today is a migrant. The WHO estimates that 8 per cent of the European population are migrants (World Health Organization, 2013). Migrants have poorer access to services and make less use of information and health promotion services than the general population. Strategies that are known to be effective in enhancing health literacy are:

* engaging migrant users and communities in planning
* patient navigators
* translated signage or pictograms
* use of plain language
* use of images, photographs and graphics in materials
* training for health providers.
* Health mediators as used in one project to improve the health of Roma children (www.changemakers.com/intrapreneurs/entries/improving-health-roma-childrentogether-better-health-us[accessed 09.03.15]).

Targeting risk groups

Needs assessment may help to identify populations who are underserved, and also groups at particular risk. The concept of risk groups has emerged as a means of directing health promotion activities to people who are most in need. A risk group may be defined as a population group vulnerable to certain diseases or conditions. A risk group's vulnerability may be due to genetic, lifestyle, economic, social or environmental characteristics. Normative needs derived from epidemiological research, which identifies groups with poorer than average health, are often used to establish target groups. For example, lower socio-economic groups at most risk from ill health and premature death are a commonly identified risk group. Comparative need is used to identify at-risk groups who have low take-up rates of services.

However, a focus on high-risk groups can lead to 'victim blaming'. Health problems are seen as specific to particular groups, who may also be seen as responsible through their behaviour for their own ill health (Naidoo and Wills, 2010). For example, young people are the subject of numerous targeted health promotion campaigns; yet it is not being young that is a risk, but certain activities. Gay men were barred from blood donation in many countries until recently, but similarly, it is not being gay that is a risk but certain activities. Many health promoters also reject the notion of targeting because they prefer to work in partnership with groups and communities on the issues *they* define as important.

Allocating resources

The NHS was predicated on the notion that there was an untreated pool of sickness which, once treated by a national health service, would diminish. Experience shows that there can be unlimited demand for healthcare. As healthcare is provided, so expectations rise; as technology improves, people with disabilities and chronic conditions live longer and demand more healthcare. General improvements in health and living conditions have led to people living longer and an increase in the percentage of older people in the population. It will not be possible to meet all these needs, as resources are limited.

Most healthcare workers accept that some kind of priority setting or rationing of healthcare is inevitable. There have always been waiting lists, but rationing is a more far-reaching concept. It entails decisions about how much money should be put into different forms of care or treatment. Not only does this raise issues about justice and equity, it also poses the huge dilemma about who decides the priorities for investment. Public views may be very different from those of doctors. For example, infertility treatment may have a high value to individuals but not to society as a whole. Osteoporosis screening (bone-density measurement) may be rated highly by the public but not by doctors, who have access to more information and are therefore able to question its effectiveness.

While the 'postcode lottery' of accessing drugs such as herceptin on the NHS is frequently highlighted, there are also considerable variations in local spending. This is only partly explained by the age and needs of the population and the local cost of services. For example, in 2006 Islington PCT in inner-city London was spending four times as much as Bracknell PCT on the outskirts of London on mental health, even after adjustment for needs (Kings Fund, 2006).

In Oregon, USA, a health commission of healthcare workers and the public devised a complex formula to prioritize health services, and decided there were certain services that they would not provide (www.oregonhealthdecisions.org/index.htm#welcome). Despite a free and available service in the UK, health authorities are beginning to consider particular services which will not be provided as part of the NHS. Cosmetic surgery, for example, is not provided free for cosmetic reasons alone, but may be allowed for the correction of congenital abnormalities, injuries and other special criteria determined locally. Many primary care organizations elicit public views on healthcare priorities and changing provision to primary care, day-case surgery and the care of the mentally ill in the community.

 Learning Activity 18.6 Deciding priorities

Consider the following typical costs (not actual amounts) of interventions. What factors would you take into account in deciding priorities?

Home visit by community psychiatric nurse	£50
Tonsillectomy	£250
Hip replacement	£1,000
Place in group home for someone with learning difficulties	£30,000 per year
Pregnancy termination	£200
Brief intervention of psychotherapy (10 weeks)	£1,500
Day care for an older person with mental ill health	£200 per week

Health needs assessment

Needs assessment can be carried out from the perspectives of professionals, the lay public or key informants (members of the community with a particular viewpoint, such as teachers or police officers). It can be carried out at different levels, from that of the individual to specific groups (e.g. population groups, such as older people or people with specific health problems), local geographic communities or national populations. It can inform general practice profiles, community profiles, intervention planning or service design.

Wright (1998) describes three approaches to health needs assessment.

1. Epidemiological (the focus is on the size and nature of the problem).
2. Corporate (the focus is on the views of stakeholders).
3. Community (uses a variety of methods to enable communities to identify, prioritize and decide what actions to take to meet health needs).

In all cases health needs assessment is a systematic and explicit process identifying issues affecting a population that can be addressed. Health needs assessment is:

- about health not just disease
- about needs not just demands
- an assessment not just a response.

Health needs assessment should be guided by these common questions.

- What information is needed?
- How can I find out this information?
- What am I going to do with the information when I obtain it?
- What scope is there to act on the information?

What information is needed?

The first step in a needs assessment is to define the relevant population group or community, including its demographic and social characteristics; behaviours, values and lifestyles; cultural environment; and historical circumstances. Community nurses are often involved in compiling community profiles to identify the health of a community and what resources are needed to enable it to achieve health and stay healthy. A community profile has been described as:

A comprehensive description of the needs of a population that is defined, or defines itself, as a community, and the resources that exist within a community, carried out with the active involvement of the community itself, for the purpose of developing an action plan or other means of improving the quality of life in the community.

Hawtin and Percy Smith (2007), p. 5.

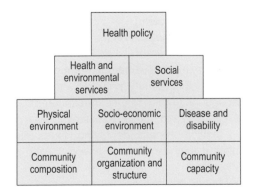

Fig. 18.4 ● Community information profile. (From Annett, H., Rifkin, S., 1990. Improving Urban Health. WHO, Geneva.)

Community profiles do not follow a standard format. Figure 18.4 shows a schematic representation of the main elements:

- the composition of the community, e.g. its age profile, social networks, the way the community is organized and its capacity in relation to skills and organizations
- socio-ecological environment, e.g. extent of economic activity and unemployment, private car ownership, housing, transport links, green areas, air pollution
- availability, effectiveness and impact of health and social service provision
- local strategies for health, e.g. health improvement programmes, regeneration projects.

Health profiles (see Chapter 3), by contrast, are compiled by the NHS and provide snapshots of people's health in an area. They show the difference in health between the specified area and other areas across five domains (communities, children and young people's health, adults' health and lifestyles, diseases and poor health, life expectancy and causes of death).

Gathering information and public participation

Routine information that is already available (e.g. census, NHS and local authority data) will give a picture of the potential needs of a community and what is available to meet those needs. It may give an idea of areas of unmet need and identify groups experiencing inequities of healthcare provision. Information on effective interventions is also available (see Chapter 20). The community's perceptions of its own health needs and expectations of services or interventions are a vital part of planning, as are the views of professionals about the nature of health needs, best practices and existing service delivery.

Since the NHS reforms of the 1990s, engaging with service users and local people is central to the provision of public health services. Planning guidance emphasizes that there will be different needs and priorities within each community. It also highlights that listening to views is as important as using epidemiological or survey data. Our companion volume (Naidoo and Wills, 2010) discusses this shift to patient and public involvement. There are many reasons for this:

- ethical – people have the right to a voice
- pragmatic – where people have identified the solution it is more likely to be appropriate and used
- political – experts and professionals may have vested interests in a particular provision and limited understanding of people's needs.

The aim of gathering information from communities is to understand issues from their perspective. As we saw in Chapter 10, interventions based on such information are more likely to be effective than if they are suggested by outside experts or professionals, whose interpretations of need may be based on general interpretations and impressions of the community.

The gathering of community knowledge can take place in different ways. Chapter 10 discusses this in more detail. There may be a formal exercise of consultation conducted in a top-down way. Frequently the consultation is confined to issues relating to patient satisfaction with services, and particularly the hotel aspects of care. Ong and Humphris (1994, 89) regard this as inadequate:

It is not sufficient to see users as consumers who are satisfied or dissatisfied with services. The place of users is in the joint definition of need, priority setting and evaluation. This approach means a paradigm shift whereby the community perspective will be used as the guiding principle for setting priorities in health care.

The term 'co-production' is used to describe a way of working whereby citizens and policymakers, or people who use services, carers and service providers, work together to create a decision or service which works for them all. Co-production is built on the principle that those who use a service are best placed to help design it. It does not view people as the passive providers of information, but as active participants in the process. Public participation in needs assessment can range from tokenistic consultation where the results may seemingly be ignored, and the timing, location and publicity for public meetings may lead to a poor turnout, to community control – as we saw in the ladder of participation in Chapter 10. Public participation needs to be carefully planned and its initiators need to be motivated to listen and include, and to act on people's views.

Many health and local authorities are using a range of methods to achieve a wider picture of community needs. These approaches represent a move away from traditional epidemiological data gathering towards techniques which reflect the importance of social and environmental factors and the involvement of the community in data collection. These include:

- public meetings and forums
- interviews with users and key informants
- focus groups
- using local media such as radio phone-ins
- community health panels and citizens' juries
- research techniques such as rapid appraisal, ethnographic studies and observation
- participatory appraisal.

Rapid appraisal is a research technique applied to both urban and rural settings. It is geared to identifying the health needs and priorities of a target population quickly and without great expense. It uses secondary data already available, and then researchers interview people with knowledge of the area to identify problems and solutions. Key informants are:

- people who work in the community and have a professional understanding of local issues (e.g. teachers, health visitors, police)
- people who are recognized community leaders and represent a section of the community (e.g. religious leaders, councillors, leaders of self-help groups)
- people who are important in informal networks and play a role in local communication (e.g. shopkeepers, bookmakers, lollipopmen and -women).

 Learning Activity 18.7 Rapid appraisal

List some of the advantages and disadvantages of rapid appraisal as a method of community needs assessment.

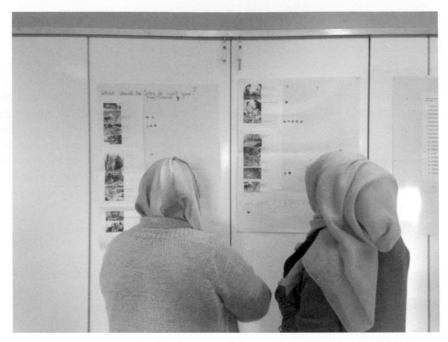

Fig. 18.5 ● Participatory appraisal ranking exercise used in a community event to assess health needs

Participatory appraisal (as shown in Figure 18.5, for example) uses members of the community as data gatherers, valuing their knowledge and experience. A range of methods may be used to capture the ways in which people describe local issues, e.g. mapping, community walks, timelines, photography and life histories. These techniques focus on mapping community assets and resources.

The advantages of participatory appraisal are:
- its underlying ethos of shared ownership of research
- it can build capacity in people undertaking the training to carry it out
- it may describe issues differently from the usual professional viewpoint
- it can focus on assets as well as deficits in the community.

The disadvantages of participatory appraisal are:
- the views of local people may not be as valued as epidemiological data
- it is time-consuming
- it may raise false expectations among the community that identified issues will be acted upon.

Collecting data where there are low levels of literacy demands different techniques. Participatory appraisal methods are highly visual and use a range of activities to elicit and triangulate the same information. Tools used in participatory interviews or group meetings include brainstorming, mapping, ranking, sequencing and diagramming. Mapping exercises, for example, can locate specific community assets or identify areas for community change. Methods of ranking or matrix scoring can indicate priorities for the development of health needs.

Whose needs count?

Moves to participation in either community affairs or healthcare cannot involve everyone, and it is important that participation does not favour those with the most influence and loudest voices.

Service users' and carers' involvement in decision-making is now a statutory requirement, including those who previously might have been excluded, such as children, people with mental ill health issues and people with learning difficulties. There are many guides as to how to involve service users and children effectively, e.g. https://www.nwleics.gov.uk/files/documents/guide_to_involving_children_and_young_people/Guide%20to%20Involving%20Children%20and%20Young%20People.pdf (accessed 11.03.15).

Learning Activity 18.8 Harder to reach

- What reasons can you think of to explain why certain groups are harder to reach?
- Can you think of groups that might be harder to reach?

Setting priorities

The traditional public health approach for setting priority areas includes the following criteria.

1. The issue should be a major cause of premature death or avoidable ill health in the population as a whole or among specific groups of people.
2. There are marked inequalities in those who suffer ill health or premature death.
3. Effective interventions should be possible, offering scope for improvements in health.

In addition, there may be locally determined priorities of specific health issues, such as diabetes, or particular population groups, such as older people.

We have seen in this chapter that people's identified needs may also be taken as the first step in the planning process. However, this subjective interpretation may be tempered by economic priorities. People may express a need for interventions or treatment whose effectiveness is in doubt, e.g. antibiotics for simple colds or ear infections. For health promoters, therefore, a simple needs assessment may not be an adequate basis for setting priorities. A range of other influences may determine what is included in a local health promotion plan:

- national targets of reducing disease
- a national theme, e.g. World AIDS Day
- a major determinant of health in the area, e.g. air pollution or poverty
- pragmatism on the basis of available skills and interests
- cost and staffing
- longer-term strategy

- existing activity
- cost-effectiveness and what is amenable to change and evaluation
- client choice
- professionals' views.

Case Study 18.3 Questions to ask when planning a needs assessment

- What defines the scope of the health need to be addressed? Are you interested in the whole population or a particular subsection, such as older people or women?
- What is the size of the problem? How many people share the health need?
- What are the views of patients, carers and the local community? What is known from previous work? Who do you need to talk to locally?
- How do your figures compare with local and national averages? How important is the problem compared with other issues?
- What interventions are already taking place? Do you have a response to the problem? What are other agencies doing?
- What has worked elsewhere? Is there any relevant literature available or projects which can be visited? Are there examples of best practice in the area in which you are interested?
- What could and should you be doing in future? Consider all options, prioritize and develop an action plan, as described in Chapter 19.

Conclusion

This book has shown that there are several tensions or 'pulls' in health promotion, identified by Beattie and described in Chapter 5. One of these 'pulls' can be illustrated in relation to the type of information used to plan interventions:

- identifying needs through participatory, bottom-up and negotiated approaches versus professionally led top-down approaches
- using types of data that are subjective, individual or community-held views versus objective, primarily epidemiological, data.

The selection of an approach and methods to measure needs will depend on the purpose and context. The process of encouraging participation in public services by identifying and understanding individual and community needs has led to attempts to make such services more flexible. So, for example, we find, as part of the nursing process, clients being encouraged to identify aspects of their situation that they deem harmful to their health. We find health organizations using a variety of methods to ascertain the views, beliefs and health behaviours of their population, in addition to the objective measures yielded by epidemiology. We find voluntary and community groups being required as part of their funding to monitor not only their clients' use of the service but also their health needs.

The public sector, including the NHS, is seeking to integrate public views into the planning process. However, most of the information used to assess needs is gathered from a professional perspective which assumes a direct relationship between certain indicators and needs, and which is embedded in a medical model of health. For example, if health statistics show an above-average incidence of coronary heart disease, local health planners may well assume a need for greater provision of cardiac treatment and rehabilitation services, and a health promotion programme to address risk factors for coronary heart disease. Health promoters have an important role to play in ensuring that needs assessment which feeds health needs into planning takes account of public views and self-defined needs, and uses indicators to measure a social model of positive health. For those with client caseloads, it is a vital task to know the health status of patients/clients and how this may differ from the broader community in order to plan appropriate interventions.

Assessing health needs is important both in terms of promoting health and in determining priorities. For health promoters the process of identifying needs is not, however, the only basis for setting priorities.

Resource constraints will limit what is available and what is deemed amenable to change. Professional views, practice wisdom and existing activity will provide boundaries to what is considered possible.

Question for further discussion

In your practice, how is need identified?

Summary

This chapter has discussed the ways in which need is defined. We have seen that perceptions of need vary according to whether these are client or professional views, and how the assessment is made – clients' expressed views, levels of service use or epidemiological and social data. The chapter concludes that need is relative, and influenced by values and attitudes as well as the historical context. It also considers the role of health promotion in identifying and meeting certain needs.

Further reading and resources

Green, J., Tones, K., Cross, R., Woodall, J., 2015. Health Promotion: Planning and Strategies, third ed. Sage, London. *A useful text illustrating approaches to promoting health. Chapter 5 discusses needs assessment.*

Health Development Agency, 2005. Clarifying Approaches to Health Needs Assessment, Health Impact Assessment, Integrated Impact Assessment, Health Equity Audit and Race Equality Impact Assessment. HDA, London. *Practical guides to assessing health needs to inform decisions and assess impact through auditing provision, access and outcomes still available through Public Health Observatory websites, e.g.* www.nwph.net/nwpho/lists/AuditTools/AllItems.html.

Robinson, J., Elkan, R., 1996. Health Needs Assessment: Theory and Practice. Churchill Livingstone, Edinburgh. *A clear and readable account of general principles and issues in health needs assessment. It looks at epidemiological approaches and locality commissioning.*

Feedback on learning activities

18.1 Need relates to the experience of a problem which requires a response.

There are two different understandings of what constitutes a health need. It can be seen as:

- a subjective, relative concept which is judged by an expert or professional and is influenced by whether the need can be met
- an objective and universal concept which is a fundamental right.

18.2 Important human needs include those shared with all living bodies, e.g. food, water and shelter, and those which are unique to humans, e.g. the need for a social network, social recognition, liberty and freedom of expression. Maslow (1943) proposed a hierarchy of needs, with the most fundamental need being physiological, followed by safety, love and belonging, esteem and self-actualization. Human needs are shared by all people, regardless of their country.

18.3 At first sight these developments may be seen as the consequence of medical advances. However, medical interventions in childbirth can also be seen as an attempt to establish doctors' control over that of midwives. The range of interventions may, on the one hand, alienate women and make childbirth an uncomfortable and distressing experience; on the other hand, the very availability of these services may create a need for them. A very different list of needs may be compiled by pregnant women, including for example:

- the same known midwife to be present through-out labour and birth
- water births
- partner to be present during birth
- home births.

These felt or expressed needs may or may not be acknowledged and met by service providers.

18.4 Increasingly, healthcare workers seek to identify clients' views and perceptions about their health as part of their assessment. What they often find is that their perception differs from that of the client. Clients' need for information is often underestimated, and in healthcare settings this may mean that information is confined to ward or clinic routines. Despite the greater emphasis on being client-centred, practitioners tend to assess needs in relation to the service they provide. Practitioners may interpret client needs as information needs because

it is possible to provide this, whereas the satisfaction of physical needs (as in Maslow's hierarchy) may seem beyond their scope.

18.5 The medical and individualistic approach is adopted because it is a well-understood part of the nurse's professional role. The nurse understands coronary heart disease prevention as focusing on risk factors, even though they may not be relevant to this situation. The patient may have other health needs, such as a concern about getting back to work or when he might be sexually active again. Assessing individual health needs means starting with the patient's own concerns.

18.6 Some of the factors you might take into account are as follows.

- Costs – the relative costs of different services, and the opportunity costs (e.g. if the money is spent on this, what is it not being spent on?).
- Numbers – how many people will benefit from the service, and will it provide the greatest good for the greatest number?
- Effectiveness – what are the likely outcomes of providing care or treatment? Will it promote health, prevent ill health or improve or cure ill health?
- Quality – what areas of health-related quality of life (physical, mental, social, well-being, perception of pain, self-care) will be most affected by the service?

18.7 Rapid appraisal is useful if virtually nothing is known about the needs and priorities of the target population. It can give a deep understanding of the problems and issues in a community and provide a sense of local ownership. But it does not provide the quantitative analysis of the size of the problem which many public health departments require. It may also be difficult to get beyond personal agendas to find out the community's views.

18.8 It is very difficult to get a cross-section of a community, and there are some groups of people who are harder to reach. These include homeless people, unemployed people, refugees, migrants and people from Black and minority ethnic groups. Some groups comprise individuals who may have a similar experience of health services because of a defining characteristic, e.g. being unemployed or homeless, but who do not have a collective voice or means of expressing their views. Other groups may be informal, with no recognized meeting place. Many groups may be wary of formal and statutory bodies.

References

Annett, H., Rifkin, S., 1990. Improving Urban Health. WHO, Geneva. Available as a scanned document online at: http://apps.who.int/iris/bitstream/10665/62112/1/WHO_SHS_NHP_88.4.pdf (accessed 11.03.15).

Bradshaw, J.R., 1972. The taxonomy of social need. In: McLachlan, G. (Ed.), Problems and Progress in Medical Care. Oxford University Press, Oxford. Available online in a collection at: http://www.york.ac.uk/inst/spru/pubs/pdf/JRB.pdf (accessed 11.03.15).

Bradshaw, J., 1994. The conceptualisation and measurement of need: a social policy perspective. In: Popay, J., Williams, G. (Eds.), Researching the People's Health. Routledge, London, pp. 45–59.

Cavanagh, S., Chadwick, K., 2005. Health Needs Assessment: A Practical Guide. Health Development Agency, London. Available at: http://www.webarchive.org.uk/wayback/archive/20140616173814/http://nice.org.uk/nicemedia/documents/hna.pdf (accessed 11.03.15).

Cohen, D., 2015. Health economics. In: Naidoo, J., Wills, J. (Eds.), Health Studies; an Introduction, third ed. Palgrave/Macmillan, Basingstoke, pp. 377–401.

Doyal, L., Gough, I., 1992. A Theory of Human Need. Macmillan, London.

Hart, T., 1971. The inverse care law. Lancet 1, 405.

Hawtin, M., Percy-Smith, J., 2007. Community Profiling: A Practical Guide, second ed. Open University, Buckingham.

Kings Fund, 2006. Local Variations in NHS Spending Priorities. Kings Fund, London.

Mara, D., Lane, J., Scott, B., Trouba, D., 2010. Sanitation and health. PLoS Medicine 7 (11), e1000363. http://dx.doi.org/10.1371/journal.pmed.1000363.

Maslow, A.H., 1954. Motivation and Personality. Harper & Row, New York.

Maslow, A., 1943. A theory of human motivation. Psychological Review 50, 370–396.

Naidoo, J., Wills, J., 2010. Public Health and Health Promotion: Developing Practice, second ed. Baillière Tindall, London.

NICE, 2003. Health Equity Audit. A Guide for the NHS. Available online at: http://webarchive.nationalarchives.gov.uk/20130107105354/http://www.dh.gov.uk/prod_consum_dh/groups/dh_digitalassets/@dh/@en/documents/digitalasset/dh_4084139.pdf (accessed 09.03.15).

Nutbeam, D., 1998. Evaluating health promotion progress, problems and solutions. Health Promotion International 13 (1), 27–44. Available online at: http://heapro.oxfordjournals.org/content/13/1/27.full.pdf+html (accessed 09.03.15).

Ong, B.N., Humphris, G., 1994. Prioritising needs with communities: rapid appraisal methodologies in health. In: Popay, J., Williams, G. (Eds.), Researching the People's Health. Routledge, London, pp. 59–85.

Parry, G., Cleemput, P.V., Peters, J., Moore, J., Walters, S., Thomas, K., Cooper, C., 2004. The Health Status of Gypsies and Travellers in England. Department of Health, London. Available online at: https://www.sheffield.ac.uk/scharr/research/publications/travellers (accessed 11.03.15).

Wright, J. (Ed.), 1998. Health Needs Assessment in Practice. BMJ Publishing, London.

World Health Organization, 1978. Report on the Primary Health Care Conference: Alma Ata. World Health Organization, Geneva. Available online at: http://www.euro.who.int/__data/assets/pdf_file/0009/113877/E93944.pdf (accessed 1.11.03.15).

World Health Organization, 1985. Targets for Health for All. WHO Regional Office for Europe, Copenhagen.

World Health Organization, 1986. Ottawa Charter. WHO, Geneva. Available online at: http://www.who.int/healthpromotion/conferences/previous/ottawa/en/ (accessed 11.03.15).

World Health Organization, 1997. The Jakarta Declaration. Leading Health Promotion into the 21st Century. Available online at: http://www.who.int/healthpromotion/conferences/previous/jakarta/declaration/en/ (accessed 09.03.15).

World Health Organization, 2013. Health Literacy: The Solid Facts. WHO, Copenhagen. Available online at: http://www.euro.who.int/__data/assets/pdf_file/0008/190655/e96854.pdf (accessed 11.03.15).

Chapter **Nineteen**

19

Planning health promotion interventions

Learning Outcomes

By the end of this chapter you will be able to:
* understand the value of careful planning and preparation
* understand what is required to translate a needs assessment into effective action
* distinguish project activities from outcomes
* identify realistic aims and objectives.

Key Concepts and Definitions

Aims are broad goals or statement of what is to be achieved.

Contingency plan is a plan for an organization to respond coherently to an unusual event.

Milestones are key events with dates that mark progress.

Objectives are specific activities that need to be done in order for the project to achieve its aims.

Outcomes are changes, effects or results.

Outputs are what is done or produced.

Plan is how to get from your starting point to your end point and what you want to achieve.

Policy is guidelines for practice which set broad goals and the framework for action.

Programme is an umbrella term for all activities.

Stakeholders are those directly affected by an intervention or whose support is necessary.

Strategy is a broad framework for action which indicates goals, methods and underlying principles. It derives from evidence, identified needs and experience. It may be used at all levels, as in a programme strategy or an implementation strategy.

Importance of the Topic

We saw in Chapter 18 how needs assessment and targeting may be carried out, and the importance of undertaking this process and being clear about the context in which it is done. This chapter builds on the discussion of the first stage of planning – needs assessment – in Chapter 18. It is important to be clear why you are carrying out an intervention or project, and what changes or improvements are expected. Funders, managers, commissioners and other stakeholders will want to know this as much as the actual activities that may take place. In determining the best approach, you may need to work with others, use the available resources to best effect and set a clear action plan of who does what and when. Planning at different levels, from broad strategic planning through project planning to small-scale health education planning, is considered in this chapter. The PRECEDE-PROCEED model (Green and Kreuter, 2005) is reviewed in detail, as it is widely used. Quality and audit issues and how these relate to planning are then considered.

Reasons for planning

Health promoters usually have no problem in finding things to do which seem reasonable. Work areas are inherited from others, delegated from more senior members of the workplace or demanded by clients. It is possible to be kept very busy reacting to all these pressures, and planning health promotion interventions may seem a luxury or a waste of time. However, there are sound reasons for planning health promotion or being proactive in your work practice. Planning is important because it helps direct resources to where they will have most impact. Planning ensures that health promotion is not overlooked, but is prioritized as a work activity.

Planning takes different forms and is used at different levels. It may be used to provide the best services or care for an individual client, as in the nursing process, or it may be for group activities, such as antenatal classes. Planning may also refer to large-scale health promotion interventions targeted at whole populations.

The degree of formality of the planning process also varies. When planning a one-to-one intervention, the process is informal and may involve no one else. Planning for a group intervention may involve liaising with other professionals as well as the target group, to find out what their aims and objectives are and what sorts of methods and resources are available and acceptable. A written plan may be produced to act as a guide and a statement of agreed outcomes and methods. Planning a large-scale intervention will usually involve more long-term collaborative activity. Often a working group (or task force or local forum) will be established early on to identify interested groups or stakeholders and gain their support and expertise. A written plan will usually be produced, outlining not only objectives and methods but also a timescale of what is to be achieved and when, funding details and a budget, who is responsible for which tasks, and how the intervention will be evaluated, any targets monitored and the findings reported back.

There has been much greater emphasis on systematic planning in recent years due to a need for greater economic accountability, more focus on targets and their achievement, and the need to include evidence as part of project development. It is particularly important for practitioners to be clear about the rationale for interventions, the goals and the approach adopted.

Health promotion planning cycle

Planning involves several key stages or logical stepping stones which enable the health promoter to achieve a desired result. The benefit is being clear about what it is you want to achieve, i.e. the purpose of any intervention. Planning entails five steps.

1. An assessment of need.
2. Setting aims – what it is you intend to achieve.
3. Setting objectives – precise and measurable outcomes.
4. Deciding which methods, interventions or strategies will achieve your objectives.
5. Evaluating outcomes in order to make improvements in the future.

Some planning models are presented in a linear fashion. Others show a circular process to indicate that any evaluation feeds back into the process, as illustrated in Figure 19.1.

This seemingly rational and simple approach describes how decisions should be made. It does not take into account that there may not be agreement on objectives or the best way to proceed, and that in real life planning is often piecemeal or incremental. There is no grand design, but circumstances dictate many small reactive decisions.

 Learning Activity 19.1 The planning cycle

What do you think would be the best starting point for planning an intervention or programme? Why?
Think of any planned activities you have been involved with. What was the starting point? Why?

In a famous quote attributed to the American 'Yogi' Berra, 'If you don't know where you're going, how are you gonna know when you get there?' This neatly sums up the challenges of planning and the importance of knowing what we hope to achieve. All sorts of assumptions underlie what we do – about what we think is the problem or situation to be addressed, about the participants and, for example, how they learn or what might motivate them, about the resources needed – and yet these are rarely made explicit. A logic model is a depiction of a project/programme showing what it

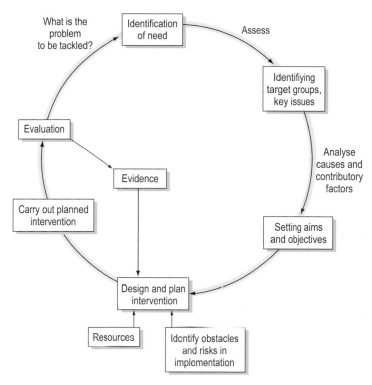

Fig. 19.1 ● Health promotion planning cycle.

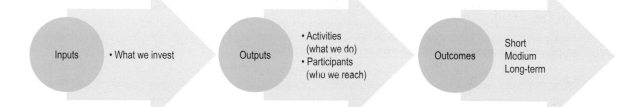

Fig. 19.2 ● The logic chain.

will do and what it will accomplish. It is, as the name suggests, a model representing the programme showing the inputs, outputs and expected outcomes. It tests the logic of that programme through a series of 'if-then' relationships that lead to the desired outcomes. These if-then relationships express the programme's theory of change, and how and why a set of activities is expected to lead to early, intermediate and long-term outcomes over a specified period. Thus if we do these activities, then this output will be achieved; if we deliver these outputs, then this purpose will be achieved; if the purpose

is achieved, then this will contribute to the goal. Flaws in the logic chain might include having a purpose that is too far away from the outputs or cannot be assessed. Figure 19.2 illustrates this logical chain of connections showing what the programme is to accomplish.

Figure 19.3 shows a simple logic model in relation to a professional development intervention for staff working with children and young people. The theory of change is that *if* there is increased professional development through education and organizational support, in the form of reasonable caseloads and

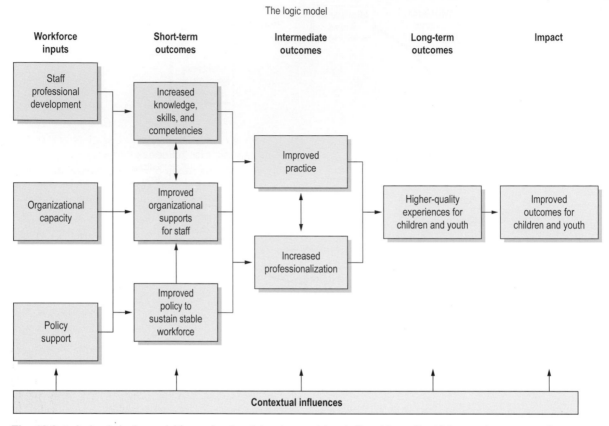

The logic model

Fig. 19.3 ● A simple logic model for professional development for staff working with children and young people. (Harvard Graduate School of Education. Harvard Family Research Project – The Evaluation Exchange XI 4 [periodical] http://www.hfrp.org/evaluation/the-evaluation-exchange/issue-archive.)

opportunities for advancement, *then* this will result in increased staff retention and improved practice, an intermediate outcome. *If* staff stay and they are more professional, *then* there will be more meaningful and enriching activities for young people, who in turn have the potential to yield positive youth outcomes.

Strategic planning

Strategy tends to be used as an umbrella term to cover a broad programme. It may therefore have several different objectives and projects. Practitioners often do not start with a blank sheet and have to work in a wider policy context where issues are determined nationally. Strategies may be local as well

as national, and involve many stakeholders. A stakeholder analysis helps to identify relevant partners and their interests regarding the issue. For example, all local authorities are required to have a strategy to tackle obesity that will include the following.

- A detailed specification of services, projects and activities.
- Identification of costs, inputs and quality standards.
- Expected outcomes. These are expressed as present-day goals rather than targets which specify how and when an objective will be measured. For example, a target for health services to improve childhood obesity, may be to increase the % of 5-16-year-olds participating in at least two hours of intensity sport per week to over 90% by a specified date.

Learning Activity 19.2 Planning a strategy

You are involved in a working group drawing up a local strategy to reduce alcohol use.
1. Who would you involve in the project planning?
2. What would influence the choice of goals that you adopt?
3. If you decided to control availability, what might be achievable outcomes?
4. What might be an appropriate activity or intervention?
5. What factors may affect what you want to achieve?

Project planning

Project planning is a smaller-scale activity, and refers to planning a specific project which is time limited and aims to bring about a defined change. Examples of small-scale health promotion projects include a project to raise the awareness among university students about meningitis, a project to train school nurses in presentation skills and a project to map safe routes to school for young children.

 Learning Activity 19.3 Carrying out a project

The strategy outlined in Learning Activity 19.2 might include a project centred on training general practitioners (GPs) and practice nurses to identify problematic use of alcohol at an early stage. This project, which is part of the overall alcohol reduction strategy, would require careful and detailed planning, including the following.
• Setting appropriate objectives. For example, would it be appropriate to set an objective of reducing problem drinking in the practice population? Why not?
• How might objectives best be achieved? For example, should training be unidisciplinary or multidisciplinary? Should the training be accredited? Who would be the best person to run the sessions? What venue, day and time would be most acceptable? How would the sessions be funded? How long will the project last?
• How would you evaluate the project? What criteria would you use to demonstrate success?

The kind of planning most health practitioners will be involved in will be on a small scale. For example, you may want to plan a health education session

with an individual client, or a series of sessions with a small group around a specific issue. Using the example above, you might want to plan a single session in detail. This would require you to:
• set detailed objectives for participants to achieve by the end of the session, for example, being aware of symptoms and behaviours (for example, poor attendance and time-keeping at work, especially in the mornings) which might be due to problematic alcohol use
• investigate the range of resources available and select resources to use in the session
• plan the session showing different activities and time allocated for each
• plan a means of evaluating the session.

Planning models

Planning, whatever the scale of the activity, requires systematically working through a number of stages that relate to the following questions.
• What is the nature of the problem?
• Who is affected?
• What are the causes and contributory factors?
• What needs to be done to tackle the problem?
• How should any intervention be carried out?
• How will we know if it is successful?

Stage 1: What is the nature of the problem?

A range of issues is important in this 'diagnosis' stage of understanding why a problem should be addressed and for whom it exists. As we saw in Chapter 18, priorities do not always arise out of the needs that may be identified in community profiles or needs assessments, but may be defined on the basis of national or local epidemiological data reporting trends in illness and deaths. Equally, the causes identified from epidemiological data may not accord with what people themselves identify as the causes. As we also saw in Chapter 18, it is important to identify what can be changed. If the problem or issue is incorrectly understood and diagnosed, then everything that flows from it will be ill conceived.

Stage 2: What needs to be done? Set aims and objectives

Aims are broad goals concerned with improving health in a particular area or reducing a health problem, for example, reducing the amount of alcohol-related ill health, and are statements of intent. Objectives need to be specific, and should be statements that define what participants will have achieved by the end of the intervention. Objectives therefore need to be measurable in some way. There is a balance to be struck between setting objectives which are realistic but also challenging. When writing objectives it is recommended that they are SMART:

specific
measurable
achievable
realistic
time-bound.

Health promotion objectives can refer to educational, behavioural, policy, process or environmental outcomes.

- Educational objectives may be divided into three categories, and are usually expressed in relation to the learner:

  knowledge objectives concerning increased levels of knowledge

  affective objectives concerning changes in attitudes and beliefs

  behavioural or skills objectives concerning the acquisition of new competencies and skills.

  These will lead to short-term outcomes.

Medium term outcomes will have:

  - Behavioural objectives, including changes in lifestyles and increased take-up of services, for example, reducing the amount of binge drinking or the prevalence of drink-driving.
  - Policy objectives, including the development or implementation of policy, for example, implementing alcohol-free policies in workplaces.
  - Process objectives include the achievement of health promotion principles, for example, participation and intersectoral collaboration.
  - Environmental objectives include changing the environment to make it more health promoting,

for example, restricting the advertising and sale of alcohol.

 Learning Activity 19.4 Setting health education objectives

What might be appropriate objectives for a project on the early identification of alcohol-related problems by GPs and practice nurses?

Objectives also reflect perspectives about the determinants of health, and values about what are the most important things to achieve. These perspectives and values may be your own or may be derived from your organization.

 Learning Activity 19.5 The role of determinants in planning

Consider the different aims that may be included in a drug prevention strategy.
1. To reduce the risks associated with drug use and enable clients who do choose to use drugs to do so safely.
2. To reduce levels of harmful drug use.
What values and views about the determinants of drug use are reflected in these different aims?

Stage 3: Identify appropriate methods for achieving the objectives

Decisions about how to go about addressing the problem will depend on objectives, but also on available evidence of effective interventions, available funding and the expertise of practitioners (see Chapter 20). Certain methods go with certain objectives but would be quite inappropriate for others. For example, participative small-group work is effective at changing attitudes, but a more formal teaching session would be more effective if specific knowledge is to be imparted. Community development is effective at increasing community involvement and participation, but would not be appropriate if local government policy change is the objective. The mass media are effective in raising people's awareness of health issues but largely ineffective in persuading people to change their behaviour. So the next stage in planning is deciding which methods are the logical choice given your objectives. You may then find you have to compromise owing to constraints of time, resources or skills, but this compromise should concern the amount of input or the use of complementary methods. It should not mean that you end up using inappropriate methods which are unlikely to achieve your objectives.

Stage 4: Identify resources and inputs

When objectives and methods have been decided, the next stage is to consider whether any specific resources are needed to implement the strategy. Resources include human resources, financial resources and materials and equipment. Funding is an important issue for larger-scale interventions which require additional inputs over and above existing services and staff. For larger-scale interventions you may need to prepare a budget, which is a statement of expected costs. This includes direct costs, which relate to the project, and fixed costs, which happen anyway.

 Learning Activity 19.6 Budgetary planning

What would you need to include in a budget plan for training sessions for GPs and practice nurses on early identification of problematic alcohol use, discussed in Learning Activity 19.4?

A budget control system regularly monitors what is spent and what remains. This is usually done by monitoring the amount of money allocated, the amount of money spent and the variance between the two (underspend or overspend) under each budget heading every month.

Stage 5: Plan evaluation methods

Evaluation must relate to the objectives you have set, but can be undertaken more or less formally. For example,

in relation to an educational session you might decide to ask participants their views at the end of the session, or spend some time noting your own perceptions of what went well and what could be improved next time. Or you might design a more formal means of evaluation, for example, a questionnaire for participants to fill in anonymously, which is timetabled into the session. Project evaluation is discussed in more detail in Chapter 20.

Stage 6: Set an action plan

This is a detailed written plan which identifies tasks, the person responsible for each task, resources which will be used, a timescale and means of evaluation. You might also include interim indicators of progress to show if you are proceeding as planned. Many factors can threaten the sustainability of a project. Being clear about the external factors underlying the structure of the project and what assumptions are being made is a key requirement of most project plans, especially where large sums of money are being allocated. For example, projects may depend on achieving community involvement or successful funding bids.

A Gantt chart (set out as an example in Figure 19.4) is a useful tool at this stage. A Gantt chart plots tasks and the people responsible for these tasks against a timescale in which these activities need to be undertaken. It portrays in a graphical form the interdependence of project tasks and how each single task contributes to the whole. Implementation is the project activity, for example, training sessions. Evaluation, review and the final completion report record project outcomes and assess whether objectives have been met. It is useful to have a time lag between completing the project and the final review in order to assess long-term as well as immediate outcomes.

Stage 7: Action, or implementation of the plan

It is often useful to keep a log or diary to note unexpected problems and how you dealt with them, as well as unintended benefits. This information can then be fed into the evaluation process. You will also

	March	April	May	June	July	August	September	October
Marketing and publicity	H and A							
Recruit participants		A						
Plan sessions				H	H			
Accreditation			H and A					
Pre-course needs assessment questionnaire				H and R				
Prepare materials, collect resources					H and A			
Check venue, timing, refreshments						A		
Action: training sessions							H	
Post-course sessions								H and R
Evaluation report								H and R

Three workers are involved:

H is a health promotor
A is an administrative officer
R is a researcher.

Fig. 19.4 ● A Gantt chart.

want to plan for documentation and dissemination of the project findings, whether this is in the form of a report, a newsletter or a presentation.

Planning models

Log frames (logistical frameworks) are widely used in international development projects to identify the activities of a programme and any inherent risks that might delay completion. A log frame is not the same as the logic model described earlier. A logical framework takes the form of a table. The rows describe the four different results the project aims to achieve or contribute: objectives, outcomes, outputs and activities. The columns describe the verifiable indicators, the means of verification (i.e. what information is used to provide verification) and the assumptions and external factors that may influence the project. Log frames can be useful to ensure that activities are monitored, outcomes evaluated and means and ends are brought together. Critics argue that they are potentially inflexible and time-consuming to produce.

PRECEDE-PROCEED model

Figure 19.5 illustrates the PRECEDE-PROCEED planning model, one of the earliest and best-known models which has now been revised and simplified (Green and Kreuter, 2005). PRECEDE stands for 'predisposing, reinforcing and enabling causes in educational diagnosis'. This model recognizes the multiple determinants of health and starts with an assessment of the quality of life, which is the ultimate goal. Health contributes to quality of life. The model then works 'backwards' in a sequence of diagnostic phases to identify the environmental and organizational factors that influence health behaviour, including health service utilization. It considers the *predisposing factors*, those personal factors such as individual motivation, knowledge attitudes and beliefs; *reinforcing factors*, the attitudes and behaviours of role models, peers and employers; and *enabling factors*, resources and skills that either support or hinder change in behaviour or environment. As well as diagnosing what needs to be addressed, the capacity for implementation of a proposed programme is also considered.

Learning Activity 19.7 Using a log frame

Complete the log frame below.

Project	Indicators of achievement	Means of verification	Important risks and assumptions
Objectives			
To reduce the harmful effects of binge drinking among young women			
Outcomes			
To raise awareness of using safe taxi companies to get home			
Outputs			
Purse cards with taxi numbers			
Posters in bar and club toilets			
Tannoy announcements in bar and club toilets			
Activities			
Working with specified taxi companies to recruit women drivers			
Working with bar and club owners			

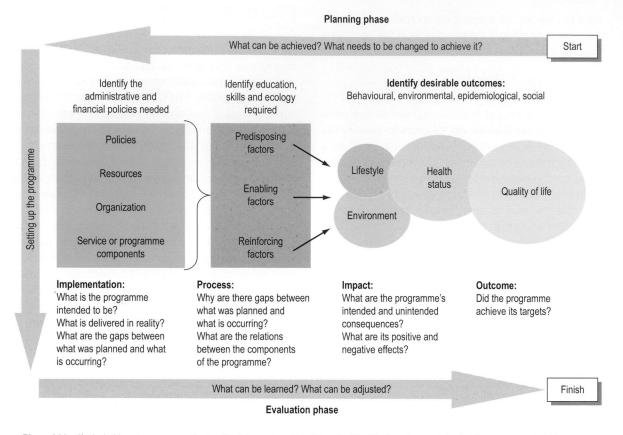

Phase 1 Identify desirable outcomes regarding health status and quality of life – the identification of a population's felt concerns and problems relating to their quality of life, e.g. unemployment, crime.

Phase 2 Identify desirable outcomes regarding lifestyle and environment – the identification of a population's health practices, e.g. service utilization, self-care and management, lifestyles and environmental factors.

Phase 3 Identify required education, skills and ecology, e.g. beliefs, values and attitudes that affect motivation to change; skills and resources, social factors, e.g. income; social norms and social support.

Phase 4 Identify the administrative and financial policies that are needed. How well does the implementation of the programme meet these needs?

Phase 5 Implementation of the intervention follows logically from the previous phases. The management and administration of the intervention are also considered at this stage. Administrative diagnosis includes assessment of resources and organizational relationships, and the production of a timetable.

Phase 6 The impact and outcomes of the programme are used in the evaluation of the intervention, although Green et al. (2005) stress that this should be an integrated activity addressed throughout the planning process.

Fig. 19.5 ● PRECEDE-PROCEED planning model. (Green, L.W., Kreuter, M.W., 2005. Health Program Planning: An Educational and Ecological Approach. fourth ed. McGraw-Hill Higher Education, NY.)

The model may be broken down into phases, as shown below. Priority targets for intervention are established through each phase of the assessment process (phases 1–4) on the basis of their causal importance in the chain of health determinants, their prevalence and their changeability. The results of this assessment process guide the development of the intervention (phase 5). The evaluation (phase 6) then tracks the impact of the intervention on factors identified as important targets in the assessment process.

Phases of the PRECEDE-PROCEED model

Phase 1. Identify desirable outcomes regarding health status and quality of life – the identification of a population's felt concerns and problems relating to their quality of life, for example, unemployment, crime.

Phase 2. Identify desirable outcomes regarding lifestyle and environment – the identification of a population's health practices, for example, service utilization, self-care and management, lifestyles and environmental factors.

Phase 3. Identify required education, skills and ecology, for example, beliefs, values and attitudes that affect motivation to change; skills and resources; and social factors, for example, income, social norms and social support.

Phase 4. Identify the administrative and financial policies that are needed. How well does the implementation of the programme meet these needs?

Phase 5. Implementation of the intervention follows logically from the previous phases. The management and administration of the intervention are also considered at this stage. Administrative diagnosis includes assessment of resources and organizational relationships, and the production of a timetable.

Phase 6. The impact and outcomes of the programme are used in the evaluation of the intervention, although Green and Kreuter (2005) stress that this should be an integrated activity addressed throughout the planning process.

The intention is that using the PRECEDE-PROCEED model will guide the health educator to the most effective type of intervention. Using knowledge drawn from epidemiology, social psychology, education and management studies, the health educator can arrive at an optimum intervention. The model is said to be based on a complementary mix of expertise drawn from these different disciplines. In practice, the model is often modified and is rarely used as illustrated (see Green's own website for an account of the application of the model, http://www.lgreen.net/precede.htm). For example, it is unusual to begin the process of planning with an agenda as open as 'quality of life'. Priority topics, target groups or settings are more often identified at the outset. For example, English public health white

papers have focused on specific diseases. So in practice PRECEDE often begins at the behavioural diagnosis rather than the needs assessment phase.

The PRECEDE-PROCEED model may be criticized on several grounds. PRECEDE as a health education planning model mirrors the medical world. The planning process is dominated by experts. The general public may be involved in identifying problems, but the ways and means of tackling these problems are to be determined by experts. The focus is on achieving behavioural change at the level of individuals or groups. The social, political and environmental context of health is systematically screened out by the model in phases 2 and 3. To some extent this may be explained by PRECEDE being a health education rather than a health promotion planning model. A model developed specifically for health education cannot be expected to apply to other forms of health promotion, but for most people education, even if it does not include changing the environment, does include clarifying values, beliefs and attitudes, facilitating self-empowerment and supporting autonomy. Using the PRECEDE-PROCEED model subordinates these activities to the primary aim of behaviour change. It could be argued that PRECEDE-PROCEED is a model dominated by social psychology and behavioural perspectives rather than educational perspectives, and that the label is therefore misleading. PRECEDE-PROCEED is, however, a highly structured planning model which ensures that certain issues are considered. If the objective is behaviour change, then PRECEDE-PROCEED is a useful model to follow.

Quality and audit

Assessing the quality of practice through quality assurance, quality management or audit is an important aspect of professional practice. It helps to improve standards, identify cost-effective activities, demonstrate worth to outside agencies and ensure that activities meet stakeholders' requirements. In the UK a strategic process to identify and understand healthcare needs has been in place since 1990. Its purpose is to decide how to spend available resources and to secure and monitor appropriate services, engaging in activities that lead to improved population health, reduced health inequalities and improved access, quality, experience and outcomes of care for service users. Currently the process is conducted by clinical commissioning groups, which assess local needs, determinants of health and inequalities. This introduction of commissioning of services and placing of contracts has highlighted the need for specification of quality. There has also been an increased emphasis on audit of public sector activities, and clinical audit is well established. Targets have been set, for example, a reduction in accident and emergency and ambulance attendance waiting times, and in infections acquired in hospital. Such targets are not popular with everyone, and have been criticized as distorting clinical priorities. Indeed, the UK government has referred to the 'bonfire of the targets'. Setting targets is about measuring performance in relation to a level of service or activity level. Quality is less concerned with number crunching than with how the activity is perceived by recipients. There is now more emphasis on quality through specifications such as CQUINS (commissioning for quality and innovation). Continuous quality improvement, total quality management and the use of external standards all aim to improve services and also provide answers to the variability in programme development. Quality in healthcare relates to:

- safe care (avoidance of harmful interventions)
- effectiveness (care which conforms with best practice)
- enhancement of the patient/user experience.

The core principles of quality interventions in health promotion have been defined (Speller et al., 1994) as:

- equity – that users have equal access to and/or equal benefit from services
- effectiveness – that services achieve their intended objectives
- efficiency – that services achieve maximum benefit for minimum cost
- accessibility – that a service is easily available to users in terms of time, distance and ethos
- appropriateness – that a service is that which the users require
- acceptability – that services satisfy the reasonable expectations of users

- responsiveness – that services adapt to the expressed needs of users.

Quality expresses a notion of 'fit for the purpose', but also conveys a notion of excellence. Quality assurance or audit is a systematic process through which desirable levels of quality are described, the extent to which these levels are achieved is assessed and follow-up action is taken to achieve optimum levels of quality. Quality assurance is an ongoing process of continual assessment and improvement of practice, and therefore differs from evaluation, which focuses on outcomes at a specific point in time. A quality system may include elements of quality assurance and quality management.

Quality is about doing things in the correct manner. The criteria in the European Quality Instrument for Health Promotion (EQUIHP) for supporting the development of interventions, benchmarking and evaluation (Bollars et al., 2005) are listed below. EQUIHP states that indicators of quality relate to appropriate design, good management and practice that accords with core principles.

 Case Study 19.1 European Quality Instrument for Health Promotion

1. Framework of health promotion principles
This approach embraces the principles of health promotion, including a positive and comprehensive approach to health and attention for the broad determinants of health, participation, empowerment, equity and equality.
2. Project development and implementation
   a. Analysis – the project is based on a systematic analysis of the health problem and its determinants, and of the context in which it will be implemented.
   b. Aims and objectives – the aims and objectives of the project are clearly defined.
   c. Target group – the group of people the project intends to influence is clearly defined.
   d. Intervention – the strategies and methods for an effective intervention are clearly outlined.
   e. Implementation strategy – there is a clear description of the way the intervention will be carried out.

f. Evaluation – the effects (effect evaluation) and quality (process evaluation) of the intervention will be assessed.
3. Project management
   a. Leadership – a person has been designated who is ultimately responsible for and capable of managing the project.
   b. Planning and documentation – the working plan and organization of the project are firmly established.
   c. Capacity and resources – the expertise and resources that are necessary to implement the project successfully are available.
   d. Participation and commitment – the ways in which various parties will be involved in and committed to the project is clearly outlined.
   e. Communication – the way in which all the participants (target group and stakeholders) will be informed about the project is clearly established.
4. Sustainability
   The continuation of the project is ensured.

---

http://ec.europa.eu/health/ph projects/2003/action1/docs/2003_1_15_a10_en.pdf.

Audit is a systematic process of scrutinizing a service or programme in order to improve performance. Audit may focus on a particular aspect, for example, organization and management or training. Part of the purpose of an audit is to build a picture, providing evidence of gaps and areas for improvement by comparing what is done with agreed best practice. A key part of an audit is to see if a service meets the needs of its users, so it may involve gathering and acting on local people's views. Audit may involve an internal review or scrutiny by an independent external auditor (e.g. the Audit Commission or Office for Standards in Education, Children's Services and Skills [OFSTED] inspectors of schools).

Conclusion

There are sound reasons for adopting a planning model to structure health promotion interventions. Recognizing that health is a complex socially determined concept means that activities to promote health require careful planning, and often collaboration and working together with different agencies. Activities at different levels all benefit from planning, although the factors which need to be considered will vary according to the level of planned intervention.

A systematic approach will ensure that what is done:
• is relevant to agreed strategic objectives
• involves key stakeholders at the important stages of the project
• is relevant to the real problems and issues of target groups/beneficiaries
• has feasible objectives and can be realistically achieved
• measures and verifies successes
• ensures that benefits generated by projects are likely to be sustainable.

Planning provides a standard framework in which projects/programmes/interventions are developed, implemented and evaluated. The planning cycle ensures that the results of a project are fed back into new projects and programmes. Many health promotion projects fail because they are ill conceived, have simple educational or behavioural objectives which fail to analyse causes, take a narrow reductionist view of health and/or do not take account of existing evidence.

In reality, planning health promotion is a more complex process than planning models suggest. This is because rational decision-making is only one factor in determining what happens. Many other factors are also important, including historical precedent, enthusiasms of key people and the political context. So it is unlikely that any health promotion intervention proceeds exactly along the lines indicated by a planning model, but this does not mean models are not useful. Models help structure activities and can act as a checklist to ensure that important stages are not missed out. They are there to be modified in the light of experience, not to act as straitjackets.

Chapter 20 goes on to discuss the evaluation stage. Evaluating interventions and being able to determine to what extent health promotion is successful in achieving its objectives are the key to establishing health promotion as a central plank of health work.

Questions for further discussion

- What factors would you take into account when planning a health promotion intervention? How could you assess the quality of your health promotion work?

Summary

This chapter has clarified the terminology used in the planning process and discussed the reasons for planning health promotion interventions. Planning happens at different levels, and an account of this has been given. Two planning models which have been developed specifically for health promotion have been discussed in greater detail. The assessment and evaluation of planning have been discussed through reference to quality assurance and audit cycles.

Further reading and resources

Davies, M., Kepford, J., 2006. Planning a health promotion intervention. In: Davies, M., Macdowall, W. (Eds.), Health Promotion Theory. Understanding Public Health Series. OUP, McGrawHill, Maidenhead. *A useful short summary of some key factors to take into account.*

Ewles, L., Simnett, I., 2010. Promoting Health: A Practical Guide, sixth ed. Baillière Tindall, Edinburgh. *Chapter 7 gives further details and a practical guide to Ewles and Simnett's model. Chapter 8 discusses project planning in more detail.*

Green, J., Tones, K., Cross, R., Woodall, J., 2015. Health Promotion. Planning and Strategies, second ed. Sage, London. *Chapter 4 provides a readable and detailed discussion of systematic approaches to planning, and discusses various planning models.*

Taylor, V. (Ed.), 2012. Leading for Health and Wellbeing. Sage, London. *Chapter 7 focuses on leading at a local level including performance management. Chapter 8 focuses on project management.*

 ## Feedback to learning activities

19.1 Figure 19.1 suggests that the planning cycle begins with a needs assessment through which the programme's focus and any specific target groups may be identified. The underlying causes and contributory factors that led to the problem and the areas that will need to be addressed are then identified.

19.2
1. *Who would you involve?* Identifying likely partners and developing a team. This is likely to include elected councillors, licensed victuallers, magistrates, police service and voluntary agencies dealing with alcohol-related problems.
2. *What would influence the goals?* An analysis of the current situation would identify the issues that present the greatest demand on resources, or possibly the issue that is most amenable to change.
3. What might be achievable outcomes? Where do we want to go? Objectives might include:
   - reducing the promotion of alcohol
   - reducing alcohol-related antisocial behaviour
   - protecting young people from alcohol-related harm.
4. *Activities or interventions. How do we get there?* A possible activity might be an awareness workshop for local councillors, banning advertisements for alcohol on local authority premises, promoting health practitioners' awareness via sessions for GPs and practice nurses on early identification and referral, use of local by-laws to prevent drinking in public, and sessions in youth clubs and community centres.
5. *What factors may affect what we want to achieve? What may stop us getting there?* The local council may not be supportive of a proactive policy on licensing. The alcohol industry may be a powerful economic force locally.

19.3
- An objective of reducing problem drinking is unrealistic and too long term for a single intervention project.
- Unidisciplinary training has the advantage of practitioners understanding each others' roles and being less competitive, but most issues benefit from a multidisciplinary approach, as this enables mutual understanding of the extent of the problem.
- Criteria to evaluate the success of the project could include data on staff involvement in the pro-

ject, for example, take-up of training and number of accredited staff by the end of the project. Data on reducing problem drinking in the practice population, although the ultimate goal of the project, are more problematic to collect (e.g. does one rely on self-reports, or require independent corroboration through measures such as blood and liver function tests?). Even if reduced problem drinking is verified, attributing this to the project is also problematic. Ideally, there needs to be a control population to ensure any positive results are attributable to the project.

19.4 A training session might have the following educational objectives.

1. Increasing participants' knowledge of the range of harmful effects and symptoms associated with problematic alcohol use.
2. Increasing participants' knowledge of the extent of problematic alcohol use and its association with social and demographic factors, for example, gender, age, employment status, occupation.
3. Investigating participants' attitudes towards alcohol and cultural depictions of alcohol use. Identifying the range between social drinker and alcoholic, with the many stages in between. Recognizing social, media and peer pressures to drink which contribute to many people's problematic usage of alcohol.

4. Enabling participants to use an assessment tool effectively to identify problematic alcohol use.
5. Enabling participants to use the stages of change model to identify problem drinkers and appropriate interventions.

19.5 The first aim is a harm-reduction one, where the focus is on the prevention of harm rather than the prevention of drug use itself, and on people who continue to use drugs. It recognizes the complex interplay of social factors that influence vulnerability to drug-related harm, including poverty, social inequality and discrimination. The activities may include needle exchanges, peer education and counselling. The second aim is simply a disease-reduction approach, where the focus may be on education or enforcement activities controlling supply.

19.6 Direct costs include:
- staff costs – salaries, superannuation, employer's National Insurance payments, annual increments
- capital costs, for example, computers
- costs of specific activities, for example, rental of community centre for training, buying resources to use in the training
- telephone, postage, photocopying
- travel and subsistence
- training and conferences to support staff development.

  Fixed costs include overheads to cover accommodation, heating, lighting, telephone rental, etc.

19.7

Project	Indicators of achievement	Means of verification	Important risks and assumptions
Objectives			
To reduce the harmful effects of binge drinking among young women	Reduction in hospital admissions to accident and emergency and other wards due to the effects of alcohol	Hospital statistics	That the harmful effects of binge drinking are health related (as opposed to safety related, e.g. driving under the influence of alcohol) That hospital admission will be sought by women under the influence of alcohol
Outcomes			
To raise awareness of using safe taxi companies to get home	Increase in use of safe taxi companies by women under the influence of alcohol	Taxi records	That young women have available resources (money) to use taxis, and that there are no public transport options for the journey home

Continued

Project	Indicators of achievement	Means of verification	Important risks and assumptions
Outputs			
Purse cards with taxi numbers	Publication and distribution of cards advertising taxis	Data confirming publication and distribution of cards	That women will use the cards to order taxis, and that they have the money to pay for taxis
Posters in bar and club toilets	Production and placement of posters in bar and club toilets	Spot checks in bars and clubs to verify placement of posters	That women will read the posters and act on the information displayed in them
Tannoy announcements in bar and club toilets	Playing tannoy announcements in bar and club toilets	Monitoring tannoy announcements in bar and club toilets	That women will hear and process the information given in the announcements
Activities			
Working with specified taxi companies to recruit women drivers	Data on the sex of taxi drivers employed by taxi companies	Taxi companies' records on the sex of their drivers	That women will feel safer with women taxi drivers, and be more likely to use taxi companies which can provide women drivers on request
Working with bar and club owners			

References

Bollars, C., Kok, H., Van den Broucke, S., et al., 2005. European Quality Instrument for Health Promotion with User Manual Woerden: NIGZ. Available online at: http://ec.europa.eu/health/ph_projects/2003/action1/docs/2003_1_15_a10_en.pdf (accessed 11.03.15).

Ewles, L., Simnett, I., 2010. Promoting Health: A Practical Guide, sixth ed. Baillière Tindall, London.

Green, L.W., Kreuter, M.W., 2005. Health Program Planning: An Educational and Ecological Approach, fourth ed. McGraw-Hill Higher Education, NY.

Speller, V., Evans, K., Head, M., 1997. Developing quality assurance standards for health promotion in the UK Health Promotion International. Perspectives 12, 215–224. Available online at: http://heapro.oxfordjournals.org/content/12/3/215.full.pdf (accessed 22.09.15).

20

Evaluating health promotion interventions

By the end of this chapter you will be able to:
- understand the importance of evaluation in project management
- assess critically the challenges of evaluating complex interventions
- understand the differences between process, impact and outcome evaluation
- distinguish appropriate methods to evaluate projects
- discuss how evaluation can build an evidence base for health promotion.

Key Concepts and Definitions

Evaluation The assessment of the worth or value of something.

Evidence-based practice The explicit use of clinical expertise, patients' values and the best research evidence in decision-making regarding patient care.

Cost-effectiveness Economical in terms of the money spent for goods or services received.

Acceptability Adequate to satisfy a need, requirement or standard.

Equity The state or quality of being just or fair.

Outcome An end result or consequence.

Impact The immediate effect.

Importance of the Topic

Evaluation is an integral aspect of all planned activities, enabling an assessment of the value or worth of an intervention. Evaluation also performs several other roles. For practitioners, evaluation helps develop their skills and competencies. For funders, evaluation demonstrates where resources can be most usefully channelled. For lay people, evaluation provides an opportunity to have their voices heard. There are additional reasons why evaluating health promotion is a key aspect of practice. As a relatively new discipline, there is great pressure on health promotion to prove its worth through evaluation of its activities. In addition, there is a drive to ensure that all practice is evidence-based. This affects health promotion as well as more clinical activities. In a situation where resources will always be limited, demonstrating the cost-effectiveness of interventions is important. There are thus many factors leading to a demand for evaluation of health promotion practice.

Evaluating health promotion is not a straightforward task. Health promotion interventions often involve different kinds of activities, a long timescale and several partners who may each have their own objectives. Health promotion may be seen as belonging within the health services, where the dominant evaluation model is quantitative research centred on experimental trials, with randomized controlled trials (RCTs) as the preferred evaluation tool. Health promotion has had to argue its case for a more holistic evaluation strategy encompassing qualitative methodologies and taking into account contextual features.

The focus of this chapter is on evaluating health promotion interventions. Evaluation of research studies is also part of the health promoter's role and remit, and readers are referred to Chapters 2 and 3 in our companion volume (Naidoo and Wills, 2010) for a detailed discussion of this topic. This chapter considers what is meant by evaluation, the range of research methodologies used in evaluation studies, its rationale, how it is done and its role in building the evidence base for health promotion.

Defining evaluation

Evaluation is a complex concept with many definitions that vary according to purpose, disciplinary boundaries and values. A comprehensive definition is 'the systematic examination and assessment of features of a programme or other intervention in order to produce knowledge that different stakeholders can use for a variety of purposes' (Rootman et al., 2001, p. 26). This definition is useful, because it also flags up the importance of the purpose of evaluation and the fact that there can be many different reasons to evaluate. Evaluation can provide information on:

- the extent to which an intervention met its aims and goals
- the manner in which the intervention was carried out
- the cost-effectiveness of the intervention.

It is important to be clear at the outset about the purpose of evaluation, as this will determine what information is gathered and how it is obtained. The value-driven purpose of evaluation distinguishes it from research (Springett, 2001). Evaluation uses resources which might otherwise be used for programme planning and implementation, so a clear purpose is necessary to legitimate and protect this use of resources.

 Learning Activity 20.1 The role of evaluation

You have a limited budget (from lottery money) and a tight timescale to deliver a community health promotion intervention designed to improve nutrition. Stakeholders include the funders, local schools, social housing and sheltered accommodation providers, community associations, primary healthcare staff, social care staff and the community. Your proposed plan of action includes an evaluation, and you have suggested earmarking 5 to 10 percent of your budget and time for this purpose. A coalition of some of the stakeholders has approached you requesting that you omit the evaluation and concentrate all your resources on the intervention. How would you respond? What arguments might you use to defend the proposed evaluation?

From a practitioner's perspective, evaluation is needed to assess results, determine whether objectives have been met and find out if the methods used were appropriate and efficient. These findings can then be fed back into the planning process in order to progress practice. Evaluations of interventions are used to build an evidence base of what works, enabling other practitioners to focus their inputs where they will have most effect. From a lay perspective, evaluation helps to clarify expectations and assess the extent to which these have been met. Evaluation may also help determine what strategies had most impact, and why. Without evaluation, it is very difficult to make a reasoned case for more resources or expansion of an intervention. Even when a programme is rolling out an established and effective intervention, specific local features may have an unanticipated impact that will only become apparent in an evaluation. There are sound reasons for evaluating all interventions, although more innovative projects will require more substantial and costly evaluation.

The rationale for evaluation includes the following reasons.

- To assess how resources were deployed (*effort*).
- To assess whether what has been achieved was an economically sound use of resources (*efficiency*).

- To measure impact and outcomes, and whether the intervention was worthwhile (*effectiveness*).
- To assess the intervention's or programme's contribution to equity (*equity*).
- To judge the adequacy, feasibility and sustainability of the delivery of the intervention or programme (*feasibility*).
- To assess the overall benefits of the intervention (*efficacy*).
- To inform future plans.
- To justify decisions to others.

Why evaluate?

Evaluation uses resources that could otherwise be used to provide services. Given that services are always in demand, there needs to be a strong rationale for devoting resources to evaluation rather than service provision. New or pilot interventions warrant a rigorous evaluation, because without evidence of their effectiveness or efficiency, it is difficult to argue that they should become established work practices. Other criteria that can be used to determine if evaluation is worth the effort relate to how well it can be done. If it will be impossible to obtain cooperation from the different groups involved in the activity, it is probably not worthwhile trying to evaluate. If evaluation has not been considered at the outset but is tacked on as an 'afterthought', the chances are that it will be so partial and biased as to be not worth the effort.

Evaluation is only worthwhile if it will make a difference. This means that the results of the evaluation need to be interpreted and fed back to the relevant audiences in an accessible form. All too often, evaluations are buried in inappropriate formats. Work reports may go no further than the manager, or academic studies full of jargon may be published in little-known journals.

 Learning Activity 20.2 What to evaluate

A well-man clinic is introduced in a primary healthcare practice. The aim is to monitor the health of middle-aged men and provide information and advice enabling them to adopt healthier lifestyles, so that in the longer term health risks such as high blood pressure or smoking are reduced. Over a period of time, the practice nurse invites all men aged 50 to 65 into the practice for a half-hour session where she checks vital statistics (weight, blood pressure), asks about lifestyle (e.g. diet, smoking, alcohol and drug use, sexual activity, exercise) and gives individually tailored information and advice about adopting a healthier lifestyle. This intervention takes up a significant proportion of her time and workload.

How would you evaluate this programme?

What to evaluate

Health promotion objectives may be about individual changes, service use or changes in the environment. A range of possible objectives associated with smoking-reduction interventions, each of which would need evaluation, might include:

- increased knowledge, e.g. harmful effects of passive smoking
- changes in attitudes, e.g. less willingness to breathe in others' smoke
- changes in behaviour, e.g. stopping smoking
- acquiring new skills, e.g. learning relaxation methods to reduce stress
- introduction of healthy policies, e.g. funding to enable general practitioners to prescribe nicotine replacement aids for people on low incomes
- modifying the environment, e.g. banning tobacco advertising and promotion, banning smoking in cars carrying children
- reduction in risk factors, e.g. reduction in number of smokers and amount of tobacco smoked per person
- increased use of services, e.g. take-up rates for smoking-cessation clinics, number of calls made to quit-smoking telephone helplines
- reduced morbidity, e.g. reduced rates of respiratory illness and coronary heart disease
- reduced mortality, e.g. reduced mortality from lung cancer.

Although all these factors relate to health, they are quite separate, and there is no necessary connection between, say, increased knowledge and behaviour change. It is therefore inappropriate to evaluate a given objective (e.g. increased physical activity) by measuring other aspects of an intervention (e.g. number of leaflets taken at a health fair or number of people reporting that they would like to exercise more). It is important to choose appropriate indicators for the stated objectives. This issue is discussed further in Chapter 19, which emphasizes the use of a logic model to identify appropriate indicators.

Process, impact and outcome evaluation

Evaluation is always incomplete: it is impossible to assess every element of an intervention. Instead, decisions are taken about which evaluation criteria to prioritize, and also sometimes which objectives are to be assessed. A distinction is often made between process, impact and outcome evaluation. Process evaluation (also called formative or illuminative evaluation) is concerned with assessing the process of programme implementation. Outcomes can be immediate (impacts), intermediate or long term (outcomes). Impact and outcome evaluations are both concerned with assessing the effects of interventions.

Chapter 19 identified that evaluation may refer to various features of an intervention or project.

- *Effectiveness* and the extent to which it achieves its intended outcomes. Does the intervention work? Are any changes achieved as a result of the intervention or project? Does the intervention or project work better than alternatives?
- *Efficacy* and the extent to which it achieves maximum benefit for minimum cost. Does the project provide value for money? Is the project more cost-effective than other interventions?
- *Acceptability* and the extent to which it meets needs. Do people respond to or take up the service? Are people satisfied with what is offered?
- *Equity* and the extent to which it ensures equal access and ability to benefit. Does the intervention enable equal access for those in need? Do people with greater needs gain greater benefits?
- *Quality.* Is the project or intervention delivered in the best possible way? Is it sustainable? Is it feasible? What are the barriers to implementation?

Process evaluation

Process evaluation may be from the perspective of participants and/or practitioners and/or other stakeholders such as funders. Stakeholders' perceptions and reactions to health promotion interventions and facilitating or inhibiting factors may be sought. More objective data, such as whether targets were met and timescales and budgets adhered to, can also be included. The aims of process evaluation are practical – can the intervention be repeated, can it be refined, and can it be reproduced in similar or different settings with similar or different target groups?

There are four main questions in process evaluation.
1. Is the programme reaching the target group (programme reach)?
2. Are participants satisfied with the programme (programme acceptability)?
3. Are all the activities of the programme being implemented (programme integrity)?
4. Are all the materials and components of the programme of good quality (programme quality)? (Hawe et al., 1994; Nutbeam, 1998).

Process evaluation employs a wide range of qualitative or 'soft' methods: examples are interviews, diaries, observations and content analysis of documents. These methods tell us a great deal about that particular programme and the factors responsible for its success or failure, but they are unable to predict what would happen if the programme were to be replicated in other areas. Because process evaluation does not use 'hard' scientific methods, its findings tend to be more easily dismissed as unrepresentative. However, process evaluation is crucial to health promotion. We need to understand how health promotion interventions are interpreted and responded to by different groups of people and whether the intervention itself is health promoting, and for this we need process evaluation.

Impact and outcome evaluations

Evaluation of health promotion programmes is usually concerned to identify their effects and any changes achieved as a result of an intervention. The effects of an intervention may be evaluated according to its:

- *impact* – the immediate effects or outputs, such as increased knowledge or shifts in attitude
- *outcome* – the longer-term effects, such as changes in lifestyle.

A challenge for an evaluation is picking out what changes have taken place, and which changes are attributable to the intervention. A common expectation is that health promotion will contribute to a reduction in morbidity and mortality. Yet any such effect is likely to be small, and may not appear for some years. The timing of an evaluation will affect what data can be collected and how confident we can be that the effects are due to the intervention. This is illustrated in the following learning activity.

Learning Activity 20.3 When to evaluate: Impact and outcomes of a cardiovascular disease reduction programme

A programme to reduce cardiovascular disease may have the following five effects.

1. Improves people's knowledge of the risk factors for coronary heart disease and stroke.
2. Increases people's motivation and intention to take up risk factor screening opportunities.
3. Persuades more people to attend screening clinics.
4. Increases media coverage of coronary heart disease and stroke.
5. Reduces premature mortality rate from cardiovascular disease.

Which of these outcomes could be evaluated immediately, after 6 months, after 12 months or after 5 years?

Impact is normally taken to be the immediate outcomes of an intervention or project. For example, a health promotion programme for secondary schools may include as the last session a review of the programme. Students may be invited to identify how they have changed since the programme began and how they think the programme will affect their future behaviour.

Outcome evaluation is more difficult, because it involves an assessment of longer-term effects. Using the same example given above, outcome evaluation

may be used to determine whether the programme did affect students' behaviour one year later. One way of ascertaining this would be to compare participants' health-related behaviour (e.g. relating to smoking, alcohol and exercise) before and after the programme, but there are bound to be changes in students' behaviour over one year, irrespective of any health promotion programme. So it would be better to compare the students to another group of similar students who did not receive the programme, to see if the same changes occur in both groups. The second or control group of students is necessary to avoid the danger of attributing all behaviour change to the health promotion programme and therefore overestimating its influence. Pre- and post-studies and experimental studies are the most reliable ways to determine effects.

Learning Activity 20.4 Outcome versus output: What is the difference?

What is the difference between an outcome and an output?

Outcome evaluation is more complex and costly than impact evaluation. Going back a year later to the same students and getting new information from them will take up time and resources, as will obtaining a matched group of students to use as the control group. However, despite these problems, outcome evaluation is often the preferred evaluation method because it measures sustained changes over time. Results using data on impact or outcome are often expressed numerically, and this again increases credibility. Quantitative or 'hard' data are seen as more concrete or factual than the 'soft' data used in process evaluation.

Evaluation research methodologies

Evaluation covers many different activities undertaken with varying degrees of rigour and reflectiveness. At its simplest level, evaluation describes what any competent practitioner does as a matter of course – that is, the process of appraising and assessing work activities, e.g. 'How did that consultation go?' or 'Did the patient understand what I said?' This includes the process of informal feedback or the reviewing of health promotion interventions. Evaluation also refers to a more formal or systematic activity where assessment is linked to intentions: evaluation may be of a defined project or intervention, or a series of interventions as part of a programme. Depending on what you want to know, evaluation may focus on:

- assessing effectiveness (e.g. RCTs, non-randomized designs, case control studies)
- understanding the change process – a process evaluation, generally using qualitative methods, can provide insight into why an intervention fails/works
- assessing cost-effectiveness – an economic evaluation using cost-benefit or cost-effectiveness analysis.

Learning Activity 20.5 Evaluation research methodologies

A hospital nurse has set up a project to help cardiac patients to stop smoking. The intervention involved the identification of a key worker who was allocated time to interview patients to assess their smoking behaviour and draw up individual plans. After discharge, patients were followed up by a weekly telephone call for 6 weeks. How could this project be evaluated so that any success in terms of smoking cessation in the target group could be shown to be due to the project? What would be the strengths and limitations of the methods you identify?

Evaluation is often more formally conducted as research using a variety of different methods. The classic scientific method of proof, the experiment, relies on controlling all factors apart from the one being studied, and can best be achieved under laboratory conditions. However, this is clearly impossible and unethical to achieve where people's health is concerned. The RCT is the next most rigorous scientific method of proof, and involves randomly allocating people to an intervention or control group. Random allocation means that the two groups should be matched in terms of factors such as age, gender and social class, which

are all known to affect health. Any changes detected in the intervention group are then compared to those found among the control group. Changes which occur in the intervention but not the control group can then be attributed to the health promotion programme.

In the well-man clinic example in Learning Activity 20.2, an RCT study would involve randomly allocating all men in the target group to either the intervention group (invited for screening) or the control group (not invited). The two groups would then be compared after the intervention had taken place. If the intervention group showed statistically significant improvements in health status or health-related behaviour over and above those recorded for the control group, the intervention would be deemed to be effective (Figure 20.1).

The degree of scientific rigour necessary to conduct an RCT is hard to achieve in real-life situations. Most health promotion programmes have spin-off effects, and indeed are designed to do so. It is impossible to isolate different groups of people or to ensure that programmes do not 'leak' beyond their set boundaries. However, the RCT design does mean that changes detected in the input group may be ascribed to the health promotion programme with a greater degree of confidence.

Evaluation research may also use qualitative methods to focus on understanding the processes involved in change. This kind of evaluation provides details on what is happening in interventions and which features have been effective. This is achieved through the use of qualitative methodologies and methods, and the case study is one example of this approach. The health promotion intervention is the 'case' that is intensively studied using a variety of methods. This enables the evaluator to get a detailed picture of how the intervention has affected the people involved. Case studies are typically small scale and findings are expressed in descriptive rather than numerical terms. Each case study is unique, and findings cannot be generalized to other situations. Its strength as a method is that there is a high degree of confidence that identified effects are real and result from the programme. In the well-man clinic example in Learning Activity 20.2, a qualitative case study approach might involve in-depth interviews with a sample of men who took up the screening opportunity and the practice nurse.

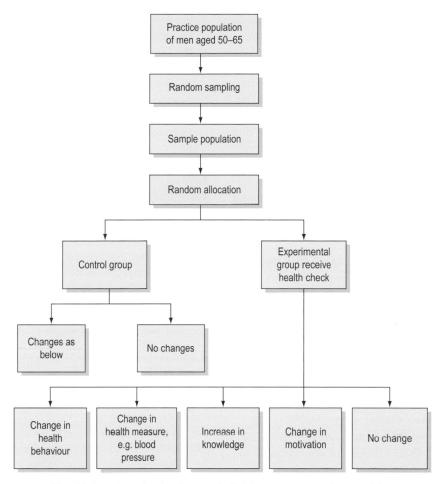

Fig. 20.1 • A randomized controlled trial to assess a well man clinic.

The interviews would aim to explore what motivated the men to accept the invitation to attend the clinic, how they found the experience and how (if at all) it has affected them.

Both the RCT and the case study are methods which can be used to investigate the effects of health promotion interventions. There are many other methods, e.g. surveys which aim to identify significant trends, and observational studies which track cohorts over time. In practice, methods often overlap or are combined. The RCT fits into a scientific, quantitative medical model of proof, has higher status and is generally regarded as more respectable and credible than the case study.

Evaluating complex interventions

Many health promotion interventions are complex, involving multiple stakeholders and many different programme components, and have an effect at individual, organizational, service or population level. Interventions may also be context specific, i.e. taking account of, and trying to use, specific features of the context. Community programmes such as SureStart are examples of complex interventions. The goals may include not just direct effects but triggering changes that will impact on the context and magnify the effects.

The use of scientific methods of evaluation, such as experimental trials, to evaluate such interventions is therefore inappropriate. Instead of screening out all factors apart from the intervention to identify if something 'works', evaluation of complex interventions seeks to unpack and examine the 'trigger' effects of the intervention. Pawson and Tilley (1997) describe this process as looking inside the black box to explore what is happening at the inputs/outcomes interface. Outcome and process evaluations need to take place together. Pawson and Tilley's (1997) realist approach to evaluation provides a means of doing this, and may be summarized as:

$$context + mechanisms \rightarrow outcomes$$

In other words, an evaluation seeks to understand the following.

- How does an intervention lead to the outcome, and what is the mechanism by which change is produced?
- What factors may account for why change takes place, and are there factors that may explain the intervention's differential effects?

The realist approach is one of the 'theory-driven' approaches to evaluation. It assumes evaluation follows the classic scientific methodology of beginning with hypotheses and then trying to use empirical evidence to support, falsify or choose between theories. There are five steps in the theory-of-change approaches to evaluation.

1. Identify long-term goals and the assumptions behind them.
2. Backwards mapping to reveal the necessary preconditions to achieve goals.
3. Identify the initiative's interventions that will lead to the desired changes.
4. Develop outcome measurement indicators to assess the initiative.
5. Write a narrative to explain the logic of the initiative.

As complex interventions are interventions that contain a number of components, so there are several dimensions of complexity in evaluating such programmes:

- the interactions between the components of the intervention/s

- the number of groups or organizational levels targeted by the intervention
- the number and variability of outcomes
- the degree of flexibility or tailoring of the intervention.

A good theory of change is, however, according to early work at the Aspen Institute, 'plausible, doable and testable' (Connell and Kubisch, 1998).

 ## Case Study 20.1 Realist evaluation

Realist evaluation is an approach that aims to find out the factors influencing outcomes and why an intervention works differently in different contexts (Pawson and Tilley, 1997). (Pawson explains realist evaluation at https://www.youtube.com/watch?v=xJSehOBa75I.) This is important, as it helps us understand how an intervention can be consistently replicated. A realist evaluation tries to understand what works, for whom, in what respects, to what extent, in what contexts and how? The evaluation's principal task is to extract and test the theories of change that describe how the intervention is expected to lead to its effects and what mechanisms will generate what outcomes. For a programme to 'work', it needs to operate successfully at a number of different levels.

So the evaluation of health education programmes, for example, would need to understand the following.

- Ideas – are the programme ideas persuasive, is the information fresh, interesting?
- Individuals – are the teachers/presenters effective; are the audience/students interested?
- Institution – programmes can be delivered in schools, colleges or prisons by tutorials, lectures, virtual learning environments or social media. Does the medium make a difference?
- Infrastructure – supposing that the subject has advanced in skills and learning, do the surrounding culture, economy and environment value the learning?

The evaluation design begins by formulating hypotheses about potential programme mechanisms. The next part of the design is to formulate hypotheses about the contexts that might make a difference to the action of the mechanisms. The different hypotheses make predictions on 'for whom and in what circumstance the programme will succeed (and fail)'.

Evaluating cost-effectiveness

Part of the reason for evaluation is to determine whether desired results were achieved in the most economical way and whether allocating resources to health promotion can be justified. There are many different ways of calculating the economic pluses and minuses of health promotion. Cost-benefit analysis is a way of calculating whether, and to what extent, something is worth doing. Cost-benefit analysis relies on pricing both the inputs and the benefits of a health promotion programme. An attempt is then made to calculate the cost of each benefit. This is known as a cost-benefit ratio. Putting a price on health outcomes or benefits is a very difficult exercise. One approach to this problem is to compare the cost-benefit ratio for a health promotion intervention with the cost-benefit ratio for some other health intervention. It is often assumed that prevention is cheaper than cure and that health promotion saves money, but this is not necessarily the case.

 Case Study 20.2 Cost-effectiveness of smoking cessation

The value-for-money tool (www.thensmc.com/resources/vfm) helps calculate the cost-effectiveness of social marketing and behaviour change programmes. Smoking cessation saves money by:

- not having to treat people with smoking-related diseases on the National Health Service
- not having to pay sickness benefit and disability pensions to people with smoking-related diseases
- increased production in industry because fewer employees are off sick.
  Other benefits that are less easy to cost include:
  - less exposure to second-hand smoke
  - the effect of smoking cessation on the uptake of smoking among children and young people.

Smoking cessation spends money by:

- paying retirement pensions to people who live longer
- paying unemployment benefits for people in the tobacco production and retail industries made unemployed due to a fall in demand
- loss of government revenue from tobacco taxation
- costs of pharmacotherapies.

Once a decision has been made to implement an intervention, economic analysis can help to determine the most efficient way of resourcing it. Efficiency refers to the maximum benefit that can be derived from the least cost. Cost-effectiveness is a comparison in monetary terms of different methods used to achieve the same outcomes. 'Cost-effectiveness analysis addresses *technical* efficiency in the sense that it can tell us the best way to do something but not whether or not that something is worth doing' (Cohen 2015, p. 393). Opportunity costs refer to what is sacrificed or foregone when resources are allocated to something, e.g. a health promotion project.

Economic appraisal is an important element in evaluation, because there are always competing claims for limited resources. Using economics to make health-related decisions might seem a distasteful idea, and people may shy away from attempts to put a value on people's health, well-being or life. But the reality is that people, societies and governments are constantly making choices and decisions that are influenced by economic considerations. It is therefore important to make the decision-making process transparent, and to include economic principles and concepts in evaluation studies. A review of evidence used to support the decisions made by the National Institute for Health and Care Effectiveness (NICE) found that the majority of public health interventions are highly cost-effective (Owen et al., 2012).

How to evaluate: The process of evaluation

In order to evaluate, decisions need to be taken about what information is needed and how it will be gathered. This needs to be done at the outset of an intervention, to ensure that relevant data are gathered at the appropriate time. There are several stages in an evaluation.

1. Describe the programme, and clarify aims and objectives.
2. Identify issues and questions of concern to all stakeholders.
3. Design the information-gathering process.
4. Collect the data.

5. Analyse the data.
6. Make recommendations.
7. Disseminate findings.
8. Take action.

Many commentators (Thorogood and Coombes, 2010; Morgan, 2006) have argued that the evaluation process should adhere to health promoting principles, i.e. evaluation should involve the participation of all stakeholders and be an empowering experience.

Evaluation therefore involves several key aspects that need to be considered. These aspects may be summarized as: what to measure; who evaluates; how to evaluate, including how to gather and analyse data; and what to do with the results, or putting the findings into practice. Each of these key aspects will now be considered.

What to measure

Deciding what to measure to assess the effects of health promotion is not easy. In theoretical terms, the many meanings and definitions of the concept 'health' result in a lack of consensus about how best to evaluate it. For those who subscribe to the medical model of health, data concerning morbidity, disability and mortality are appropriate measures to use for evaluation purposes. For those who adopt a more social model of health, a much broader range of measures (including, for example, measures of socio-economic status or the quality of the environment) will be appropriate. For people who have prioritized an educational approach, measures of knowledge and attitude change will be paramount.

The golden rule must be to measure the objectives set during the planning process (for more details on objectives, see Chapter 19 on programme planning). Although this sounds straightforward, in practice it can be difficult, and a surprising number of evaluation studies violate this principle. Different stakeholders might have different objectives, and the evaluation needs to take this into account. The objectives set may concern areas where there is a lack of consensus over appropriate measurement. For example, process objectives such as increased multiagency collaboration or increased community involvement are difficult to measure.

To collect relevant data would require a special effort because they are not measured routinely. Changes in people's attitudes or beliefs are particularly problematic to measure.

The success of a health promotion intervention is not solely about achieving behavioural changes or reductions in disease rates. For example, a needle-exchange scheme should not be judged solely by a reduction in the rate of human immunodeficiency virus (HIV) infection among drug users. Other markers of success, such as the take-up rate, are also important. In many cases, expecting a clear change in morbidity from a behaviour change would be unrealistic. Although there is a link between needle sharing and HIV infection, there are other risk factors, and expecting risk reduction from this initiative might be unwise.

As we saw in Chapter 19, by using a logic model you will have a theory of change which explains how and why a set of activities – be they part of a project or a comprehensive initiative/complex intervention – is expected to lead to early, intermediate and long-term outcomes over a specified period. The research evidence and knowledge from practitioners and participants will have informed the programme. For example, the evaluation of an antenatal education programme with the overall goal of preparing new parents for parenthood and giving children a good start in life will have a range of outcomes to measure.

- Short term: knowledge; behaviours during pregnancy, e.g. diet, smoking.
- Intermediate: birth outcomes, e.g. reduction in clinical interventions, birth weight, mood.
- Longer term: reduction in postnatal depression, cognitive development and later educational achievement.

The logic model will:

- make explicit hypothesized links between determinants of health and health outcomes, such as whether knowledge about pain during childbirth is associated with less use of pain relief or whether preparation for parenthood is associated with greater parental input in early childhood such as reading, leading to educational achievement
- examine theoretical plausibility and mechanisms of action of an intervention

- identify key effect mediators or moderators, such as the capability of the person delivering the antenatal education
- specify intermediate outcomes and potential harms, including differential effects among population subgroups and, in this example, the potential difference in take-up.

A programme may have several different objectives, some of which are easier to measure than others. It then becomes tempting to measure the easiest objectives and extrapolate from these findings. But if the measurements are of different classes of events (e.g. combining behavioural, environmental and attitudinal objectives), it is not legitimate to do this.

 Learning Activity 20.6 Indicators of success

A programme has been launched with the objective of reducing child accidents. Key stakeholders include community and hospital-based health practitioners, community groups (parents' and neighbourhood groups) and local authority staff, including environmental health officers and health and safety officers. Various indicators have been suggested as suitable means of evaluating the programme:

- take-up of campaign literature
- campaign awareness
- sales of child-safety equipment
  - making changes to the home environment to improve safety, e.g. installing stair gates
  - making changes to the local environment, e.g. traffic-calming measures
- reduction in the number of accidents to children
- reduction in the number of severe accidents to children that require hospitalization.

For each indicator discuss the following.
Is it appropriate?
Is it feasible?
Who would measure it?

A balance needs to be struck between setting the threshold for success too high, leading to interventions that are unjustly deemed to be ineffective, and setting the threshold too low, leading to a judgement that health promotion is not worth the effort.

Striking the correct balance involves knowing what changes are likely to take place in the absence of the intervention, and then setting a realistic goal of what additional change is feasible and represents an efficient use of resources.

 Learning Activity 20.7 What constitutes evidence of success?

A smoking-cessation programme is launched which includes clinics for those wishing to give up smoking. A clinic run by a health promoter attracts 20 clients who attend all six sessions. At a six-month evaluation, 25 percent of the participants have stopped smoking. Is this success?

When to evaluate

The first challenge is the timing of an evaluation, as this can affect its results. If an evaluation is seeking to determine the outcomes of an intervention, a longer timescale is desirable. However, this has problems. Health promotion is a long-term process and contexts and settings are constantly changing, so it can be difficult to be sure that any changes detected are due to the health promotion input, and not to any other factor. Health-related knowledge, attitudes and behaviour are constantly changing, regardless of health promotion programmes. Societies and environments are also changing in response to many different factors. One solution to this problem might be to evaluate sooner and use a shorter timescale; but to do so might mean that longer-term sustained outcomes are missed. The best solution is to evaluate over different time periods, but this requires more resources.

Who evaluates

Success means different things to different groups of people, or stakeholders, all of whom have their own agendas and interests. Different stakeholders have unequal power to impose their evaluation agendas on others. Different groups of people engaged in health promotion interventions will each have invested something, but may well be looking for different results. For example, funders of a project may be looking for efficiency or results which can be interpreted as cost-effective. Practitioners may be looking for evidence that their way of working is acceptable to clients and achieves the objectives set. Managers may be looking for evidence of increased productivity, measured by performance indicators. Clients may be looking for opportunities to take control over some health-related aspects of their lives. It is therefore important to be clear at the outset about whose perspectives are being addressed in any evaluation. A starting point is simply to acknowledge that different vested interests are involved, and try to identify them. The ideal is then to go on to represent the views of the different stakeholders by collecting data from each group. This process is called pluralistic evaluation (Smith and Cantley, 1985). Using the process of methodological triangulation, which employs a wide range of data sources, an overall picture may be built up. Pluralistic evaluation which takes into account different stakeholders' views is more complete, although the findings may be complex and lack clarity. Pluralistic evaluation is a means of building capacity and empowering clients and service users as well as practitioners. In practice, pluralistic evaluation may appear too complex and costly, and evaluation is often carried out by external researchers or insider practitioners. The former tend to be larger scale in remit and potentially more objective.

 Learning Activity 20.8 Insider or external evaluation?

A dental health project has been launched, and needs to be evaluated. There are two choices, either an 'in-house' evaluation conducted by the people involved in running the project, or an external evaluation conducted by outside researchers. What are the pros and cons of each option?

How to evaluate: Gathering and analysing data

The process of evaluation involves making decisions about what methods to use to gather and analyse relevant data. Each of these stages is discussed separately.

Gathering data

Practical difficulties arise when trying to obtain data and to combine different forms of data to provide an overall picture. Some relevant data are already available and accessible, for example on morbidity and mortality. Others already exist and may be obtained, for example policy documents or health surveillance data. However, some data will need to be collected and, particularly in areas such as attitude change or empowerment, there are no easy or accepted means of doing this.

A wide range of data, both qualitative and quantitative, may be used in evaluation studies. Guiding principles when selecting methods of data collection are to use appropriate and feasible tools. 'Appropriate' means gathering data that will help meet the objectives of the evaluation. 'Feasible' means gathering data within budgetary and time constraints (see Learning Activity 20.6). Process evaluation often uses qualitative data, whereas outcome evaluation is more likely to use quantitative data. However, both forms of data may be applicable in various ways at different times.

The medical model of research dominant within healthcare settings prioritizes the RCT as the most rigorous form of quantitative methodology. However, as we have seen in this chapter, RCTs may be inappropriate for evaluating health promotion interventions, where the context is an important and acknowledged element. RCTs may also be misleading and unnecessarily expensive (Morgan, 2006). The call for evaluation to be a health promoting process in itself also mitigates against the use of specialist quantitative methodologies such as RCTs. For participation in an evaluation to be empowering, stakeholders need to be able to understand, contribute to and oversee the process.

Evaluation seeks to assess process and effect, and it is therefore vital to have baseline data to use for comparison purposes. Unless baseline data are collected, it will be impossible to state that impacts or outcomes are due to the intervention. Planning needs to take account of this, and allocate sufficient resources to allow for the collection of pre- and post-intervention data.

Analysing the data

There are various ways of analysing data, depending on whether the data are quantitative or qualitative, what kind of intervention or study was carried out and what resources and expertise are available. There are many excellent textbooks that discuss data analysis in depth (e.g. Bowling, 2014), and the reader is referred to these for a more detailed discussion of methods. However, data analysis is not just a question of methodological awareness and expertise. Values also impact on data analysis processes. The assumption is that faced with a certain set of findings, everyone would agree on their significance or meaning, but this is not necessarily the case. There may also be dispute about which findings are relevant or significant. Data analysis should be an inclusive and capacity-building exercise for all participants, enabling everyone to have a say about what data are significant and why.

Building an evidence base for health promotion

Evaluation helps build a basis of research to demonstrate which health promotion interventions succeed in meeting objectives and how they should be implemented. Evaluation therefore identifies effective health promotion practice which others can adopt.

Evidence-based health promotion has been defined as 'a public health endeavour in which there is an informed, explicit, and judicious use of evidence that has been derived from any of a variety of science and social science research and evaluation methods' (Rychetnik et al., 2004). Although this suggests that any research evidence would be used, there are accepted levels of evidence referring to a hierarchy of study designs that have been grouped according to their susceptibility to bias, as illustrated in Table 20.1. The hierarchy indicates which studies should be given most weight in an evaluation where the same question has been examined using different types of study. Because evidence-based practice is concerned with questions about the effectiveness of interventions, it suggests that some research designs are more valid and reliable than others in demonstrating this. The hierarchy of evidence thus privileges the RCT because it can show that an intervention causes an effect. It is therefore known as the 'gold standard'. This view about what counts as evidence excludes qualitative research designs which provide understanding of the attitudes, beliefs, behaviours and contextual issues which influence whether and how public health interventions should be implemented.

Evidence-based practice is firmly established in medicine and nursing, where RCTs of alternative treatment protocols are used to establish which form of treatment is most effective for most people. In health promotion, creating evidence-based practice is more problematic.

Table 20.1 Hierarchy of evidence

Level	Description	Example
One	Strong evidence from at least one systematic review of well-designed RCTs	Meta-analyses
Two	Evidence from at least one properly designed RCT of appropriate size	Articles in peer-reviewed journals
Three	Evidence from well-designed trials without randomization: cohort, time series or matched-case controlled studies	Articles in peer-reviewed journals
Four	Evidence from well-designed non-experimental studies from more than one centre or research group	Articles in peer-reviewed journals
Five	Opinions from respected authorities, based on clinical evidence, descriptive studies or reports from committees	NICE guidelines Evidence-based local guidelines, procedures and care pathways Government committees
Six	Opinions from colleagues	Colleagues, peers, local reports

Learning Activity 20.9 Evidence-based health promotion

Why might it be difficult to establish evidence-based health promotion practice?

Predictability, repeatability and falsifiability are the criteria by which results are assessed in evidence from medicine, and these are based on widely recognized scientific principles. Predictability is said to be met when a properly implemented intervention will bring about an expected outcome every time. Repeatability, sometimes referred to as replicability, means the intervention can be repeated and achieve the same results wherever and whenever it is carried out. To be falsifiable, the intervention must be capable of being disproved as an effective intervention. Once implemented, the intervention is validated if rigorous evaluation research demonstrates that it works, and is falsified if it is shown to be ineffective or harmful. As we have seen in this chapter, such conditions are almost impossible in the real world and, as realist evaluation approaches show, context will be key to influencing outcomes.

In biomedical sciences it is easier to show that if x (the exposure/intervention) precedes y (the effect) and there is a statistical association between x and y, and if a reduction of x will lead to a reduction of y and there is not a z confounding the association, then causation is imputed. Health promotion operates in an environment where numerous cultural, social, economic and political factors interact. Given a complex context where the links among the elements of an intervention are interrelated, causality, more often than not, cannot be directly established.

This does not mean that there is no evidence on which to base health promotion work. Meta-analyses or systematic reviews of research studies pool together findings from different studies in effectiveness reviews. Effectiveness reviews are a means of building up a knowledge base which can tell us what are reasonable expectations of success in health promotion. For example, the EPPI Centre's systematic review on children and healthy eating (Thomas et al., 2003) sought to answer the following questions.

1. Which interventions to promote healthy eating among children aged four to ten are effective for increasing fruit and vegetable intake?
2. Which barriers do they target, and which facilitators do they build on?
3. What experiences/ideas do children and their parents have about what helps or stops them from eating fruit and vegetables?
4. To what extent do interventions build on these experiences/ideas?

An independent national body in the UK, NICE, is devoted to providing evidence-based guidance on the promotion of good health and the prevention and treatment of ill health. NICE publications include guides on a range of interventions to promote health, from preventing harmful drinking (PH 24) to community engagement (PH 9) and domestic violence and abuse (PH 50) (https://www.nice.org.uk/guidance/published?type=ph).

Learning Activity 20.10 Certainty and uncertainty

Think of an intervention that you have developed or implemented. How confident were you that you were right?

Often decisions are made even when we are not certain or sure of the outcomes. We may believe something to be true but may not know, and these are the assumptions that the logic models discussed in Chapter 19 are supposed to highlight. Figure 20.2 illustrates this, showing how confidence and certainty impact on decision-making and how their absence means much of what we do may be just muddling through.

Learning Activity 20.11 In the absence of evidence

Should an intervention not be undertaken if there is no evidence base to support it?

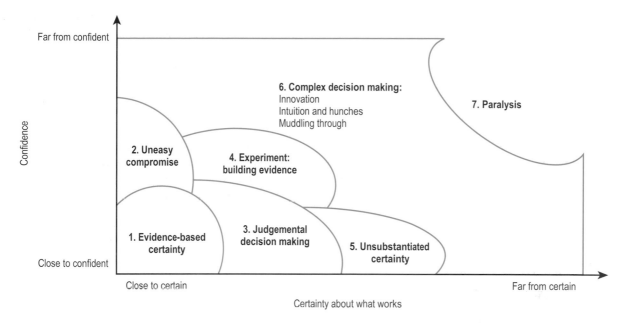

1. There is evidence clearly linking actions to outcomes, e.g. guidelines
2. There is some evidence but disagreement or lack of evidence as to its acceptability or applicability
3. There is a lack of certainty about the effect of actions and a lack of evidence
4. There is confident decision-making based on theoretical plausibility and assumptions but no evidence
5. We need to be seen to be doing something!
6. The majority of decisions are made here – a lack of evidence so decisions are made based on other considerations
7. Nothing is done because there is no evidence

Fig. 20.2 ● Certainty and uncertainty. (Stacey, R.D., 2002. Strategic Management and Organisational Dynamics: The Challenge of Complexity, third ed. Prentice Hall, Harlow.)

Being evidence-informed is challenging for practitioners for many reasons.

- There may be such a range of questions before a decision can be made that it is hard to find evidence that is relevant.
- Pertinent evidence about a programme or intervention may not be available.
- The information may be difficult to get hold of, as it is published in academic journals which may not be widely read.
- Information may be difficult to interpret, or poorly reported so that it provides very little detail.
- There may be just too much information.
- There may be differences of opinion.
- Information may be contradictory, with published research differing from the experiences of practitioners.

This chapter has advocated the importance of evaluating what we do to provide 'proof' of making a difference, and to make decisions explicit and transparent. But it has also shown how logic and theory can provide plausible explanations of what might work alongside existing evidence. Simply relying on existing evidence has limitations:

- it can be restrictive, devaluing expert opinion and ignoring the context
- the scientific model demands good-quality (well-reported) studies, not necessarily good-quality interventions
- the scientific model relies on the experiment to demonstrate effectiveness, but there are other considerations for health promoting interventions, such as efficiency, acceptability, quality and equity.

What to do with the evaluation: Putting the findings into practice

Dissemination of findings is important to publicize good practice and also to flag up interventions that were not as successful as had been anticipated. Knowing what does not work is as valuable as knowing what does, but there is a great emphasis on producing and publicizing positive results. As Hawe et al. (1994) state: 'Sometimes to avoid "failure", health promoters may avoid evaluation... At any one time many of the current initiatives may turn out to be those that fail to produce intended results. There is no shame in this... Stigma should not be attached to programmes that fail, only to those programmes that fail to learn from these experiences or to those programmes that fail to evaluate.'

Putting findings into practice can take many forms. The results of evaluation should ideally feed into an ongoing cycle of action and reflection, allowing more knowledgeable and reasoned interventions to take place. Evaluation may also enable stakeholders to progress activities and gain more support to do so. Evaluation helps to establish the cost-effectiveness of health promotion and contributes towards its evidence base.

Numerous studies of knowledge translation (e.g. Clar et al., 2011) cite difficulties in getting evidence into practice:

- lack of time
- lack of availability of research results
- information overload and lack of comprehensibility
- lack of relevance.
  So policymakers and practitioners rely on:
- single studies
- experts
- policy statements.

Making research and evaluation findings more accessible to policymakers, increasing opportunities for interaction between policymakers and researchers, addressing structural barriers such as research receptivity in policy agencies and a lack of incentives for academics to link with policy, and increasing the relevance of research to policy are all ways in which there can be greater synergy between research, evaluation and practice.

Conclusion

Evaluation contributes to the accountability and development of evidence-based health promotion practice, and so is an important aspect of the health promoter's work. This involves evaluating health promotion activity with which you are involved. The purpose of an evaluation is to know what works and to understand the nature of the change/outcomes. There are often pressures to adopt unrealistic measures of success, such as reduced mortality rates or demonstrable cost benefits. Most health promoters are engaged in more modest activities which seek to achieve changes in knowledge, behaviour, attitudes, service take-up or the policy process. These are more appropriate outcomes to use for evaluation purposes.

Evaluation is a practical activity which feeds into the theoretical debate about the nature and purpose of health promotion. This debate cannot be confined to professionals, or those who hold managerial or financial power. It must include the public, who are the targets of health promotion activity. This is why pluralistic evaluation, which enables participants to have a voice in determining effectiveness, is so important.

Evaluation is not a simple activity, and it consumes resources which might otherwise be spent on doing health promotion. The decisions about whether, when and how to evaluate are therefore important. The question of evaluation should be considered at the outset of any planned health promotion intervention. If it is to be done, it should be done in the best possible way. If this is not feasible, then it is better to admit the impossible and not attempt to evaluate. Ongoing monitoring may be the best one can do. This is acceptable, but there is a distinction between routine monitoring of activities through the use of performance indicators and a more thoroughgoing evaluation. It is important not to confuse the two, and to be clear about which it is you are doing.

Question for further discussion

- Think of a health promotion activity you have undertaken. What factors would you wish to consider in its evaluation?

Summary

This chapter has looked at how evaluation is defined, the different kinds of research methodologies used in evaluation research and why health promotion needs to be evaluated. Different kinds of evaluation have been identified, including process, impact, outcome and whole-systems evaluation. The process of evaluation, including principles and stages, has been outlined. The importance of demonstrating the cost-effectiveness of health promotion and the role of evaluation in building an evidence base for health promotion have been discussed.

Further reading and resources

Douglas, J., Sidell, M., Lloyd, C., Earle, S., 2007. Evaluating public health interventions. Ch. 11. In: Earle, S., Lloyd, C.E., Sidell, M., Spurr, S. (Eds.), Theory and Research in Promoting Public Health. Sage Open University, London, pp. 327–354. *A succinct chapter that includes a detailed discussion of how evaluation criteria can be to public health and health promotion interventions.*

Green, J., South, J., 2006. Evaluation. Open University Press, Maidenhead. *A very readable account of the theoretical underpinnings of evaluation and the practicalities of doing evaluation. The real-life challenges and complexities of evaluation are discussed in depth.*

Rootman, I., Goodstadt, M., Hyndman, B., McQueen, D.V., Potvin, L., Springett, J., Ziglio, E. (Eds.), 2001. Evaluation in Health Promtoion: Principles and Perspectives. WHO, Denmark. Available online at: http://www.euro.who.int/__data/assets/pdf_file/0007/108934/E73455.pdf (accessed 18.03.15). *A very thorough and comprehensive account of the theoretical and methodological issues relating to the evaluation of health promotion interventions.*

Thorogood, M., Coombes, Y. (Eds.), 2010. Evaluating Health Promotion. Practices and Methods, third ed. Oxford University Press, Oxford. *A useful guide that helps to explore the processes of implementation and evaluation methods.*

NICE produces guidance documents and effectiveness reviews on a variety of topics, including public health and health promotion issues such as obesity and nutrition, exercise and smoking cessation: www.nice.org.uk.

👍👎 Feedback on learning activities

20.1 Evaluation is an important part of a project or programme. It allows progress to be tracked and implementation issues to be identified, helps to identify whether or not the project was worth doing and enables adaptive management during a project. Evaluation provides accountability to the funders of a project, and also contributes to ongoing learning about why things do or do not work in practice.

20.2 There are many different ways of evaluating the well-man clinic. Monitoring lifestyle behaviours over a period of time could establish whether or not the clinic led to a reduction in unhealthy behaviours. This would be costly, and it would be difficult to follow up the participants. Monitoring vital statistics regularly could establish whether or not health improvements were being made. Monitoring of before and after data might also provide an incentive to maintain healthy changes to lifestyles. Recording the cost of providing the clinic and costing the health improvements

gained, possibly using a value-for-money tool (www.thensmc.com/resources/vfm), could provide data about the cost-effectiveness of the intervention. Noting how the sessions have been received by the men, or soliciting their comments or those of peers and colleagues, is part of the evaluation process. Asking the men what they wanted from participating in the programme and whether they achieved their goals would be a participatory form of evaluation. Comparing the socio-economic status of participants and non-participants would help determine if the programme was reinforcing or challenging social and health inequalities.

20.3 An immediate post-programme evaluation may identify the first and second effects, or the impact of the intervention. The third and fourth effects may only be apparent at a later evaluation, e.g. after six months, and are called outcomes. Twelve months after the programme, the increased attendance at screening clinics may no longer be discernible and

Continued

attendance figures may have reverted to pre-programme levels. A reduction in the mortality rate may not be discernible for five years or more, by which time it will be difficult to attribute it to the health promotion programme. The assessment of the overall success or failure of a programme is therefore influenced by the timing of the evaluation, which in turn is influenced by the amount of funding available. Longer-term evaluation tends to be more expensive, while immediate evaluation costs may be absorbed within programme budgets.

20.4 Outputs are the activities undertaken as part of the intervention or programme (e.g. how many pregnant women attend a smoking-cessation clinic). Outcomes are the changes as a result of an intervention or programme (e.g. the outcome of the programme will be to increase the number of tobacco-free pregnant women).

20.5 An RCT would involve each smoking patient on arrival in the ward being randomly allocated to either the experimental group (who receive the interview) or the control group (who do not receive the interview but get a care plan and general leaflet). Differences in the success rates of the two groups could be attributed to the interview intervention. This evaluation method is scientific and rigorous.

Case study evaluation would interview patients about their involvement in the project and examine their knowledge, attitudes and reported behaviour. This evaluation method is qualitative and less rigorous, but more insightful regarding the process of involvement in the project.

20.6

	Appropriateness	Feasibility	Who would measure it
Take-up of campaign literature	No direct link to a reduction in child accidents	Yes	Campaign staff or staff located in venues offering campaign literature, e.g. health visitors
Sales of child-safety equipment	Yes, but also affected by income so does not reflect equity	Yes	Producers or sellers of child-safety equipment
Changes to the home environment, e.g. stair gates	Yes	Uncertain	Health visitors might be able to monitor changes for under-five-year-olds
Changes to the local environment, e.g. traffic-calming measures	Yes	Yes	Environmental health officers or local traffic staff
Reduction in the number of accidents to children	Yes	Minor accidents are not routinely recorded or reported	Health visitors or hospital staff could monitor changes in the number of serious accidents to children
Reduction in the number of accidents requiring hospitalization	Yes	Yes	Hospital staff

20.7 The health promoter may be pleased with these results. People attend clinics often as a last resort, and 6 months is a reasonable time period to assess long-term behaviour change. However, the health promoter's manager may point out that 20 percent is an average success rate for people trying to quit, regardless of what methods are used. Clinics are time-consuming and 20 people is not a large group: 25 percent being quitters means five people, four of whom might have quit using other less intensive or expensive methods. So one additional ex-smoker might be the result of the smoking-cessation clinic.

20.8

Insider evaluation

Pros	Knows background to project
	Cheaper
	Acceptable to everyone
Cons	Too involved in project
	No research expertise
	Biased to prove success

Outside evaluation

Pros	Unbiased attitude
	Research expertise
	Fresh perspective
Cons	Expensive
	May appear threatening
	Unfamiliar with project

20.9 There are several reasons why proving that an evidence base exists for health promotion is problematic. These include knowing when to evaluate, knowing what constitutes success, being able to attribute results to interventions and the inappropriateness of using RCTs.

20.10 Although we talk of evidence-based practice, often interventions are implemented in the absence of evidence. In our companion book, *Developing Practice in Health Promotion* (Naidoo and Wills, 2010), Chapter 3 discusses the challenges of evidence-based practice for health promotion and describes how any decision about what to do is made up of a balanced consideration of:
- what we know (evidence)
- what we think might plausibly work (theory)
- what we think we ought to do (principle)
- what we think we can do (resources).

20.11 Where it is available, external evidence can inform, but can never replace, the expertise of individual practitioners. It is this expertise that decides whether the external evidence is applied to the target group of an intervention at all, and, if so, how it should be used for achieving effectiveness. In other words, for an effective intervention, other critical areas in addition to evidence need to be taken into consideration – for example, the needs and expectations of direct service recipients, the interests of other key stakeholders and the competency of a practitioner in planning and evaluation. More confidence in decision-making may come from the decision being evidence based, and knowing that what you do is based on sound and robust research.

But practitioners can also feel more confident and secure in their decisions if they believe that the values underpinning the intervention are just, and a cognitive processing of theory suggests that the intervention 'makes sense' – that it should plausibly work.

References

Bowling, A., 2014. Research Methods in Health: Investigating Health and Health Services, fourth ed. Open University, Maidenhead.

Clar, C., et al., 2011. What are the effects of interventions to improve the uptake of evidence from health research into policy in low and middle-income countries? Systematic Review. Dfid, UK. Available online at: http://r4d.dfid.gov.uk/PDF/Outputs/SystematicReviews/SR_EvidenceIntoPolicy_Graham_May2011_MinorEditsJuly2011.pdf (accessed 17.03.15).

Cohen, D., 2015. Health economics. In: Naidoo, J., Wills, J. (Eds.), Health Studies: An Introduction, third ed. Palgrave Macmillan, Basingstoke, pp. 378–399.

Connell, J.P., Kubisch, A.C., 1998. Applying a theory of change approach to the evaluation of comprehensive community initiatives: progress, prospects and problems. In: Fulbright-Anderson, K., Kubisch, A.C., Connell, J.P. (Eds.), New Approaches to Evaluating Community Initiatives Vol. 2: Theory, Measurement and Analysis. Aspen Institute, Washington DC. Available online at: http://www.dmeforpeace.org/sites/default/files/080713%20Applying%2BTheory%2Bof%2BChange%2BApproach.pdf (accessed 17.03.15).

Green, J., South, J., 2006. Evaluation. Open University Press, Maidenhead.

Hawe, P., Degeling, D., Hall, J., 1994. Evaluating Health Promotion: A Health Worker's Guide. Maclennan and Petty, Sydney.

Morgan, A., 2006. Evaluation of health promotion (Chapter 14). In: Davies, M., Macdowall, W. (Eds.), Health Promotion Theory. Open University Press, pp. 169–187.

Naidoo, J., Wills, J., 2010. Public Health and Health Promotion: Developing Practice, third ed. Baillière Tindall, London.

Nutbeam, D., 1998. Evaluating health promotion – progress, problems and solutions. Health Promotion International 13 (1), 27–44. Available online at: http://heapro.oxfordjournals.org/content/13/1/27.full.pdf+html (accessed 22.09.15).

Owen, L., Morgan, A., Fischer, A., Ellis, S., Hoy, A., Kelly, M., 2012. The cost effectiveness of public health interventions. Journal of Public Health 34 (1), 37–45. Available online at: http://jpubhealth.oxfordjournals.org/content/34/1/37.full.pdf+html (accessed 23.09.15).

Pawson, R., Tilley, N., 1997. Realistic Evaluation. Sage, London.

Rootman, I., Goodstadt, M., Hyndman, B., McQueen, D.V., Potvin, L., Springett, J., Ziglio, E. (Eds.), 2001. Evaluation in Health Promotion: Principles and Perspectives. WHO, Denmark. Available online at: http://www.euro.who.int/__data/assets/pdf_file/0007/108934/E73455.pdf (accessed 18.03.15).

Rychetnik, L., Hawe, P., Waters, E., Barratt, A., Frommer, M., 2004. A glossary for evidence based public health. Journal of Epidemiology and Community Health 58, 538–545. Available online at: http://jech.bmj.com/content/58/7/538.full.pdf+html (accessed 23.09.15).

Smith, G., Cantley, C., 1985. Assessing Health Care: A Study in Organisational Evaluation. Open University Press, Milton Keynes.

Springett, J., 2001. Appropriate approaches to the evaluation of health promotion. Critical Public Health 11 (2), 139–152.

Stacey, R.D., 2002. Strategic Management and Organisational Dynamics: The Challenge of Complexity, third ed. Prentice Hall, Harlow.

Thomas, J., Sutcliffe, K., Harden, A., Oakley, A., Oliver, S., Rees, R., Brunton, G., Kavanagh, J., 2003. Children and Healthy Eating: A Systematic Review of Barriers and Facilitators. EPPI-Centre, Social Science Research Unit, Institute of Education, University of London, London. Available online at: http://eppi.ioe.ac.uk/EPPIWebContent/hp/reports/healthy_eating02/Final_report_web.pdf (accessed 18.03.15).

Thorogood, M., Coombes, Y., 2010. Evaluating Health Promotion: Practices and Methods, third ed. Oxford University Press.

Glossary

Acceptability: Adequacy to satisfy a need, requirement or standard.

Advocacy: The combined efforts of individuals and groups to gain political, social or organizational support for a specific health programme or goal.

Aims: Broad goals or statement of what is to be achieved.

Attitudes: How a person feels about something, including affective and cognitive components.

Autonomy: A person's ability to be independent and free and make his or her own decisions.

Behaviour change: Purposeful changes in behaviour and activity that individuals make to promote, maintain and protect their health.

Beneficence (doing good): Actions taken to benefit and help other people.

Biomedicine: A discipline that focuses on the causes of ill health and disease within the physical body; it is associated with the practice of medicine and contrasts with a social model of health.

Brief intervention: A short, time-limited intervention to raise awareness of, and assess, a person's willingness to address a lifestyle issue.

Capacity building: Developing sustainable skills, structures, resources and policies to embed and multiply health gains.

Collaboration: Working together towards agreed goals; usually refers to different agencies working together to achieve a synergistic effect (intersectoral collaboration).

Communication: Use of media, mass media, multimedia, social media and new technologies to raise awareness and convey information and messages about health issues.

Community: A group of people with a shared culture, values and norms; people may belong to several different communities focused around different aspects of life, e.g. workplace, neighbourhood, faith or leisure interests.

Community action: Campaigns and activities undertaken collectively by people who identify themselves as a community in terms of geography or shared interests.

Community development: Action taken to develop community infrastructures and capacity to articulate and meet needs.

Community profile: A representation (written or graphical) of information regarding the characteristics of a place or community.

Contingency plan: A plan for an organization to respond coherently to an unusual event.

Cost effectiveness: Economical in terms of the money spent for goods or services received.

Curriculum: Lessons and academic content taught in a school or in a specific course or programme.

Determinants of health: Factors that have an impact on health status, including personal, social, economic and environmental factors (see social determinants of health).

Disease: An objective malfunctioning of some part of the body, detectable through medical testing and monitoring.

Disease prevention: Measures taken to prevent disease or slow its progress, e.g. reducing known risk factors, screening or pre-symptomatic intervention.

Employer: A person or business that employs one or more people and in return gives that person or people wages or a salary.

Empowerment: A process of gaining greater control over the decisions and actions that affect one's health; this involves developing skills and confidence, articulating needs and strategies, and taking action to meet needs.

Enablement: Taking action through partnerships to mobilize resources for health.

Epidemiology: Scientific study of the distribution and causes of health and disease in defined populations.

Equity: Fairness in the distribution of resources for health on the basis of needs.

Ethics: A branch of philosophy that focuses on defining moral principles and what concepts and behaviours are morally right or wrong.

Evaluation: Assessment of the worth or value of something.

Evidence-based practice: Practice based on the best available current, valid and relevant evidence derived from formal research and systematic investigation into the causes of health and ill health and the impact of interventions.

Globalization: Worldwide connections and networks of people and organizations that span national, geographic and cultural borders and boundaries.

Government: The group of people with the authority to govern a state or country.

Health: Defined by the World Health Organization as a positive concept emphasizing social and personal resources as well as physical capabilities.

Health behaviour: Action purposefully taken by individuals to promote, protect or maintain their health.

Health education: Communication of health-related information and development of the attitudes, skills and confidence necessary to enable people to take action to improve their health.

Health impact assessment (HIA): A systematic process designed to assess the impact of an intervention or policy on the health of a defined population.

Health in all Policies (HiaP): A commitment since 2006 that all policies across different sectors will systematically take into account the health implications of decisions.

Health inequalities: Avoidable and unfair differences in health status between groups of people who share the same socio-economic status or gender.

Health literacy: The cognitive ability, personal skills and motivation to access, understand and use health information to promote health.

Health needs assessment (HNA): An assessment of a population to determine if and how their health can be improved.

Health promotion: A broader concept than health education, encompassing not just individual action but also social, political and environmental action to change the determinants of health and thereby improve health; it is the process of enabling people to increase their control over, and improve, their health.

Health-promoting hospital: A hospital which not only provides medical care but also seeks to develop its health-promoting capacity, including its organizational structure and identity, active participation of staff and patients, its physical environment and its role within the community.

Health-promoting school: A school that constantly strengthens its capacity as a healthy setting for living, learning and working, and seeks to provide a healthy environment that engages all parties (children, parents, teachers, communities).

Health protection: Social, organizational, fiscal or legal measures taken to prevent disease and protect the health of individuals and communities; may refer to actions to control communicable diseases.

Health psychology: A discipline that seeks to understand the psychological and behavioural processes in health, illness and healthcare.

Health system: All public and private organizations, institutions and resources needed to improve, maintain and restore health.

Healthy pharmacy: A pharmacy which not only provides pharmaceutical services but also proactive health advice and interventions within the community it serves.

Healthy prison: A prison in which the staff, ethos and regime of the environment build up and reinforce the health and well-being of prisoners.

Healthy public policy (HPP): A policy that has a clear concern for health, well-being and equity; also used to describe the role of government in creating the conditions that support health.

Ideology: A set of ideas or beliefs which underlies and justifies the actions of governments, corporations or religious groups, or attempts to undermine these entities.

Ill health: A state of poor health when there is some disease or impairment, but not usually serious enough to curtail all activities.

Illness: The subjective state of being unwell and unable to function normally; illness may or may not coexist with disease.

Impact: The immediate effect of a force, intervention or event.

Indicator: Health indicators are quantifiable characteristics of a population (e.g. life expectancy) which may be used to justify public health interventions.

Inequalities: Variations that are not fair or just.

Inequity: A lack of equity or fairness.

Integrated care: Joined-up care across health and social care boundaries.

Life skills: Personal cognitive, social and physical skills that enable people to control and direct their lives.

Lifestyles: The pattern of personal behaviours adopted by people as a result of the interplay of individual, social, economic and environmental living conditions.

Locus of control: A person's belief in the control s/he has over her/his life.

Media advocacy: Use of media to promote a policy change.

Mediation: Health promotion cannot be achieved by the health sector alone, so its success will depend on mediation between all sectors of government as well as independent organizations (media, industry, etc.).

Medical model: A model of health based on scientific medicine, encompassing positivist methodologies and concepts of health and sickness rooted in physical changes that can be measured and quantified.

Medium/media: A channel of communication, e.g. social media.

Message: What is being communicated.

Milestones: Key events with dates that mark progress.

Model: A simplified description or graphic representation of reality (processes, organizations, beings); models are often used to hypothesize the outcomes of specific inputs or processes.

Morality: Principles and beliefs about what is right and wrong, or good and bad behaviour.

Morbidity: The incidence of disease or illness in a specified population.

Mortality: The number of deaths at a given time and location; the mortality or death rate is typically expressed as the number of deaths per 1000 individuals per year.

Motivational interviewing: Counselling technique used to assess motivation to change.

Need: Something which is required or essential rather than merely desired or wanted.

Needs assessment: A systematic process to identify needs or the gap between existing and desired conditions.

Neighbourhood: A geographically defined community within a larger area (city, town, suburb or rural area); there is often a high level of social interaction and networking between people in a neighbourhood.

Neoliberal: An economic or political approach that favours the free market and deregulation.

Non-maleficence (doing no harm): Actions that are not intended to harm other people.

Objectives: Specific activities or goals that need to be achieved for an intervention or project to achieve its aims.

Ottawa Charter: Charter produced by the first seminal World Health Organization conference on health promotion in 1986, outlining core health-promoting areas for action (developing personal skills, strengthening communities, reorienting services, building healthy public policy and creating supportive environments) and strategies (enablement, mediation and advocacy) that are still widely cited and used today.

Outcomes: Changes in the health status of individuals, groups or societies that are attributable to planned health promotion interventions, policies or services.

Outputs: What is done or produced.

Participation: The active involvement of people in interventions, research or evaluation, enabling people's views and opinions to be heard, valued and integrated into action and leading to feelings of ownership and commitment.

Personal skills: Individuals' knowledge, attitudes, skills and feelings of self-efficacy that enable them to take action.

Personal, social, health and economic (PSHE): Educational provision introduced as part of the UK schools' national curriculum in 2000; PSHE promotes healthy living by providing young people with knowledge, understanding, attitudes and practical skills.

Place-based approach: The bringing together of different stakeholders, including the local community, to address the issues of a specific location (usually a disadvantaged and deprived area).

Plan: How to get from your starting point to your end point, and what you want to achieve.

Policy: Guidelines for practice which set broad goals and the framework for action.

Politics: achieving and exercising control over human communities, e.g. states.

Power: The ability or right to control people or things.

Prisoner: A person held in custody while on trial or serving a custodial sentence for criminal offences.

Programme: activities included in an intervention

Prevention: The action of stopping something from happening; disease prevention means actions taken at primary, secondary or tertiary levels to prevent disease occurring or worsening.

Primary care: The day-to-day care provided by health workers in the community; primary care workers are usually the first point of contact for patients and provide continuing care as well as coordinating other specialist care as required.

Public health: Organized efforts by society to protect and promote the health and well-being of populations and prevent illness, injury and disability.

Quality of life: The subjective assessment individuals make of their position in life, encompassing physical, social, psychological, spiritual, independence and environmental factors; quality of life is affected by cultural, social and personal expectations.

QALY: Quality-adjusted life year is a measure that combines the quality and quantity of life lived; it is used as a measure of the impact of disease and in assessing the value of medical interventions.

Rate: A measure, quantity or frequency, typically one measured against another quantity or measure.

Risk behaviour: Behaviour that is proven to be associated with an increased risk of ill health or disease.

Risk factor: Social, economic or biological status, behaviour or environment that is proven to be associated with an increased risk of ill health or disease.

Self-efficacy: A person's beliefs in his/her ability to succeed.

Settings: Places where people conduct their everyday lives and where personal, organizational, social and environmental factors interact to affect health.

Social capital: Social support, trust and neighbourliness that result from social networking and community participation, and contribute to health and well-being.

Social class: A group of people united through having the same educational, social or economic status, e.g. working class.

Social determinants: Economic and social factors (e.g. income, social class, gender) that have a profound effect on health; these differences are not natural, but are created and maintained by social and economic policies and legislation.

Social justice: A concern with equality and democracy, encompassing measures taken to narrow the gap in income, wealth and power that exists between different groups in society.

Social marketing: The use of commercial marketing techniques (e.g. advertising, media coverage) to achieve beneficial health-related behaviour changes.

Social model: A model of health based in the social sciences which explains variations in health in relation to socio-economic factors.

Social norms: The behaviour and beliefs appropriate for a social group.

Social policy: Planned government activities to regulate society.

Socio-economic status (SES): An economic and sociological measure of a person's work experience and of an individual's or family's economic and social position in relation to others, based on income, education and occupation.

Stakeholder: Any person or organization with a direct interest in an intervention; refers to both the people implementing an intervention and those receiving it.

Strategy: Broad framework for action which indicates goals, methods and underlying principles.

Supply: Provide or make available something which is wanted or essential.

Sustainability: Meeting the needs of the present generation in a way that does not compromise the ability of future generations to meet their needs; sustainable health promotion actions are embedded in services and structures so their positive effects continue beyond the life of the programme or intervention.

Theory: an idea or proposition, often using general principles, used to explain something specific.

Want: A lack or deficiency of something.

Well-being: The positive feeling that accompanies a lack of ill health and illness, and is associated with the achievement of personal goals and a sense of being well and feeling good.

Wellness: The optimal state of health of individuals and groups.

Work: A job or paid employment; this includes unpaid or voluntary work, education and training, and caring.

Worker: A person employed to carry out specific functions, usually in return for a wage or salary.

Workplace: The physical environment where work takes place.

Further reading

Health promotion glossary. WHO, Geneva or visit http://www.who.int/healthpromotion/about/HPR%20Glossary%201998.pdf.

Smith, B.J., Tang, K.C., Nutbeam, D., 2006. WHO health promotion glossary: new terms. Health Promotion International 21, 340–345. *The World Health Organization has produced a comprehensive and detailed glossary of health promotion terms that is regularly updated. See Nutbeam, D., 1998.*

Other useful glossaries

Hubley, J., Copeman, J., 2013. Practical Health Promotion, second ed. Polity, Bristol. http://www.polity.co.uk/healthpromotion/student/glossary/.

Laverack, G., 2013. A-Z of Health Promotion. Palgrave Macmillan, Basingstoke.

Index

Note: Page numbers followed by "*b*", "*t*", and "*f*" refer to boxes, tables, and figures respectively.